Epidemiology and prevention: a systems-based approach

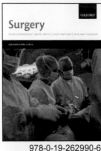
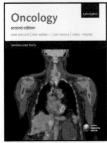
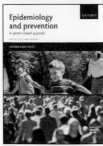
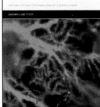

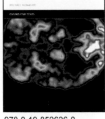

Epidemiology and prevention: a systems-based approach

Edited by

John Yarnell

Reader, Public Health Medicine and Primary Care,
Department of Epidemiology and Public Health,
Queens University, Belfast

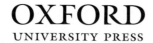

OXFORD
UNIVERSITY PRESS

OXFORD
UNIVERSITY PRESS

Great Clarendon Street, Oxford OX2 6DP

Oxford University Press is a department of the University of Oxford.
It furthers the University's objective of excellence in research, scholarship,
and education by publishing worldwide in

Oxford New York

Auckland Cape Town Dar es Salaam Hong Kong Karachi
Kuala Lumpur Madrid Melbourne Mexico City Nairobi
New Delhi Shanghai Taipei Toronto

With offices in

Argentina Austria Brazil Chile Czech Republic France Greece
Guatemala Hungary Italy Japan Poland Portugal Singapore
South Korea Switzerland Thailand Turkey Ukraine Vietnam

Oxford is a registered trade mark of Oxford University Press
in the UK and in certain other countries

Published in the United States
by Oxford University Press Inc., New York

© Oxford University Press, 2007

British Library Cataloguing in Publication Data

Data available

Library of Congress Cataloging in Publication Data

Data available

Typeset by CEPHA Imaging Pvt. Ltd., Bangalore, India
Printed in Great Britain
on acid-free paper by
Ashford Colour Press, Gosport, Hampshire

ISBN 978-0-19-853014-5 (Pbk.)

3 5 7 9 10 8 6 4 2

Preface

This book has the specific aim of making epidemiology and public health more relevant to medical and dental undergraduates and is, to our knowledge, the first textbook that uses a systems-based approach required by the curriculum in Queen's University Belfast, and those of several other universities, at least in the United Kingdom. We have also attempted to emphasize the prospects for preventing disease, often understated in a largely clinically driven curriculum, although we appreciate that to address this issue adequately would probably require a further textbook.

This book, which represents the collective efforts of contributors within or associated with the Department of Epidemiology and Public Health, Queen's University Belfast, covers all material we consider to be essential for the teaching of Epidemiology to medical and dental undergraduates. It may also be useful to those in other health-related undergraduate courses, and to non-medically qualified postgraduate students studying epidemiology. The book has been extensively researched and referenced but, for reasons of space, all references have been placed on an accompanying website, for further study and for additional teaching material.

The first five chapters introduce the reader to epidemiological methods and tools; they include chapters that provide introductions to data analysis and to screening. These chapters are not intended to be digested in one reading by beginners, but should be used for reference when reading the systems-based chapters. Words of special relevance to epidemiology are highlighted in colour and are defined in the Glossary.

The systems-based presentation generally follows the order prescribed in the International Classification of Diseases, and brief epidemiological reviews of the major diseases and disorders are provided. It is not our purpose to review diseases exhaustively, and by no means do we attempt to replace the standard textbooks of clinical medicine; it is the application of epidemiological principles to diseases in general that we wish to highlight. Opportunities for prevention and further research are noted where appropriate.

The final chapters of the book, which includes a chapter on oral health, cover other topics that feature prominently in the undergraduate curriculum: these include social and behavioural factors in disease; genetic epidemiology; clinical epidemiology and evidence-based practice; and, finally, public-health practice.

We have written this book with a particular emphasis on self-directed learning. We would encourage students to pursue the references as we have suggested, the web addresses and to pose questions for themselves and for their teachers whenever possible. Only by such interaction will epidemiology become relevant to the student's future practice.

Acknowledgements

This book would not have been written without the active encouragement of the Department of Epidemiology and Public Health, Queen's University Belfast. We thank all the contributors, but particularly Dr Anna Gavin, who convened a series of contributors' meetings in the early stages of the project, and Professor Alun Evans, Dr Dermot O'Reilly, Professor Peter McCarron, and Dr Chris Patterson who acted as associate editors. Professor Liam Murray and Dr Elizabeth Reaney also provided valuable assistance, and we thank Dr Pascal McKeown for reviewing Chapter 18. The patient, skilled assistance of Mrs Heather Porter, who compiled the book from the numerous drafts, and the excellent technical support of Mrs Rosie Kearney, Mr Joe Clint, and Angie Scott deserve special thanks. Finally to Gitanjali for her patience during the last two years.

Disclaimer

Oxford University Press makes no representation, express or implied, that the drug dosages in this book are correct. Readers must therefore always check the product information and clinical procedures with the most up to date published product information and data sheets provided by the manufacturers and the most recent codes of conduct and safety regulations. The authors and the publishers do not accept responsibility or legal liability for any errors in the text or for the misuse or misapplication of material in this work.

There are instances where we have been unable to trace or contact the copyright holder. If notified, the publisher will be pleased to rectify any errors or omissions at the earliest opportunity.

Contents

Copyright permissons

Figures

Fig 1.1 McKeown, T. (1976). *The Modern Rise of Population*. London: Edward Arnold. Reproduced by permission of Edward Arnold.

Fig 1.2 Rothman, K. J. (1976). 'Reviews and Commentary: Causes'. *American Journal of Epidemiology*, **104** (6): 587–92, by permission of Johns Hopkins Bloomberg School of Public Health.

Fig 1.3 Rose, G. (1985). 'Sick Individuals and Sick Populations'. *International Journal of Epidemiology*, **14** (1): 32–8, by permission of International Epidemiological Association.

Fig 3.1 Reprinted from Bang A. T., Bang R. A., Baitule S. B., Reddy M. H. and Deshmukh M. D. (1999). 'Effect of home-based neonatal care and management of sepsis on neonatal mortality: field trial in rural India'. *The Lancet*, **354**: 1955–61, copyright (1999), with permission from Elsevier.

Fig 5.1 Vainio, H. and Bianchini, F. (2002). *Breast Cancer Screening. IARC Handbook of Cancer Prevention* (vol. 7). Lyon: IRAC Press, www.who.int.

Fig 5.2 Gerstmann, B. B. (1999). *Epidemiology Kept Simple: An Introduction to Classic and Modern Epidemiology*. New York, NY: Wiley-Liss.

Fig 5.3 Reprinted from Cowie, M. R., Struthers, A. D., Wood, D. A., Coats, A. J., Thompson, S. G., Poole-Wilson, P. A. and Sutton, G. C. (1997). 'Value of Natriuretic Peptides in Assessment of Patients with Possible New Heart Failure in Primary Care'. *The Lancet*, **350**: 1349–53, copyright (1997) with permission from Elsevier.

Fig 6.1 Yeghiazarians, Y., Braunstein, J. B., Askari, A. and Stone, P. H. (2000). 'Medical Progress: Unstable Angina Pectoris'. *New England Journal of Medicine*, **342**: 101–14, adapted with permission 2006, copyright © 2000 Massachusetts Medical Society. All rights reserved.

Fig 6.2 Reprinted from Walker, R. W., McLarty, D. G., Kitange, H. M., Whiting, D., Masuki, G., Mtasiwa, D. M., Machibya, H., Unwin, N. and Alberti, K. M. (2000). 'Stroke Mortality in Urban and Rural Tanzania'. *The Lancet*, **355**: 1684–87, copyright (2000), with permission from Elsevier.

Fig 6.3 Reprinted from Prospective Studies Collaboration (2002). 'Age-Specific Relevance of Usual Blood Pressure to Vascular Mortality: A Meta-Analysis of Individual Data for One Million Adults in 61 Prospective Studies'. *The Lancet*, **360**: 1903–13, copyright (2002) with permission from Elsevier.

Fig 8.1 Allison, D. B., Fontaine, K. R., Manson, J. E., Stevens, J. and VanItallie, T. B. (1999). 'Annual Deaths Attributable to Obesity in the United States'. *Journal of the American Medical Association*, **282**: 1530–38. Copyright © 1999, American Medical Association. All rights reserved.

Fig 8.2 Cole, T. J., Bellizzi, M. C., Flegal, K. M. and Dietz, W. H. (2000). 'Establishing a Standard Definition for Child Overweight and Obesity Worldwide: International Survey'. *British Medical Journal*, **320**: 1240–3, reproduced with permission from the BMJ Publishing Group.

Fig 8.3 The Diabetes Control and Complications Trial Research Group (1993). 'The Effect of Intensive Treatment of Diabetes on the Development and Progression of Long-Term Complications in Insulin-Dependent Diabetes Mellitus'. *New England Journal of Medicine*, **329**: 977–86. Adapted with permission 2006, Copyright © 1993 Massachusetts Medical Society. All rights reserved.

Fig 8.4 Pharoah, P. O. D. and Connolly, K. J. (1987). 'A Controlled Trial of Iodinated Oil for the Prevention of Endemic Cretinism: A Long-Term Follow-Up'. *International Journal of Epidemiology*, **16** (1): 68–73, by permission of International Epidemiological Association.

Fig 9.1 Stanghellini, V. (1999). 'Three-Month Prevalence Rates of Gastrointestinal Symptoms and the Influence of Demographic Factors: Results from the Domestic/International Gastroenterology Surveillance Study (DIGEST)'. *Scandinavian Journal of Gastroenterology*, **34** (Suppl. 231): 20–8. Taylor and Francis Ltd, http://www.tandf.no/gastro.

Fig 9.2 Pounder, R. E and Ng, D. (1995). 'The Prevalence of *Helicobacter pylori* Infection in Different Countries'. *Alimentary Pharmacology and Therapeutics*, **9** (Suppl. 2), 33–9.

Fig 9.3 Office for National Statistics (2001). Mortality Statistics – Cause. Review of the Registrar General on Deaths by Cause, Sex and Age, in England and Wales, 2000. Mortality Data Series DH2 no. 27. London: ONS. Reproduced under the terms of the Click-Use Licence.

Fig 9.4 Reprinted from Russel, M. G. (2000). 'Changes in the Incidence of Inflammatory Bowel Disease: What Does It Mean?' *European Journal of Internal Medicine*, **11**: 191–6. Copyright (2000), with permission from European Federation of Internal Medicine.

Fig 9.5 Chief Medical Officer (2001). *The Annual Report of the Chief Medical Office of the Department of Health*. London: Department of Health. Reproduced under the terms of the Click-Use Licence.

Fig 10.1 Source: Reaney *et al.* (unpublished data).

Fig 11.1 Annegars, J. F. (2004). 'Epilepsy', in L. M. Nelson, C. M. Tanner, S. K. Van Den Eeden, V. M. McGuire (eds.), *Neuroepidemiology. From Principles to Practice*. Oxford: Oxford University Press. By permission of Oxford University Press.

Fig 12.1 WHO (2001). The World Health Report 2001, www.who.int.

Fig 13.1 Reprinted from Sprangers, M. A., de Regt, E. B. and Andries, F. (2000). 'Which Chronic Conditions Are Associated with Better or Poorer Quality of Life?' *Journal of Clinical Epidemiology*, **53** (9): 895–907. Copyright (2000), with permission from Elsevier.

Fig 13.2 Symmons, D. P., Barrett, E. M., Bankhead, C. R., Scott, D. G. and Silman, A. J. (1994). 'The Incidence of Rheumatoid Arthritis in the United Kingdom: Results from the Norfolk Arthritis Register'. *Rheumatology*, **33** (8): 735–9, by permission of British Society for Rheumatology.

Fig 13.3 World Health Organization (1994). *Assessment of Fracture Risk and its Application to Screening for Postmenopausal Osteoporosis*. WHO Technical Report Series No. 843. Geneva: World Health Organization, www.who.int.

Fig 13.4 Reprinted from Andersson, G. B. J. (1999). 'Epidemiological Features of Chronic Low Back Pain'. *The Lancet*, **354**: 581–5. Copyright (1999), with permission from Elsevier.

Fig 14.1 Office of National Statistics (1998), www.statistics.gov.uk. Reproduced under the terms of the Click-Use Licence.

Fig 14.2 US Census Bureau (2005). International Database, IDB Summary Demographic Data, http://www.census.gov/ipc/www/idbsum.html.

Fig 14.3 Reproduced from Royal College of Obstetricians and Gynaecologists (2001). *Why Mothers Die 1997–99*, with the permission of the Confidential Enquiry into Maternal and Child Health.

Fig 14.4 Reproduced from Botting, B., on behalf of the Editorial Board (2001). *Trends in Reproductive Epidemiology and Women's Health*, p. 331, with the permission of the Confidential Enquiry into Maternal and Child Health.

Fig 14.5 Office of National Statistics (2004), www.statistics.gov.uk. Reproduced under the terms of the Click-Use Licence.

Fig 14.6 Reproduced from Maternal and Child Health Research Consortium (2001). Confidential Enquiry into Stillbirths and Deaths in Infancy, p. 22, with the permission of the Confidential Enquiry into Maternal and Child Health.

Fig 15.1 Reprinted from Key, T. J., Allen, N. E., Spencer, E. A. and Travis, R. C. (2002). 'The Effect of Diet on Risk of Cancer'. *The Lancet*, **360**: 861–8. Copyright (2002), with permission from Elsevier.

Fig 15.2 Cancer Research UK, World age-standardized incidence and mortality rates for prostate cancer for selected countries, estimates for the year 2002, 2006, April.

Fig 17.1 Source: Cabinet Office, Prime Minister's Strategy Chair (2004). Alcohol Harm Reduction Strategy for England. London: Cabinet Office. Reproduced under the terms of the Click-Use Licence.

Fig 17.2 Reprinted from Ezzati, M., Lopez, A. D., Rodgers, A., Vander Hoorn, S. and Murray, C. J. L. (2002). 'Comparative Risk Assessment Collaborative Group: Selected Major Risk Factors and Global and Regional Burden Of Disease'. *The Lancet*, **360**: 1347–60. Copyright (2002), with permission from Elsevier.

Fig 17.3 World Health Organization (1999). *Health 21. The Health for All Policy Framework for the WHO European Region.* European Health for All Series No. 6. From European health for all database, WHO Regional Office for Europe, Copenhagen, Denmark.

Fig 18.1a Mange, A. P. and Mange, E. J. (1999). *Basic Human Genetics* (2nd edn). Sunderland, MA: Sinauer Associates.

Fig 18.1b Source: OMIM (2005).

Fig 18.2 Strachan, T. and Read, A. P. (2004). *Human Molecular Genetics* (3rd edn). London: Garland Science.

Fig 18.3 Strachan, T. and Read, A. P. (2004). *Human Molecular Genetics* (3rd edn). London: Garland Science.

Fig 18.5 Strachan, T. and Read, A. P. (2004). *Human Molecular Genetics* (3rd edn). London: Garland Science.

Fig 18.6 Reprinted by permission from Macmillan Publishers Ltd: *Nature Genetics*, **36**: 233–9, copyright 2004.

Fig 19.1 Reproduced with permission from Kidd, E. A. M., Smith, B. G. N. and Watson, T. F. (2003). *Pickard's Manual of Operative Dentistry* (8th edn). Oxford: Oxford University Press.

Fig 19.2 Petersen, P. E. (2003). 'The World Oral Health Report 2003. Continuous Improvement of Oral Health in the 21st Century – The Approach of the WHO Global Oral Health Programme'. Geneva: World Health Organization, www.who.int.

Fig 19.3 Whelton, H., Crowley, E., O'Mullane, D., Donaldson, M., Cronin, M. and Kelleher, V. (2006). 'Dental Caries and Enamel Fluorosis among the fluoridated population in the Republic of Ireland and non fluoridated population in Northern Ireland in 2002'. *Community Dental Health*, **23**: 37–43.

Fig 19.4 Reproduced with permission from Kidd, E. A. M. (2005). *Essentials of Dental Caries* (3rd edn). Oxford: Oxford University Press.

Fig 20.2 Ashenden, R., Silagy, C. and Weller, D. (1997). 'A Systematic Review of the Effectiveness of Promoting Lifestyle Change in General Practice'. *Family Practice*, **14**: 160–76. By permission of Oxford University Press.

Fig 21.1 BMJ Books, 1-11.

Fig 21.2 Stevens, A., Raftery, J., Mant, J. and Simpson, S. (eds.) (2004). *Health Care Needs Assessment: The Epidemiologically Based Needs Assessment Reviews.* Oxford: Radcliffe Publishing, http: www.hcna.radcliffe-oxford.com.

Boxes

Box 1.4 Bradford Hill, A. (1971). *Principles of Medical Statistics* (9th edn). London: *The Lancet.* Reproduced by permission of Edward Arnold.

Box 2.1 McCarthy *et al.* (2003). *British Medical Journal*, **326**: 624, reproduced with permission from the BMJ Publishing Group.

Box 2.4 Mays, N. and Pope, C. (eds.) (1996). *Qualitative Methods in Health Care.* London: BMJ Publishing Group. Reproduced with permission by Blackwell Publishing.

Box 3.1 Adapted from Silman, A. J. (2002). *Epidemiological Studies: A Practical Guide* (2nd edn). Cambridge: Cambridge University Press.

Box 4.2 British Medical Journal, 314: 779–82.

Box 4.4 British Medical Journal, 316: 1498.

Box 5.2 Modified from: UK National Screening Committee (2003), www.nsc.nhs.uk. Reproduced under the terms of the Click-Use Licence.

Box 5.4 Fletcher, R. H., Fletcher, S. W., Wagner, E. H. (1996). *Clinical Epidemiology. The Essentials* (3rd edn). Philadelphia, PA: Lippincott, Williams and Wilkins.

Box 8.1 Truswell, A.S. (1999) *ABC of Nutrition* (3rd edn). London: BMJ Books. Golden, M. H. N. and Golden, B. E. (2000). 'Severe Malnutrition' in J. S. Garrow, W. P. T. James and A. Ralph (eds.), *Human Nutrition and Dietetics* (10th edn). Edinburgh: Churchill Livingstone, with permission from Elsevier.

Box 8.2 Garrow, J.S. (2000) 'Composition of the Body' in J. S. Garrow, W. P. T. James and A. Ralph (eds.), *Human Nutrition and Dietics* (10th edn). Edinburgh: Churchill Livingstone.

Box 8.4 Davidson, S., Passmore, R., Brock, J. F. and Truswell, A. S. (1979). *Human Nutrition and Dietetics* (7th edn). Edinburgh: Churchill Livingstone, with permission from Elsevier.

Contributors

Dr Karen Bailie, Director of Northern Ireland Clinical Research Support Centre, Belfast.

Mr James Briggs, School of Dentistry, Royal Group of Hospitals, Belfast.

Dr Gordon Cran, Senior Lecturer in Medical Statistics, Queen's University, Belfast.

Professor Helen Dolk, Professor of Epidemiology and Health Services Research, University of Ulster.

Dr Michael Donnelly, Reader in Public Health Medicine and Primary Care, Queen's University Belfast.

Professor Alun Evans, Professor of Epidemiology, Queen's University, Belfast.

Professor Ruth Freeman, Professor of Dental Public Health, Queen's University, Belfast.

Dr Brian Gaffney, Chief Executive, Health Promotion Agency for Northern Ireland.

Dr Anna Gavin, Director of Northern Ireland Cancer Registry, Senior Lecturer, Department of Epidemiology and Public Health, Queen's University, Belfast.

Dr Stanley Hawkins, Reader and Consultant Neurologist, Department of Medicine, Queen's University, Belfast.

Dr Jacqueline James, Senior Lecturer/Consultant in Pathology, Queen's University, Belfast.

Dr Brian Johnston, Consultant Gastroenterologist, Royal Group of Hospitals, Belfast.

Professor Frank Kee, Professor of Public Health Medicine, Queen's University, Belfast.

Professor Gerard Linden, Professor of Periodontology, Queen's University, Belfast.

Professor Peter Maxwell, Professor of Renal Medicine, Queen's University, Belfast.

Professor Peter McCarron, Professor of Epidemiology, Department of Epidemiology and Public Health, Queen's University, Belfast.

Professor Liam Murray, Professor of Cancer Epidemiology, Department of Epidemiology and Public Health, Queen's University, Belfast.

Dr Sinéad McGilloway, Senior Lecturer in Psychology, National University of Ireland at Maynooth.

Dr William Moore, Specialist Registrar, Queen's University, Belfast.

Dr James Morrow, Consultant Neurologist, Honorary Clinical Lecturer and Clinical Director of Neurosciences, Royal Victoria Hospital, Belfast.

Dr Dermot O'Reilly, Senior Lecturer, Queen's University, Belfast.

Dr Jackie Parkes, Senior Lecturer, School of Nursing and Midwifery, Queen's University, Belfast.

Dr Christopher Patterson, Reader in Medical Statistics, Queen's University, Belfast.

Dr Elizabeth Reaney, Specialist Registrar in Public Health Medicine, Department of Health, Northern Ireland.

Dr Maureen Scott, Consultant, Department of Health, Northern Ireland.

Dr Brian Smyth, Communicable Disease Surveillance Centre (Northern Ireland), Belfast City Hospital.

Dr David Stewart, Director of Public Health, Eastern Health Board, Northern Ireland.

Epidemiological Enquiry and Methods

CHAPTER 1

Epidemiology: from Hippocrates to the human genome

This chapter describes a brief history of epidemiology, some important epidemiological terms and how epidemiology can contribute to the understanding of causes of disease and to its prevention.

1.1 A Short History

Epidemiology (Greek *epi*, upon; *demos*, the people) adopts a population approach to the study of the distribution and determinants of disease. Characteristically, this is nowhere better demonstrated (Lilienfield and Lilienfield 1980) 🖳 than in Hippocrates' *On Airs, Waters, and Places*: 'Whosoever wishes to investigate medicine properly should proceed thus ... and consider the mode in which the inhabitants live, and what are their pursuits, whether they are fond of eating and drinking to excess, and given to indolence, or are fond of exercise and labour, and not given to eating and drinking.' According to Porter (1997), 🖳 Hippocrates was a School rather than one man whose teachings were widely disseminated in the Greek-speaking world between the fifth and third centuries BC. During this era the task of **hygiene** was to maintain a 'balanced constitution' to prevent disease; this was perpetuated in the prolific work of Galen in the second century AD and in Arabic medicine, which continued the Greek tradition into the Middle Ages.

The Black Death (bubonic/pneumonic plague) came to Europe spreading from city to city. It killed about a quarter of Europe's population within a few years in the fourteenth century; it continued to wreak destruction over the next two centuries and public health developed out of the need to control the disease. Physicians recognized its **contagious** nature but failed to link it with rats and fleas; the only weapons against plague were **quarantine**, isolation of patients, and burial of corpses; but **health boards** were created in many cities to initiate and regulate these public-health measures to limit the spread of the disease. Epidemics of smallpox and syphilis were common in Europe and some medical scientists took 'heroic' measures to investigate the causes of disease. In an attempt to understand gonorrhoea, in 1767 John Hunter took pus from an infected patient and inoculated his own penis with it in two places; sure enough, he contracted gonorrhoea. Unfortunately for Hunter, several weeks later the characteristic lesion of syphilis (large pox) developed. Because the original patient was harbouring both diseases Hunter ended up with one more disease than he had bargained for.

During the nineteenth century cholera spread from India carried by merchant ships and overland both westwards and further east. The first major epidemic hit London in 1832 with 7000 deaths (Porter 1997). 💻 The London Epidemiological Society was formed in 1850 largely to combat the successive outbreaks of cholera in London and other cities in Britain. In the 1850s John Snow, an anaesthetist practising in Soho, London, recognized from the geographic distribution of cholera cases that the disease was linked with water likely to have been contaminated by sewage. Sanitary reform, the provision of clean drinking water, and disposal of sewage became established in the major cities of Britain and Europe. By the end of the nineteenth century, particularly in Germany, the microscope had been developed to an extent that allowed the identification of the bacteria responsible for anthrax, cholera, and tuberculosis; with the development of these laboratory and immunological tools, the science of infectious disease epidemiology was able to start in earnest (Chapter 16). A myriad of bacteria were being discovered and it was clear that many of these caused no disease. Two pioneers in bacteriology and microscopy formulated the Henle–Koch postulates to assist the process of linking specific bacteria with particular diseases; these postulates are shown in Box 1.1 and are particularly relevant for bacterial infections. Although they serve as a useful yardstick for all infectious diseases, viruses and parasites can be host-specific, and evidence of infection is more readily obtained from immunological tests of

---

BOX 1.1 THE HENLE–KOCH POSTULATES

1 The organism must be found in all cases of the disease.

2 It must be isolated from patients with the disease and grown in pure culture.

3 When the pure culture is inoculated into susceptible animals or man, it must reproduce the disease.

---

antibody formation which have been developed during the twentieth century.

Many of the early definitions of epidemiology, for example 'disease as a mass phenomenon' (Greenwood 1934) 💻 or 'the study of disease in populations' (Stamler 1958) 💻 are discussed in detail elsewhere (Lilienfeld 1978). 💻 A history and key concepts in the development of epidemiology are well summarized by Lilienfeld and Lilienfeld (1980). 💻

By the end of the first quarter of the twentieth century with improvements in nutrition and living conditions, particularly for the poor, infectious diseases began to wane in the more advanced industrialized countries, and chronic diseases such as lung cancer and heart attack (coronary disease) began to emerge as important causes of death and illness. Coronary disease was not new, but had previously been confined to the better off. Heberden described the disease in 1772 and Samuel Black noted in 1819 that 'the primary and original cause of the disorder (angina pectoris) is ossification of the coronaries' (Evans 1995). 💻 He went on to describe and contrast the distribution of the disease in the Irish and in the French, and these he linked with contrasting lifestyles.

By the 1950s the epidemics of heart attack and lung cancer, notably in men, were well developed and widely recognized by the leading medical authorities, particularly in the United States of America (USA) and Great Britain. **Epidemiological studies** were developed to investigate the causes of these diseases and **prospective studies** such as those among British doctors clearly established the link between tobacco smoking and both lung cancer and coronary disease (Doll and Hill 1954; Doll *et al.* 1994). Epidemiologists became interested in both the prevention and treatment of disease. In the 1960s Cochrane showed that fewer than half of routine medical and surgical treatments were based on scientific evidence, and the discipline of **evidence-based medicine** was born (Cochrane 1972) (Chapter 20). To establish causality there is a hierarchy of different types of epidemiological study, both observational and **experimental** (see Chapter 3), and often a painstaking procession up these echelons. Sometimes it is possible to bypass a step, sometimes it is impossible to proceed at all. Often people who criticize epidemiology do not understand its strengths and weaknesses: the method applied must be appropriate to the situation. If not, to criticize is rather like blaming a carthorse for being useless at flat racing. In an otherwise excellent book, *Cancer: The Evolutionary Legacy*, Greaves (2000) draws attention to the limitations of epidemiology but praises the Linxian Study (Blot *et al.* 1993), which is a population-based nutritional interventional study in a poor region of China designed by epidemiologists to attempt to reduce the high incidence of gastric cancer in that region. Although the first well-known recorded experiment in curative/preventive medicine was performed by James Lind, who allocated six types of treatment to 12 sailors with scurvy on HMS *Salisbury*'s return to Plymouth in 1747 (the treatment with citrus fruits was effective), only recently has its methodology been developed and ratified with the growth of evidence-based medicine (see Chapters 4 and 20) and the 'gold standard' of the **randomized controlled trial** (RCT) become established. The methodology was originally applied widely in crop trials, and subsequently in medicine, but human beings proved altogether more difficult to study than plots of wheat. In certain circumstances, where evidence is lacking, or the studies required are just too costly or impracticable to conduct, causality may be ascribed by applying several criteria (see section 1.3 and Box 1.4) all of which have certain limitations: it is simply the best we can do in the circumstances until new evidence is accumulated or new techniques of investigation become available.

At the beginning of the twenty-first century **epidemiology is a broad-based population science**, drawing on many disciplines from biology and sociology to biostatistics and philosophy of science which investigates the **causes of human disease** and **methods for their control.** Past and future epidemiology has been discussed by others (Davey Smith and Ebrahim 2001) but the need for scientific rigour cannot be overstated. The science of molecular biology and the human genome offer many opportunities for epidemiology to contribute to the disciplines of genomics and proteomics (Day *et al.* 2001), while the broad scope of epidemiology ensures that its future evolution and development will remain at the forefront of the battle against human disease.

1.2 Defining and Measuring Disease in Populations

Most doctors in most branches of medicine tend to use the word **disease** rather loosely. Literally, 'dis-ease' means the body not at ease or in harmony with itself and we can all recognize this state of body or mind. Usually this is self-limiting, but if it does not resolve and becomes an **illness** we may seek the opinion of a general practitioner, who, in turn, would try to decide if it could be a specific disease entity requiring treatment, which may warrant a full diagnostic workup. Hospital specialists and other medical scientists such as pathologists, microbiologists, immunologists and radiologists tend to work with disease entities where the **natural history** (the causes and unhindered clinical progression) of the disease is generally well described and treatment options are known. The scope of epidemiology has become so broad that epidemiologists have to work at a number of different levels of diagnostic certainty which are described in Box 1.2.

A disease entity may have a single **cause**, such as a bacterium or virus, or a combination of causes which have been well defined. Even for the infectious diseases, however, there is still the issue of **host susceptibility/resistance** for most agents. For many infectious diseases a minimum of three components is required for disease: a susceptible host, an infectious agent, and an environment favourable for the reproduction and growth of the infectious agent. Most diseases are defined solely on the typical clinical history, symptoms, and signs, with or without the assistance of laboratory or other diagnostic facilities. If the cause of a particular disease is not understood, then the disease may possibly comprise more than one disease entity: this is termed **disease heterogeneity. Disorder** tends to be used for malfunction of particular systems, for example

BOX 1.2 **DEFNITIONS OF DISEASE AND DISORDERS IN MEDICAL RESEARCH**					
Causal research:	Disease entity				
Applied epidemiology and	Specific conditions:	Disease Syndrome	Disorder	Condition	Trait
health services research:	Non-specific conditions: Disability		Illness	Sickness	

cardiovascular disorder, endocrine disorder, etc. **Condition** is usually a state of the body or of an organ, for example overweight or obesity. **Trait** indicates a predisposition to disease ranging from a specific genetic trait to a personality or psychological trait predisposing to mental illness. The term **syndrome** (a collection of symptoms and signs occurring together) is widely used (and abused) in medical practice. Some syndromes are well established as disease entities: for example Wernicke's syndrome (encephalopathy), a complex of neurological signs associated with thiamine deficiency and alcoholism; whereas others are either poorly defined, for example chronic fatigue syndrome (myelo-encephalopathy, ME); or even artificially created by doctors, for example metabolic syndrome. **Disability** (formerly handicap) implies a malfunctioning of a particular body system, for example mental disability. **Illness** refers to the subjective state of an individual or unspecified disease state whereas **sickness** usually signifies a dysfunctional state or, in sociology, as the 'sick role', the social consequences of illness. **'Sickness absence'** is much studied by epidemiologists and other health-care researchers, but it is notoriously difficult to standardize definitions of disorders, conditions, or illnesses that have been described either by the patient or by their doctor as a 'cause' of absence from work.

Measurement of disease

How the epidemiologist attempts to measure the level of a disease in a population depends to a certain extent on the purpose of the measurement or the study, which is dealt with in Chapter 2; but for basic, descriptive purposes two types of measurement are important. The **prevalence** of a disease counts the **number of cases** in a given population. This can be at a particular point in time; **point prevalence** (often referred to simply as prevalence); **period prevalence**, measured over a period of time; and **cumulative prevalence**, which refers to the total number of episodes of disease accumulated during the individual lifespan of each member of the population. Although prevalence is described above as a number it is most often used in the sense of **prevalence 'rate', 'ratio', proportion, or percentage**, in which instance the number of cases is divided by the population size. Clearly the type of measurement used very much depends on the natural history of the disease in question. Some diseases, such as measles for example, may occur once in an individual and confer lifelong immunity. Other diseases may be episodic in nature and occur during different periods in the lifespan, such as epilepsy and recurrent

heart attacks; **point prevalence** and **attack rates** are the measurement of choice for these conditions. Yet other diseases may be chronic and long-term in nature (for example multiple sclerosis, diabetes mellitus). Some diseases carry a very high **case-fatality** (80–100 per cent) whereas others may be rarely life-threatening. It is helpful in the descriptive epidemiology of a new disease to be able to count the number of cases and to describe their distribution according to *who* has acquired the disease, *where* they have acquired it and *when* (i.e. distribution of disease by **person**, **place**, and **time**: see Chapter 3).

The other important measure of disease is **incidence**, which is the number of **new cases** of disease occurring in a specified period of time. The **attack rate** or cumulative incidence refers to the number of new episodes of disease in a given time period. Again, incidence is frequently used as shorthand for **incidence rate**, which relates it to a given population (its size used as the denominator) and enables different populations to be compared. Typically incidence rates would be calculated per annum. **Incidence rate** is a measurement that tends to be used in **longitudinal** studies in which people are followed up for new cases of disease over a period of years. Proxy indicators of disease (traits, diagnostic and screening tests) are discussed in Chapter 5, but prevalence and incidence measurements of these indicators are largely identical to those for disease entities. Box 1.3 shows the main types of measure used in epidemiological studies.

1.3 **Models of Causation and Determinants of Disease**

As noted by Rothman (1998), epidemiology is an 'embryo' among the sciences. Although this 'embryo' has had major public health successes, such as establishing a link between contaminated water supplies and cholera, or tobacco smoking and lung cancer, the methodology and theoretical basis of epidemiology continue to develop and expand. The concept of **cause** is a critical issue in the philosophy of scientific method and medical sciences are no exception to this. Epidemiology seeks to examine 'causes' of disease in whole populations and is fortunate today in having available basic medical sciences such as microbiology, biochemistry, pathology and immunology (non-epidemiologists may have a different perspective on this!). At first sight the 'cause' of an infectious disease is straightforward: the single infectious agent associated with the clinical manifestation of the disease. However, the reality is

---

BOX 1.3 MEASURING DISEASE: PREVALENCE AND INCIDENCE

	Prevalence		Incidence	
Point	**Period**		**Proportion**	**Rate**
Number of cases of disease in a population at a particular point of time	Number of cases in a population during a specific period of time		Proportion of people in a population developing a disease in a given time period	Rate at which new disease events occur in a population

		Attack rate or cumulative incidence	**Incidence (density)***
Prevalence rate		New cases or episodes developing in study period ÷ population at risk at beginning of study period	New cases developing in study period ÷ person – years at risk
Number of cases ÷ Population at risk (often P%)			

- New and old cases included
- Follow up not required
- Diseases of long duration will inflate prevalence with age
- Preferred measure to assess burden of disease in population

- New cases or episodes of disease only
- Follow up of whole population required
- Duration of disease will not inflate incidence
- Preferred measure to assess risk of disease and cause and effect

*Commonly referred to as incidence rate

---

different: for most infectious diseases infectivity rates are low, i.e. many individuals can be exposed to the agent but do not develop the clinical disease. Tuberculosis was a major cause of death in Europe, and remains so in the developing world, but factors such as malnutrition, overcrowding and smoking are strongly associated with the likelihood of clinical disease (synonym: risk factors, see Chapter 3). McKeown (1976) has shown, by simple examination of trends in mortality from major infectious diseases, the crucial role of external factors (social and environmental) entirely separate from the infectious agent itself in 'causing' their decline (Fig. 1.1).

For an infectious disease the infectious agent is clearly a factor *necessary* for the development of a disease. Such a factor is known as a **necessary cause**. If an agent causes a clinical disease in 100 per cent of individuals exposed to it (which is rare, but infectivity is high in some infectious diseases, such as anthrax or smallpox) then this is said to be a **sufficient cause**. For chronic diseases there are instances of single sufficient causes

for **monogenic disorders** but for most a combination of factors act together to produce a **combined sufficient cause (multiple causes)**. For the development of premature coronary heart disease (see Chapter 6) raised plasma cholesterol may be a necessary factor in a given population, but this is insufficient as a single causal factor for all cases of the disease. Different sets of multiple causes for coronary heart disease are illustrated by using Rothman's pie charts as shown in Figure 1.2. It is the task of the epidemiologist to examine as many potentially causal factors as possible and to quantify their likely contribution to the development of the disease. It should be noted that 'causal' factors may be related to each other and not show truly independent effects, but it may be helpful to define all possible causes to create the maximum potential for prevention. (For further discussion see Poole (2001) and Davey Smith and Ebrahim (2001).)

Bradford Hill, a medical statistician who worked with Doll on the link between tobacco smoking, lung cancer, and other important diseases, and who was also a

BOX 1.4 CRITERIA USED IN OBSERVATIONAL EPIDEMIOLOGICAL STUDIES TO DISTINGUISH 'CAUSAL' FROM NON-CAUSAL ASSOCIATIONS

- **Strength**: relative risk of lung cancer in smokers is 10 times that in non-smokers.

- **Consistency**: similar results in several studies from different countries possibly using different methodologies.

- **Specificity**: specific exposures (often occupational) may be associated with specific diseases.

- **Temporality**: did the putative cause precede the onset of the disease?

- **Biological gradient**: risk of respiratory cancers and of cardiovascular diseases increases with amount of cigarettes smoked and number of years of smoking.

- **Plausibility**: a biological mechanism should exist.

- **Coherence**: evidence from different sources provides biological 'coherence' to the overall hypothesis.

- **Experimental evidence**: from 'natural' or observed preventive experiments (without evidence from a scientifically conducted intervention study).

- **Analogy**: comparison with other diseases caused by similar biological mechanism.

Adapted from: Bradford Hill, A. (1971). *Principles of Medical Statistics* (9th edn). London: The Lancet.

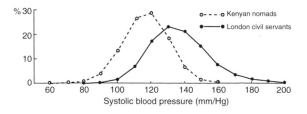

Fig. 1.3 Distributions of systolic blood pressure in middle-aged men in two populations.
Source: Rose, G. (1985). 'Sick Individuals and Sick Populations'. *International Journal of Epidemiology*, **14(1)**: 32–8.

and the UK or US. This is currently reflected in the respective mortality rates (which are closely linked to incidence) for coronary heart disease in the two populations; 54/17 in Japan, and 229/80 in the UK and 230/90 in the US in 2000, data are for men/women per 100 000, age-standardized to the European standard population (see Chapter 2). Population cholesterol levels are closely linked to dietary factors, which are culturally determined (see Chapter 6).

Despite the relatively slow progress in tobacco control there are many other legislative and advisory measures in place to help maintain the environment free of major hazards to our health. Throughout Western Europe the European Union has been instrumental in raising standards of water and air quality, but the agricultural policies and the prevailing legislation failed to prevent the spread of **bovine spongiform encephalopathy (BSE)** into the human population. In the UK the newly formed Health Protection and Food Standards Agencies have a watchdog role for environmentally caused diseases (see Chapter 21).

Secondary prevention of disease denotes the interruption of the full development of the natural progression of the disease and the restoration of normal health. This activity covers a broad spectrum of the natural history cycle from the beginning, in the case of pre-symptomatic disease, for example screening for early breast tumours or carcinoma *in situ* of the cervix, to the early treatment of myocardial infarction by thrombolytic therapy, which minimizes the area of myocardial damage. Secondary prevention is also used in the sense of preventing the recurrence of the disease. In Europe, for example, the European Society of Cardiology has formulated guidelines on secondary prevention after a series of European-wide surveys, which showed that many patients with myocardial infarction were poorly followed up, and that many clinicians had failed to check and modify cardiovascular risk factors on discharge from hospital (De Backer *et al.* 2003).

Tertiary prevention denotes the prevention of the major consequences of the natural history of a disease once its effects in a patient have become established. Examples in medical practice are: the rehabilitation of patients with long-term disability from coronary heart disease or stroke with exercise and psychological support; the long-term management and treatment of chronic diseases such as schizophrenia or Alzheimer's disease. Epidemiologists and biostatisticians have a role, along with clinicians, in developing effective treatments and efficient management of these diseases and to

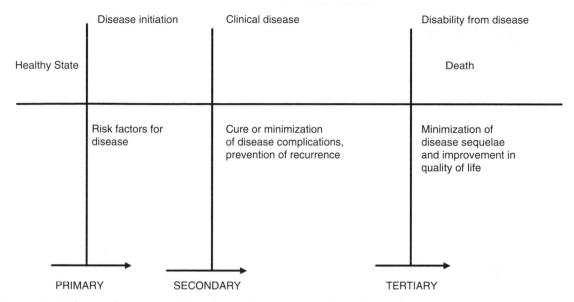

Fig. 1.4 Principal features of primary, secondary and tertiary disease prevention during the natural, uninterrupted progression of a disease.

promote primary, secondary and tertiary prevention at all stages of disease progression whenever the scientific information and evidence allow this. Further discussion of these topics is to be found in Chapters 5 and 21. The main features of primary, secondary and tertiary prevention are shown in Figure 1.4.

Consideration of the principles shown in this figure provide a framework for clinical practice and for research questions for specific diseases. This framework is also useful in the design of screening programmes, which may be at the primary or secondary (and occasionally tertiary) level of disease prevention (see Chapter 5 and Figure 5.1).

Further Reading

Gerstman, B. B. (1999). *Epidemiology Kept Simple. An Introduction to Classic and Modern Epidemiology.* New York, NY: Wiley-Liss.

McMahon, B. and Trichoupolos, D. (1996). *Epidemiology. Principles and Methods.* (2nd edn). Boston, MA: Little, Brown and Company.

References

References for this chapter can be found at www.oxfordtextbooks.co.uk/orc/yarnell. Where possible, these are presented as *active links* which direct you to an electronic version of the work. If you are a subscriber to that work (either individually or through an institution), and depending on your level of access, you may be able to peruse an abstract or the full article if available. 🖳

are widely read and highly influential internationally in changing established views of disease treatment and prevention, for example the *New England Journal of Medicine*, the *Journal of American Medical Association*, and *Archives of Internal Medicine* published in the USA, and *The Lancet* and *British Medical Journal* published in the UK. Articles in such journals will usually have been peer-reviewed by experts in the field to ensure, as far as possible, that the methodology is sound and the conclusions valid. An abstract published by such journals provides the busy clinician or medical student with an outline which should include: **the purpose of the study, its most important features, and why the authors feel that the findings are important**. An example of such an abstract is given in Box 2.1.

Whatever the purpose of the study, previous similar studies should be reviewed in detail as they will often indicate the choice of study design or help to refine hypotheses. A thorough electronic search using several key words in a major database, such as that held by the American Library of Medicine (PubMed) and freely available to any internet user, is the minimum necessary for any epidemiological study. Techniques for searching the medical literature will be described in more detail in Chapter 20.

2.2 Sources of Data and Uses of Routine Health Data

Public health activities rely on accurate population health data. Here we provide a brief overview of the major sources of **official or routine health data** that can be used to assemble a detailed picture of population health. Fuller discussion of routine health statistics and surveys available in the UK (Kerrison and Macfarlane 2000), in the USA (Luck 2002), and internationally (World Health Organization 2003) is to be found elsewhere. Web-based sources of routine data are shown in Box 2.2.

BOX 2.1 EXAMPLE OF ABSTRACT STRUCTURE IN A MEDICAL JOURNAL

Title Central overweight and obesity in British youth aged 11–16 years: cross-sectional surveys of waist circumference.

Objective To compare changes over time in waist circumference (a measure of central fatness) and body mass index (a measure of overall obesity) in British youth.

Design Representative cross-sectional surveys in 1977, 1987, and 1997.

Setting Great Britain.

Participants Young people aged 11–16 years surveyed in 1977 (boys) and 1987 (girls) for the British Standards Institute ($n = 3784$) and in 1997 (both sexes) for the national diet and nutrition survey ($n = 776$).

Main outcome measures Waist circumference, expressed as a standard deviation score using the first survey as reference, and body mass index (weight (kg) / height (m)²), expressed as a standard deviation (SD) score against the British 1990 revised reference. Overweight and obesity were defined as the measurement exceeding the ninety-first and ninety-eighth centile, respectively.

Results Waist circumference increased sharply over the period between surveys (mean increases for boys and girls, 6.9 and 6.2 cm, or 0.84 and 1.02 SD score units, $p < 0.0001$). In centile terms, waist circumference increased more in girls than in boys. Increases in body mass index were smaller and similar by sex (means 1.5 and 1.6, or 0.47 and 0.53 SD score units, $p < 0.0001$). Waist circumference in 1997 exceeded the ninety-first centile in 28 per cent ($n = 110$) of boys and 38 per cent ($n = 147$) of girls (against 9 per cent for both sexes in 1977–87, $p < 0.0001$) whereas 14 per cent ($n = 54$) and 17 per cent ($n = 68$), respectively, exceeded the ninety-eighth centile (3 per cent in 1977–87, $p < 0.0001$). The corresponding rates for body mass index in 1997 were 21 per cent ($n = 80$) of boys and 17 per cent ($n = 67$) of girls exceeding the ninety-first centile (8 per cent and 6 per cent in 1977–87) and 10 per cent ($n = 39$) and 8 per cent ($n = 32$) exceeding the ninety-eighth centile (3 per cent and 2 per cent in 1977–87).

Conclusions Trends in waist circumference during the past 10–20 years have greatly exceeded those in body mass index, particularly in girls, showing that body mass index is a poor proxy for central fatness. Body mass index has therefore systematically underestimated the prevalence of obesity in young people.

Source: McCarthy *et al.* (2003). *British Medical Journal*, **326**: 624, reproduced with permission from the BMJ Publishing Group.

Basic epidemiological tools

This chapter introduces the basic tools of epidemiology. Sources of data, both routinely available and collected specifically for particular studies, are reviewed. Qualitative and preliminary studies are discussed.

2.1 Purpose of the Study

As implied in Chapter 1, epidemiology has come to embrace a broad range of studies seeking to answer questions about disease in humans, usually by studying whole or sub-populations, but sometimes only patient groups. Increasingly epidemiology is described in sub-specialities, for example social, genetic, and clinical epidemiology, the latter emphasizing the use of epidemiological (and statistical) methods in clinical settings in hospital and general practice, particularly for diagnosis and clinical decision-making (alternative choices of treatment or care) (see Chapter 20). Silman (2002) has suggested that six aspects of human disease fall into the remit of epidemiology: **disease definition, occurrence, causation, outcome, management, and prevention**, as defined individually in Chapter 1. Epidemiologists tend to ask questions about disease occurrence, causation, definition, and prevention; clinicians often ask about the effectiveness of therapy, management, and outcome. Many published human studies fall under the general umbrella of epidemiology, but this is often not mentioned specifically in the abstract or text, and an epidemiologist may not be included among the authors. Clinicians now have the opportunity to undertake epidemiological training and to work alongside biostatisticians. Certain journals

Vital statistics (births, deaths, and marriages)

Most countries record each birth and death, making such registries of vital statistics an ongoing census of the population. A census is a prerequisite for establishing a **demographic profile**, which provides a picture of the age structure of a particular country or population. As **fertility rates** (number of births per 1000 women aged 15–44 years (sometimes 49 years) in a defined geographical area) are usually also available, future estimates of population growth and structure can be made. Some country profiles are shown in Chapter 14 (Fig. 14.2). The UK decennial census is discussed later in this chapter.

Mortality data

In most countries recording of death is a statutory requirement for all age groups. **Infant mortality** (death rates in the first year of life) is commonly used as an indicator of the general health and the effectiveness of the preventive health-service infrastructure that we take for granted in modern industrialized societies. Other indicators of population health include mortality in children under five years of age and mortality under 65 years of age. **Life expectancy data** are derived directly from *current* mortality rates (these data project life expectancy at any given age) and tend to underestimate life expectancy as mortality rates continue to improve for most countries.

In the UK, most death certificates are completed by doctors (a small percentage are also completed by coroners), according to standardized protocols proposed by the World Health Organization (WHO). Box 2.3 shows the layout of the medical certificate of cause of death. It is divided into two parts: Part 1 lists the conditions that led directly to death, with the condition that started the morbid train of events (the underlying cause of death) entered last in the list. Conditions that contributed to, but did not directly cause death are entered in Part 2. These conditions are then coded according to the International Classification of Disease (ICD).

Routine mortality statistics are therefore based on identifying a single underlying cause of death. To derive the most useful information from the death certificates, even when it has been badly completed, ICD incorporates selection rules and modification rules, which apply to particular conditions, combinations, or circumstances.

In the UK, accuracy of death certification may be enhanced by the fact that certification is done by a doctor or coroner in 99.9 per cent of cases; nevertheless, death certificates are usually completed in hospitals by junior doctors often without instruction. Inspection of the causes of death in Box 2.3 will indicate the potential for miscoding if the 'underlying cause' is inappropriately placed.

There have been ten versions of the ICD since its inception in 1900. Each revised classification has been developed to incorporate advances in medical knowledge and understanding of the disease process. ICD-10 now includes 8000 unique codes which comprise a letter that denotes a broad chapter or system of disease and two or three numbers that further refine the classification (for example 'I' represents all circulatory disease; I21 represents acute myocardial infarction).

While mortality data are very accurate in terms of the number and timing of events they are somewhat less robust when specifying cause of death. They are also subject to changes in investigation, diagnostic and coding practices which can render comparisons between areas and across time problematical. Perhaps surprisingly finding the exact cause of death can be difficult, even in modern medical environments. This level of uncertainty increases with age as older patients

---

BOX 2.3 CERTIFYING THE CAUSE OF DEATH (FROM THE UK DEATH CERTIFICATE)

CAUSE OF DEATH

*The condition thought to be the 'Underlying Cause of Death' should
apply in the lowest completed line of Part 1*

		(ICD10)*
I (a) Disease or condition directly leading to death†	*Cardiac arrest*	(I46.9)
(b) Other disease or condition, if any, leading to: I(a)	*Congestive heart failure*	(I50.0)
(c) Other disease or condition, if any, leading to: I(b)	*Acute myocardial infarction*	(I21.9)
II Other significant conditions CONTRIBUTING TO THE DEATH but not related to the disease or condition causing it	*Diabetes mellitus, insulin dependent*	(E10.8)

*Coded by the Office for National Statistics (ONS).

---

often suffer from multiple pathologies and there may be a reluctance to subject them to invasive diagnostic procedures. The most accurate way to determine the cause of death, and check the accuracy of death certificates, is to perform post-mortem examinations but this has largely fallen out of fashion and is undertaken in less than 10 per cent of hospital deaths in the UK, although other countries may have higher rates. One reason for this may be the belief that current medical technology can detect most of the important medical information about a person, including the cause of death. However, studies throughout the world have repeatedly demonstrated a worrying discrepancy between the diagnosis given on the death certificate compared with that at hospital post-mortem.

It is possible that some of the increase in deaths over the twentieth century attributed, for example, to cancer has been artifactual and due to an increased clinical awareness allied to an increased availability of investigative technology. Radiological examination has become more refined (for example computerized tomography) and is now complemented by ultrasound (Doppler) and magnetic resonance imaging. Endoscopic examination is now a common outpatient procedure allowing direct examination and biopsy of suspect areas. Analyses of blood chemistry, serology, biomarkers, and cytology are becoming increasingly sophisticated and available to a wider range of doctors. All these and other diagnostic facilities will both increase the chances of diagnosing cancer, if it is present, and the accuracy of cancer coding.

Other difficulties, particularly when comparing time (secular) trends, can be caused by changes in the way

diseases are coded. In the early twentieth century 'old age' was a bona fide cause of death, and one of the most commonly certified cause of death for those aged 70 and over, up until the 1950s. Changes in coding practices after that time required a more accurate diagnosis and deaths due to bronchopneumonia, circulatory disease and, to some extent, cancers increased to fill the vacuum left by the 'demise' of 'old age' as a cause of death. The introduction of ICD-10 in the UK in 2001 further changed the coding rules used to select the underlying cause of death from the death certificate. It was associated with a 20 per cent reduction in the number of deaths attributed to pneumonia and a corresponding increase in those attributed to chronic debilitating diseases, particularly the musculo-skeletal system and various types of dementia. To facilitate comparisons over time, many countries have undertaken a 'bridging' exercise, where all deaths in one year are coded according to both ICD-9 and ICD-10 classifications, to produce estimates of the changes arising from the introduction of the new classification system.

There are additional difficulties in interpreting international mortality data which relate to different population structures in countries; in particular comparisons between rich and poor countries require standardization of the age structures in each country. WHO produces mortality rates that are standardized to the European Standard Populations (for advanced industrialized countries) and the World Standard Population (for a global estimate, which includes a large proportion of countries with young populations). Crude (overall) deaths rates for the UK or the US are higher than those for Egypt or Iraq (in the year 2000), which is entirely due to the high proportion of children and young adults in the last two countries. These issues are discussed further in Chapter 14 (section 14.1).

Morbidity data

A disadvantage of mortality data is that they do not reflect the burden of morbidity from important diseases – for example mental health problems – which seldom result in death. The ICD is also used by hospitals and primary care to record morbidity but additional classification systems also exist. WHO has a classification system for cancer, which is based on histological type rather than site. This classification may be more relevant to survival as different types of tumour may respond differently to therapy. Clinicians and epidemiologists may also use other classification systems, particularly in health-care research, where ICD codes may be inappropriate or inadequate for a particular study.

Morbidity data too, however, have their deficiencies: the definition of what constitutes a disease is often imprecise, no one source covers the range of illness episodes, and coverage and available information are often incomplete. Therefore, a wide range of sources is needed for any attempt at completeness.

Morbidity data from secondary care

In the UK, the first hospital survey was conducted in 1949. The Department of Health currently compiles the **hospital episode statistics** (HES) database, containing all patient-based records of finished consultant episodes (ordinary admissions and day cases) by diagnosis, operation, and specialty from National Health Service (NHS) hospitals in England. However, the confidentiality of such data is an issue under the Data Protection Act, and anonymized data are usually supplied for research purposes. The Scottish Morbidity Record system allows individual patient-record linkage between hospital admissions and deaths, permitting more precise investigation of disease rates (Kendrick and Clarke 1993). Pell *et al.* (2004) have used the ability to link mortality data with patient records to examine associations between diseases in pregnancy and subsequent risk of stroke. Other examples of linkage of routine data sources with other data are shown in Table 2.1.

Morbidity data from primary care

In the UK most people are registered with a general practitioner – often the first port of call for an ill patient – who deals with a wide range of health problems. A national study of morbidity statistics from general practice is performed at approximately 10-year intervals, using a sample of volunteer general practices in England and Wales. One example is the General Practice Research Database (GPRD), originally set up in 1987, from which findings are published in series MB6 from the Office of National Statistics (ONS). With longitudinal data on several million patients, this is a unique data source for research into many aspects of disease risk, management, and treatment. **Prescribing data**

TABLE 2.1 Some examples of research use of routine data

Geographical area	Study topic	Data used	Design	Reference
World	Global mortality attributable	Viral statistics. Smoking surveys	Cross-sectional	Ezzati, M. and Lopez, A. D. (2003). 'Estimates of Global Mortality Due to Smoking'. *The Lancet*, **362**: 847–52.
Country: England and Wales	Health inequality in migrants	Census and mortality statistics	Longitudinal: record linkage	Harding, S. and Maxwell, R. (1997). 'Differences in Mortality of Migrants', in F. Drever and M. Whitehead (eds.). *Health Inequalities*. Decennial Supplement Series DS, No. 15. London: Stationery Office, 108–221.
Country: England and Wales	Occupational mortality	Census and mortality statistics	Longitudinal: record linkage	Drever, F. (ed.) (1995). *Occupational Health: Decennial Supplement*. London: HMSO.

Continued

and social services at the level of small geographical areas, such as electoral wards. The data collected are confidential and only now can the 1901 census be searched by research workers after 100 years of remaining confidential.

However, the decennial census is expensive and there is a delay of two to three years before the data become available. In practice this means that good data are available for only a few years after a census, and, after this period, there is increasing reliance on estimates of the population. In recent years there have also been concerns about the completeness of the UK census, especially the enumeration of younger males in inner city areas. Intercensal population estimates are derived from knowledge of the three drivers of population change: births, deaths, and migration. For example the population of an area one year after the census$_{(t+1)}$ is equal to the original population at time (t), plus the **natural increase** (births – deaths) plus the **net migration** (immigration – emigration):

i.e. Population$_{t+1}$ = Population$_t$ + Births – Deaths + immigration – emigration

Population movement is the main reason why it is difficult to produce accurate intercensal estimates of the population, and especially so for small areas. International migration estimates are derived in the UK from the **International Passenger Survey**, which is a continuous survey that samples a selection of persons arriving at, or departing from, the main air and seaports. Tracking population movement within a country is even more difficult, though this can be assessed from changes in other data sources such as the electoral register, uptake of social security benefits, etc.

The electoral register

This is potentially an alternative source of population estimates in the UK and elsewhere. Its strength is that it is validated and updated on an annual basis in the UK. Its weakness is that it only contains lists of people who are old enough to vote and will miss people who do not want to vote or who have not been able to register, for example because they have recently changed address. Issues about data protection have placed increasing restrictions on the use of these data.

General practitioner lists

Almost everyone in the UK is registered with a general practitioner and as these data are held centrally, they can provide descriptions of the age and sex composition of small areas throughout the country. There are two

main weaknesses with these data: (i) list inflation, which arises because of the retention of people who have migrated or died (immortals or ghosts); and (ii) address inaccuracies, because practices may not be aware that the patient has changed address. However, a move to introduce a unique NHS number in the UK is likely to greatly improve the accuracy of such systems.

National insurance data

Recent years have seen an increasing use of administrative databases, such as receipt of pensions, which can be used to provide good indications of older people by age, sex and geography. The main weakness of such systems is the variability of the uptake. Some countries such as The Netherlands and Sweden have a system of continuous population registration (in which all changes of permanent residence are registered) that are so complete as to render the census obsolete. It is possible that this will become more common in other European countries in future years. In the UK, however, there is an increasing tendency to supplement the census-based area characteristics with those based on routine administrative databases, such as those for national insurance and social security benefits, which are usually well maintained.

The General Household Survey

The General Household Survey (GHS) is a multi-purpose continuous survey performed by the Social Survey Division of the ONS, which collects information on a range of topics from people living in private households in Great Britain. The survey started in 1971 and has been done almost yearly since then. From a changing sample of approximately 13000 addresses, all adults aged 16 years and over are interviewed in each responding household. Core data comprise detailed sociodemographic and health information.

Health survey for England

In 1991 this became a series of annual surveys, used to underpin and improve targeting of nationwide health policies. From a national 'representative' sample of about 20000 individuals the survey estimates the proportion of the population with specific health conditions, including psychological health, and risk factors associated with those conditions. It also examines differences between population sub-groups, and monitors targets in the health strategy. Each annual survey retains core items but may focus on a particular health topic. From 1995 the height and weight of children at different ages has become an added component, monitoring overweight and obesity, replacing the earlier national study of health and growth which was designed to evaluate trends in undernutrition. Similar surveys are performed periodically but less frequently in Scotland, Wales, and Northern Ireland. Sampling issues (how to obtain a 'representative' sample) are discussed in Chapter 4.

Using routine data in health research

Routine data have several important strengths that enable them to be used to answer pertinent health questions: these include their power and efficiency and that they are often population-based. However, they remain an under-used source of data that could enable epidemiological studies to be undertaken and have an important role in understanding and improving the health of populations. Types of epidemiological study are discussed in Chapter 3, but some examples of the research uses of routine data both from the UK and other European countries are shown in Table 2.1. A major repository for routine data is the UK Data Archive (UKDA), which allows interested individuals or groups to register and access a wide range of data sources for research purposes (see Box 2.2).

2.3 Quantitative and Qualitative Studies

Epidemiological studies are **quantitative** in nature, usually producing population estimates of disease prevalence and incidence, and, for most studies, statistical tests can be applied to examine particular hypotheses. In contrast, **qualitative studies** place an emphasis on the development of concepts rather than on numbers or statistics: that is, on the meaning, views, and experiences of research participants (or subjects), which assist the formulation of research hypotheses. Qualitative studies have their origins in disciplines such as sociology and social anthropology, and are used increasingly by epidemiologists, often in collaboration with specialists in the core disciplines. One of the ways in which qualitative research methods can be used by epidemiologists and health-care researchers is to develop questionnaires suitable for quantitative use, particularly in social and psychiatric epidemiology, and in the development of instruments (questionnaires) designed to evaluate physical and medical functioning (well-being). Several different instruments have been developed on the basis of extensive qualitative studies for use as comparators of health status in different communities and even countries (for example SF-36, Euroquol, etc., which measure several different aspects of physical and mental health) and were an essential first step in developing the weighting (adjusting) factors used to calculate quality adjusted life years (QALYS) and disability-adjusted life years (DALYS) (see Chapters 12 and 17 for examples of their use). The key terms and methods used in qualitative studies are shown in Box 2.4.

There are several reasons why we need qualitative research in health and health care. According to Black (1994), qualitative methods can be used effectively to illuminate and contribute to quantitative studies, including epidemiological research by:

- Identifying the most appropriate variables that should be measured.

- Generating hypotheses for subsequent investigation by quantitative methods.

- Increasing understanding about the way quantitatively assessed variables were defined, understood, and completed.

BOX 2.4 GLOSSARY OF TERMS USED IN QUALITATIVE RESEARCH

- **Case studies** focus on one or a limited number of settings; used to explore contemporary phenomenon, especially where complex interrelated issues are involved. Can be exploratory, explanatory, or descriptive or a combination of these.

- **Consensus methods** include **Delphi** and **nominal group techniques** and **consensus development conferences**. They provide a way of synthesizing information and dealing with conflicting evidence, with the aim of determining extent of agreement within a selected group.

- **Constant comparison**: iterative method of content analysis where each category is searched for in the entire data set and all instances are compared until no new categories can be identified. **Analytic induction**: use of constant comparison specifically in developing hypotheses, which are then tested in further data collection and analysis.

Continued

BOX 2.4 GLOSSARY OF TERMS USED IN QUALITATIVE RESEARCH (*Continued*)

- **Content analysis**: systematic examination of text (field notes) by identifying and grouping themes and coding, classifying, and developing categories.

- **Epistemology**: theory of knowledge; scientific study which deals with the nature and validity of knowledge.

- **Fieldnotes**: collective term for records of observation, talk, interview transcripts, or documentary sources. Typically includes a field diary which provides a record of the chronological events and development of research as well as the researcher's own reactions to, feeling about, and opinions of the research process.

- **Focus groups**: method of group interview which explicitly includes and uses the group interaction to generate data.

- **Hawthorne effect**: impact of the researcher on the research subjects or setting, notably in changing their behaviour.

- **In depth interviews**: face-to-face conversation with the purpose of exploring issues or topics in detail. Does not use pre-set questions, but is shaped by a defined set of topics or issues.

- **Induction**: process of moving from observations/data towards generalizations, hypotheses, or theory; **grounded theory**: hypothesizing inductively from data, notably using subjects' own categories, concepts etc; opposite of **deduction**, process of data gathering to test predefined theory or hypotheses.

- **Naturalistic research**: non-experimental research in naturally occurring settings.

- **Observation**: systematic watching of behaviour and talk in naturally occurring settings. **Participant observation:** observation in which the researcher also occupies a role or part in the setting in addition to observing.

- **Paradigm**: Framework of theory in which the investigator is operating.

- **Purposive sampling**: deliberate choice of respondents, subjects, or settings, as opposed to **statistical sampling**, concerned with the representativeness of a sample in relation to a total population. **Theoretical sampling** links this to previously developed hypotheses or theories.

- **Reliability**: extent to which a measurement yields the same answer each time it is used.

- **Social anthropology**: social scientific study of peoples, cultures, and societies; particularly associated with the study of traditional cultures.

- **Triangulation**: use of three or more different research methods in combination; principally used as a check of validity.

- **Validity**: extent to which a measurement truly reflects the phenomenon under scrutiny.

Adapted from: Source: Mays, N. and Pope, C. (eds.) (1996). *Qualitative Methods in Health Care*. London: BMJ Publishing Group. Reproduced with permission by Blackwell Publishing.

- Explaining results, particularly unexpected findings reported in quantitative studies.

Furthermore, qualitative methods, such as observation, interviews, and the analysis of documentary material, are more appropriate than quantitative methods when there is uncertainty and a lack of clarity about a health issue (such as waiting lists) or about the variables that may contribute to the subject of a study.

Two types of preliminary study likely to have qualitative aspects may be performed before large-scale quantitative investigations: **feasibility studies** can be used to examine the practical possibility of conducting a large-scale study; and **pilot studies** may be done to develop hypotheses, establish questionnaire design, or to estimate the sample size required for a main study.

References

References for this chapter can be found at www.oxfordtextbooks.co.uk/orc/yarnell/. Where possible, these are presented as *active links* which direct you to an electronic version of the work. ⌨

Epidemiological studies

In this chapter we distinguish the descriptive from the analytical approach in epidemiology, describe the main varieties of study, and what factors dictate the choice of study design. The concept of risk is developed using particular study designs and epidemiological data.

3.1 Descriptive and Analytical Studies

As discussed in Chapter 1, a fundamental aim of epidemiology is the description of the occurrence of a particular disease in the population, usually according to the **personal characteristics** of individuals (for example age, sex, occupation, etc.), **place**, and **time** of occurrence. Hence many epidemiological studies involve a description of the disease or condition in the population. Such **descriptive studies** are often quick to complete, particularly when they are based on routinely collected data, and may generate hypotheses that can be tested in analytical studies. For many diseases, particularly relatively rare ones, this basic **descriptive epidemiology** is well known from studies of prevalence and incidence in different countries; for example the descriptive epidemiology of cancers that are rare in one country but more common in others. However, analytical studies for these cancers remain largely uninformative (Chapter 15). Similarly, multiple sclerosis has a marked female–male distribution and a north–south gradient in Europe but there are few clues as to the causal factors (Chapter 11).

Descriptive studies

Several study designs are described that are particularly useful in the early stages of definition of a new disease, condition or syndrome etc. (see Box 1.2). A **case series** is simply a series of cases of disease that can be useful to raise awareness initially of a new disease or disease variant. Both acquired immunodeficiency disease syndrome (AIDS) and bovine spongiform encephalopathy (BSE) were initially described from the excess occurrence of cases of related rare diseases, which eventually led to new disease definitions, an essential first step in descriptive epidemiology. A **population prevalence** study counts the number of cases of a particular disease or condition in the general population, usually by means of a special survey or census (see Table 2.1 for examples of this). Such studies can be used to estimate cases in the population, to assess the health needs of the population and to determine trends over time (secular trends). Studies of population prevalence can also be used for analytical purposes, in which causal hypotheses are tested, provided that relevant data have been collected. Other examples of this type of study design are shown in Table 2.1 and Box 7.2, which show secular trends in childhood obesity and the international prevalence of asthma symptoms respectively.

Ecological studies

These are quite widely used in preliminary descriptive epidemiology, particularly in describing differences between different geographical areas or regions, and in different ethnic and cultural groups. In an ecological study the outcome event (usually the disease under study) is not linked to individual subjects but to groups of subjects leading to the possibility of the **ecological fallacy** (an observed relation in grouped data which is not supported by subsequent data at the individual level). Data on possible individual **confounding variables** (see section 3.2) cannot be used, often leading to inappropriate and non-causal association in ecological studies. Examples of ecological studies are given in Chapters 6 and 11.

Analytical studies

These are usually inferential or hypothetico-deductive in nature and require statistical methods of analysis: that is, the data from a sample are used to estimate characteristics or test **hypotheses** about the population from which the sample was taken (see Chapter 4). Often the hypotheses are concerned with the **associations** or relations between exposure status and disease occurrence.

An **exposure** variable may represent a risk factor or a treatment, depending on the nature of the study. In practice there can be some overlap between descriptive and analytical studies, particularly in the case of new diseases such as AIDS, legionnaire's disease and chronic fatigue syndrome in which the same data sets are used for the descriptive epidemiology and for analytical purposes. Analytical studies can be further subdivided into observational and experimental studies. In an **observational study** the exposure of a subject occurs naturally and is 'observed' or recorded by the epidemiologist; in an **experimental (or intervention) study** the exposure is 'assigned' to the **patient** by the investigator. In passing, epidemiologists tend to term volunteers or members of the public recruited from the general population '**subjects**' or '**participants**' to distinguish them from **patients** who are recruited from patient populations under clinical care.

Observational studies

These are the most common type of epidemiological study and are classified by their **designs**; some common designs are displayed in Box 3.1. The classification of these studies is based on the **time** (past, current, future) when the exposure is measured and when the disease occurrence is ascertained; this determines whether it is a **cohort** study (beginning with exposed and non-exposed groups and then studying the occurrence of the disease) or a **case–control** study (beginning with the **cases**, diseased subjects, and the **controls**, non-diseased subjects, and then investigating their exposure status). The term 'cohort' is derived from the idea of a Roman troop of soldiers marching onwards together (Latin – tenth part of Roman legion). If exposure and disease status are measured concurrently, the study is said to be **cross-sectional**. If disease information is collected currently and exposure status from past records, the study is described as **retrospective**. If exposure information is collected currently and disease status in the future, the study is described as **prospective** (or **longitudinal**). Usually case–control studies collect exposure information retrospectively and cohort studies collect disease information prospectively, but there are exceptions. The **retrospective cohort study** defines a cohort and its exposure status retrospectively from existing records typically from occupational sources. The **nested case–control** study is increasingly conducted as part of a prospective cohort study, particularly when stored biological samples are available; these can be more efficiently used in a case–control rather than in a cohort setting.

BOX 3.1 OBSERVATIONAL STUDIES

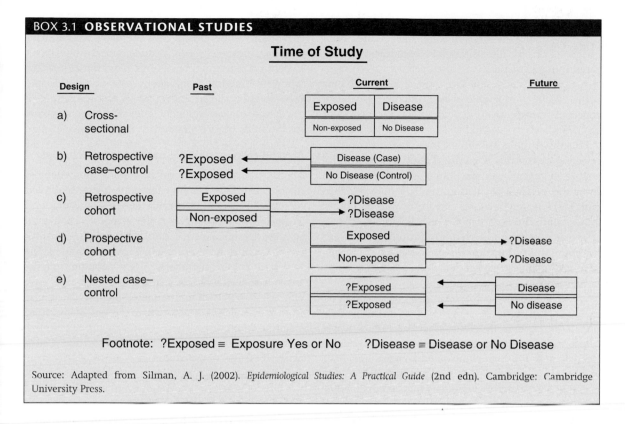

Footnote: ?Exposed ≡ Exposure Yes or No   ?Disease ≡ Disease or No Disease

Source: Adapted from Silman, A. J. (2002). *Epidemiological Studies: A Practical Guide* (2nd edn). Cambridge: Cambridge University Press.

In Chapter 6, Table 6.3 gives an example of a large case–control study, and Table 6.2 gives an example of a prospective cohort study.

Experimental or intervention studies

These are frequently performed to compare different treatments (for example drugs or surgical procedures) in which the patients (volunteers who have given **informed consent**) are receiving treatment in hospital or in primary care. Non-clinical interventions (for example dietary, behavioural, or public health) can also be investigated within a clinical setting or in the community. The gold standard for an experimental study is the **randomized controlled trial (RCT)** which compares interventions that are allocated to subjects by a randomization procedure; in addition the subject and the investigator should be '**blinded**' (unaware of the type of treatment) if possible. Examples of RCTs are given in Chapters 8 and 20. In community studies, **cluster randomized trials** are being increasingly used: the intervention is allocated to a cluster of subjects. For example all patients in a general practice list, a pharmacy, or a school may provide the sampling unit rather than an individual subject or participant. Finally, there are

designs that involve no formal randomization in the allocation of interventions to subjects: these are referred to as **quasi-experimental**. These designs are frequently used to inform public-health practice and in other situations where randomization is difficult to achieve.

3.2 Choice of Study Design

Observational studies

Several factors govern the choice of study design. These include: **the purpose of the study; previous studies; available data; and the balance between feasibility (time and costs) and validity.**

Cross-sectional and retrospective case–control studies

These are closely related and frequently overlap, as the exposure status is in practice often assessed retrospectively, based on recall by cases and controls. These studies are relatively quick and easy to undertake and are the first line of inquiry into any rare disease or newly emerging disease of uncertain aetiology. For example, human BSE, legionnaire's disease (see Chapter 16),

AIDS and severe acute respiratory syndrome (SARS) were all initially investigated using such studies. Non-infectious chronic diseases are also extensively investigated by cross-sectional or retrospective case–control studies, but usually exposures are chronic and may occur over a considerable period; thus exposure data collected retrospectively provide a concurrent test of the hypothesis in question.

Because of the possibility of **bias** (systematic error), selection of controls is a critical issue in case–control studies. In general, controls drawn by random selection from the general population, and possibly matched with cases by age and sex and for one or two other major **confounding variables** such as smoking habit or social class, are preferred. **Confounding variables are those linked both to the disease and to the exposure under investigation**. Matching effectively eliminates such variables from the comparison of exposures in cases and controls. Hospital-based controls are particularly unlikely to be representative of the general population, as selective factors operate to put people into hospital even for apparently 'random' accidents (see Chapter 17). Population-based controls are, however, cumbersome and expensive to obtain, in addition to being less likely to volunteer than other possible comparison groups. In the example of the case–control study in Chapter 6 (Table 6.3), the smoking habits of patients admitted to hospital with a heart attack (myocardial infarction) have been compared with those of their family members. The investigators ran the risk of reducing the chance of finding an association if a higher proportion of family members had similar smoking habits to the patients than was true of the general population (which is likely!). However, because of the large number of patients and controls studied, and because of the strong association, the link between heart attack and smoking habit is supported; in reality, it may have been underestimated.

Prospective or longitudinal cohort studies

These are generally considered superior to cross-sectional and retrospective case–control studies; they may be used to confirm findings from those latter studies. One advantage is that individual exposure status is known at the start of the study before the development of the disease. Hence these studies are less likely to suffer from **recall bias** that can exist in cross-sectional and retrospective case–control studies. Another advantage of the prospective approach is that multiple **end points** (or **outcome events**) can be studied, which could include fatal and non-fatal disease or the occurrence of

more than one disease: This is not usually possible in retrospective and cross-sectional case–control studies. However, prospective cohort studies are costly, difficult to perform, and time-consuming, requiring a period of follow-up ranging from about two years upwards, depending on the size of the study and the nature of the disease or diseases under study. They are unsuitable for the study of rare diseases.

Nested or prospective case–control studies

These increasingly form an important component of major prospective studies examining the development of relatively common chronic diseases or conditions. They are usually based on the availability of biological samples (blood, plasma, serum, DNA, urine, saliva, etc.) stored at the start or baseline examination of the recruited cohort members. Many potential physio-pathological risk factors can be examined in a cost-effective manner without requiring analysis of samples from the whole cohort. More than one end point can be examined if required. These studies are termed 'nested' because the exposure status is created and ascertained at the baseline examination (and subsequently 'incubated' until the end points are evaluated).

Retrospective cohort studies

In these, the exposure status of a whole cohort (for example an occupational cohort) is accurately known from historical or occupational records, and the disease status of individuals from the whole cohort is obtained in current time. Such studies are relatively quick and inexpensive to conduct.

Experimental (intervention) studies

These are widely held to be de rigeur by the medical establishment before acceptance of a new therapy or intervention. Several types of study design are possible; all have advantages and disadvantages at both the practical and scientific level. In trials of treatment in patients, a comparison group is used who receive an existing treatment or a **placebo** (dummy) treatment. In the past a control group comprising patients from a previous time period was sometimes used, termed a **historical control group**; but this approach can give misleading results. A review of empirical comparisons of randomized and non-randomized clinical trials has been reported which supports this view (Kunz and Oxman 1998). Trials involving patients can be in **parallel**, in which only one treatment is received by each patient; or they can be **crossover** trials, when a second treatment is given to a patient replacing the initial treatment, sometimes after a suitable 'washout' period. Crossover trials tend to measure alterations in symptoms or quality of life in chronic conditions. A **factorial** design can be used to compare two or more treatments, and combinations of treatments. The International Studies of Infarct Survival (ISIS) provide examples of large-scale factorial trials of treatment in acute myocardial infarction, for example ISIS-3 (1992). The process of **random allocation** of patients to treatment has been shown to be an important step in minimizing the possibility of bias in the selection of these patient groups in controlled trials. Therefore in evidence-based medicine, particularly in most patient-centred studies, the randomized controlled study is the design of choice.

When an intervention is directed at a group of individuals, randomization of the sampling unit is not always possible. As noted earlier, a cluster of subjects at a school or at a general practice can be selected as the sampling unit for random allocation, but this may not always be possible. Generally the broader the intervention strategy, particularly if mass media interventions are used, the more likely 'contamination' of control areas may occur. Two large-scale whole-population studies in which multifactorial public-health cardiovascular interventions were used over several years showed comparable net changes in each intervention area (Wales: Tudor Smith *et al.* 1998, and Kilkenny County, Ireland: Shelley *et al.* 1994) and in the respective control area. One possibility cited by these authors is that contamination of each control area occurred in these quasi-experimental studies.

In developing countries, trials of public-health intervention can be particularly important to inform and direct medical care in the absence of a well-established and resourced medical infrastructure. An example of a geographically based quasi-experimental study to reduce neonatal mortality in rural India is shown in Figure 3.1. Cluster randomized trials may be possible in rural areas in developing countries in separate communities, which are relatively isolated from each other, so that interventions do not spread into control areas unintentionally. Two examples of well-conducted cluster randomized trials to treat common sexually transmitted diseases to reduce the spread of HIV infection in rural African communities are described elsewhere (Grosskurth *et al.* 1995; Wawer *et al.* 1999).

3.3 **Risk**

The concept of risk is crucial to a basic understanding of epidemiology. An overall definition of **risk** for

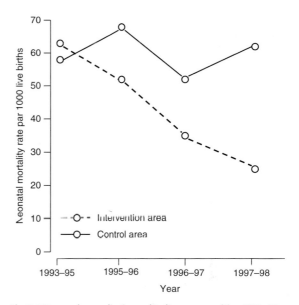

Fig. 3.1 Neonatal mortality in rural Indian communities, 1993–98: a public-health intervention study using home-based neonatal care. Source: Bang, A. T., Bang, R. A., Baitule, S. B., Reddy, M. H. and Deshmukh, M. D. (1999). 'Effect of Home-Based Neonatal Care and Management of Sepsis on Neonatal Mortality: Field Trial in Rural India'. *The Lancet*, **354**: 1955–61.

epidemiological purposes is: **the probability of the occurrence of a future adverse event such as death, a disease, or a complication of disease**. Epidemiology employs a variety of risk indices which are based on rates so that an understanding of the construction of the **rate of an event** (see Box 3.2), and in particular the role of the **reference population**, is essential.

For example **absolute risk** implies the overall risk for an individual in a given reference population. If the reference population is a whole country, region or geographically-based community, the absolute risk of a future event can only be calculated from census or vital statistics data as described in section 1.2 (Box 1.3). **Life tables** for a reference population can be calculated using actuarial methods based on current life expectancies at birth and in subsequent age groups through to the most elderly members of the population (see section 14.1). Such tables enable the average number of **life-years lost** to be calculated for a particular disease. Increasingly, life-years lost are used in public-health studies to compare particular diseases, to describe and calculate mortality that may be amenable to public-health preventive interventions (**avoidable mortality**), and to guide future

---

BOX 3.2 **DEFINITION OF A RATE**

Rate = (numerator/denominator) × multiplier, where: numerator = number of events that have occurred in a given period (for example one year); denominator = number of subjects at risk in the given period; multiplier = a convenient large number (for example 1000) used to avoid numerous decimal places. The rate is described as, for example, 'per 1000 per year'. Note that numerator and denominator must relate to the same population in terms of age group, gender, geographical area, etc.

---

public-health policies. The number of life-years lost is dependent on the average age of death for the particular disease. To enhance the usefulness of these estimates to compare different preventive approaches, life-years lost are usually adjusted for the quality of the life of an individual with a particular disease. Thus commonly used measures are: **quality-adjusted life-years (QALYs)** lost and **disability-adjusted life-years (DALYs)** lost, which are described in more detail elsewhere (Murray and Lopez 1997; Powles and Day 2002) (see also Chapters 2, 11, 12, 13, and 17).

 Absolute risk can also be calculated for the reference populations used in some types of analytical, observational, epidemiological studies (cohort and ecological studies), but not in case–control studies, unless the controls are selected randomly from the general population; nor in experimental studies, as subjects are usually **selected** to a small or large extent from a 'narrower' patient or general population. Usually this occurs because subjects have to meet entry and exclusion

criteria and may also be restricted by the severity of their illness. However, even in cohorts drawn randomly from the **study population** and where the **response rate** (the percentage of the selected sample participating in the study) is high, the sample of participants is unlikely to be wholly representative of the general population (healthier subjects may be more likely to volunteer to participate). Studies in which this has been examined have shown mortality in non-participants to be considerably higher than that among participants (Jousilati *et al.* 2005)

 The primary purpose of analytical, observational, studies, however, is not to calculate the absolute risk of disease, but to examine the relation between a particular exposure and the risk of the disease. Systematic examination of these risks for particular exposures are based on the risk of exposed individuals **relative** to the risk of non-exposed individuals and the epidemiological concept of **risk factor**. The term **risk factor** tends to be used in the epidemiological and biostatistical literature both in the widest sense as **any factor under test in a particular epidemiological study**, and in the more specific sense of **a factor that has become established in many studies to be linked causally with the development of a particular disease**. Factors that are associated with increased risk of disease but which may not be directly associated *causally* with the disease, are known as **risk markers**.

 The risk index used is dependent on the design of the study. Assuming complete follow-up, the basic information from a **cohort study** can be displayed in a 2 × 2 table. Box 3.3 details the calculations of two measures of association of exposure status and disease occurrence,

---

BOX 3.3 **RISK INDICES FOR COHORT STUDIES**

	Disease	No disease	Total
Exposed group	a (20)	b (80)	a + b (100)
Unexposed group	c (1)	d (99)	c + d (100)

Probability or risk or incidence rate (I_e) of disease in the exposed group = a/(a+b) (20/100) = 0.20.
Odds of disease in the exposed group = a/b (20/80) = 0.25.
Probability or **risk** or **incidence rate** (I_u) of disease in the unexposed group = c/(c+d) (1/100) = 0.01.
Odds of disease in the unexposed group = c/d (1/99) = 0.0101.
The risk ratio, rate ratio or **relative risk** of disease (comparing the exposed group with the unexposed group) is defined by
RR = I_e/I_u = {a/(a+b)} divided by {c/(c+d)} [20/100 divided by 1/100 = 20].
Odds ratio of disease (again comparing the exposed group with the unexposed group) is defined by
OR = {a/b} divided by {c/d} = {a × d}/{b × c} [(20 × 99) divided by (80 × 1) = 24.75] (the **cross-product ratio**).

BOX 3.4 ODDS RATIO OF DISEASE IN A CASE–CONTROL STUDY

	Disease	No disease
Exposure group	a (7)	b (3)
Non-exposure group	c (2)	d (8)
Total	a + c	b + d

Although the odds on disease in the exposed or unexposed groups cannot be calculated, the ratio of the odds of disease (comparing the exposure group with the non-exposure group) is equal to the ratio of the odds of exposure (comparing the disease group with the non-disease group) and is defined by the **odds ratio** (also called the **cross-product ratio**)

OR = {a/c} divided by {b/d} = {a × d}/{b × c}
= 7/2 divided by 3/8 = (7 × 8)/(3 × 2) = 56/6 = 9.3.

BOX 3.5 ATTRIBUTABLE RISK IN A COHORT STUDY

Using the definition of risk given in Box 3.3, the **attributable** or **excess risk** is defined as the **risk difference** (data from Box 3.3):

AR = risk of disease in the exposed group (20/100) – risk of disease in the non-exposed group (1/100)
= 0.20 – 0.01 = 0.19.

The **attributable risk** or the **attributable fraction (exposed)** or the **aetiologic fraction (exposed)** is defined as:

AR = attributable risk divided by the risk of disease in the exposed group
$I_e - I_u$ (where I_e is incidence in exposed and I_u in unexposed)
= 20 – 1 divided by 20
= 0.95 (95%)
often expressed as a percentage.

relative risk (or **risk ratio**) and **odds ratio** (the odds of exposure). Although relative risk is more easily interpretable than the odds ratio, the latter generally has better statistical properties and is the measure used in logistic regression (see Chapter 4). The **rate ratio** is a more sophisticated measure and is based on comparing the total **person-years at risk** in the two exposure groups during the study. It is used in longitudinal studies where follow-up is incomplete or subjects are studied for varying lengths of time. The **hazard ratio** is a variant of the rate ratio based on Cox proportional hazards analysis (Chapter 4).

In a case–control study there is a group of subjects with the disease (cases) and a sample of subjects without the disease (controls); the exposure status for each subject is then determined and compared in the two groups. As the exposure status of the *whole* population is not known (see Box 3.4), it is not possible to estimate the odds of disease in the exposed and non-exposed groups, nor the risk of disease in those groups, nor the relative risk unless controls are drawn randomly from the general population (which is not usually the case). However, the **odds ratio** of disease can be calculated (see Box 3.4).

The **odds ratio** is a good approximation to the **relative risk** when the proportion of diseased individuals in each group is low (for example, less than 10 per cent). This would occur whenever the disease is rare in both groups.

As will be described in subsequent chapters, many factors associated with our environment and culture (lifestyle) have been shown to be associated with the risk of common chronic diseases. For example, blood cholesterol levels, blood pressure, and smoking habit have become well-established (classic) risk factors for coronary heart disease (CHD); more recently, lack of exercise, being overweight and diabetes have also become established as risk factors. To design a strategy for intervening to reduce the incidence of CHD for example, it is helpful to be able to estimate the relative contribution of each risk factor. For an individual risk factor, this is known as the **excess** or **attributable risk** or the **risk difference**. It can be calculated from data obtained from a cohort study (see Box 3.5). An example using blood pressure as a risk factor of subsequent heart attack is shown in Table 3.1.

Calculations of excess risk rely on the risk factor in question not being associated with another risk factor for the same disease, i.e. that the risk factor is operating **independently** of other risk factors. However, this is not always the case and this will be discussed further in Chapter 17.

As described above, the **attributable risk** or **fraction** is calculated using data from a cohort study. But we have also noted that cohorts are often not entirely representative of the general population as they tend to be, firstly, from a selected age group and, secondly, to have volunteered to participate. To estimate the potential impact of an intervention on the general population it is necessary to have an estimate

TABLE 3.1 Relative and attributable risk of heart attack in a cohort of men according to their initial blood pressure

	Systolic (mmHg)	Diastolic (mmHg)	Percentage of men	Person-years of risk (PYR)[1]	Number of men developing heart attack	Heart attack rate per 1000 PYR	Relative risk ratio (compared with normal blood pressure)[2]	Excess or attributable risk per 1000 PYR[3]	Attributable risk (%)[4]
Normal (including optimal)	<130	<85	44	13,524	110	8.1 (I_o)	1	0	
High normal	130–139	85–89	20	6307	77	12.2 (I_{e1})	1.5	4.1	34
Hypertension stage I	140–59	90–99	23	6,695	115	17.2 (I_{e2})	2.1	9.1	53
Hypertension stages II–IV	≥160	≥100	13	3,628	81	22.3(I_{e3})	2.8	14.2	64

[1]Person-years of risk calculated from sum of years of follow-up for each man at each level of blood pressure.

[2]Relative risk of heart attack by blood pressure category = I_e/I_o

[3]Heart attack rate attributable to raised blood pressure = $I_e - I_o$

[4]Attributable risk per cent = Excess risk (column 8) ÷ Heart attack rate (column 6) × 100%.

> **BOX 3.6 POPULATION ATTRIBUTABLE RISK**
>
> **Population AR** = risk of disease in the total population (21/200) – risk of disease in the non-exposed population (1/100)
>
>   = 0.105 – 0.010 = 0.095.
>
> The **population attributable risk** or the **attributable fraction (population)** or the **aetiologic fraction (population)** is defined as
>
> **PAR** = population AR divided by the risk of disease in the total population, = 0.095 divided by 0.105
>
>   = 0.905 (90.5%)
>
> often expressed as a percentage.

of the level of the exposure in the general population. This is frequently done using cross-sectional surveys and enables the **population attributable risk** or **fraction** to be calculated, as shown in Box 3.6.

For an experimental study comparing two treatments with a binary outcome, the data can be summarized in a 2 × 2 table; the **risk difference** is often used as an alternative summary measure (treatment A – treatment B).

Further Reading

Gordis, L. (2004). *Epidemiology* (3rd edn). Philadelphia: Saunders.

Last, J. M. (2001). *A Dictionary of Epidemiology* (4th edn). Oxford: Oxford University Press. (This provides a comprehensive set of definitions of all technical terms that cause confusion in epidemiology: for example, relative risk, risk ratio, rate ratio, cumulative incidence, etc.)

Silman, A. J. (2002). *Epidemiological Studies: A Practical Guide* (2nd edn). Cambridge: Cambridge University Press.

References

References for this chapter can be found at www.oxfordtextbooks.co.uk/orc/yarnell. Where possible, these are presented as *active links* which direct you to an electronic version of the work. If you are a subscriber to that work (either individually or through an institution), and depending on your level of access, you may be able to peruse an abstract or the full article if available. 🖳

Data analysis in epidemiology

This chapter introduces the basic statistical terms and methods used in descriptive and analytical epidemiological reports. Where possible, examples are provided in subsequent chapters. Students are recommended to consult the references for additional reading, particularly for details of more advanced statistical techniques frequently used in modern epidemiological practice.

Introduction

The study of the distribution of a disease is generally **descriptive** in nature whereas the study of factors that are possibly associated with or cause the disease is usually **analytical**, and requires the gathering of data to test prior hypotheses. There is frequently an overlap between these approaches, particularly in health surveys. Some epidemiological studies use data from routinely collected sources (see section 2.2). However, most are based on data collected by **sampling** from **populations**. For such studies statistical methods of analysis are required. This chapter outlines the basic principles of statistical inference and briefly describes some multivariable methods that are increasingly being used in epidemiological studies. More detailed descriptions of statistical methods are given in the references listed at the end of the chapter.

4.1 Populations and Samples

The population that is to be investigated is called the **target population**, often selected or stratified by age from the **general population**. The actual population from which data are obtained is termed the **study population** and is often defined by geographical, institutional (for example schools, factories), occupational or disease criteria. How well conclusions from the study population can be applied to the target population is a matter of judgement. Whole or general population studies are often based on vital statistics that are routinely collected (see section 2.2). Otherwise such a population study is only feasible if the population is well-defined and the information required can be collected from every member of the population. In practice, however, collection of data from all members of the study population is often impossible (the decennial Census of the population is a notable exception) so that data must be obtained from a **sample** of the study population. A sample may be selected from a **sampling frame** or list of all members of a population; however, no single sampling frame is likely to be completely representative of the study population (see Chapter 2). For example, electoral or voting registers although compiled annually in the UK are voluntary and in areas with high population movements may underestimate the true population by 10–30 per cent.

The use of a sample has several practical advantages:

◆ the number of subjects is smaller, the effort and costs are less and the information is more timely;

◆ the information may be more extensive and of higher quality;

◆ a higher response rate may be achieved resulting in a reduction in **non-response bias**, which may arise if there are differences between those who choose to respond and those who do not.

To obtain useful and valid information about a population from a sample, it is important that the sample be representative of the population. This is achieved by drawing the sample **randomly** from the population: this protects against **selection bias** (a systematic difference between those selected for the sample and those in the population), and provides a theoretical basis for the application of statistical methods.

There are a variety of sampling schemes. In **simple random sampling** each member of the population has the same chance of being selected. The sample is usually selected from a list of all members of the population by means of computer-generated **random numbers**. A disadvantage of this method of sampling is that it may give practical difficulties for the data collection. Provided there are no periodic features in the list, **systematic sampling** may be more convenient: subjects are selected at regular intervals from the list (for example every tenth individual). In **stratified sampling**, a heterogeneous population is divided into strata and a sample randomly selected from each stratum. The strata are defined by one or more **categorical variables** (see section 4.2), for example gender or age group, which may have a bearing on the factors being studied. This type of sampling is recommended when the prevalence of a disease or risk factor varies across strata. Stratification then improves the precision of the analysis; it can also ensure that small subgroups of special interest (for example ethnic minority groups) are adequately represented. In **cluster sampling** the population comprises of several first-stage sampling units or clusters (for example schools, households, hospitals), each of which is made up of several second-stage units (for example classes, individuals, wards, etc.). The clusters are sampled by some suitable method; for each selected cluster, all second-stage units are then investigated. Alternatively, further sampling of the second-stage units within the selected clusters can be performed; for example, within a selected school, classes are randomly selected (**multi-stage cluster sampling**). Although these methods lead to savings in cost, effort, and time, the statistical results are less precise than those obtained using a simple random sample. Different sampling methods can be combined into a single sampling scheme, for example stratification and clustering.

In certain circumstances (for example surveys of specific groups, pilot studies) non-random sampling methods such as convenience sampling, snowball sampling, quota sampling, and focus groups are used. These methods are the stock-in-trade of market research companies sometimes employed to conduct health and social surveys, but they do not provide a suitable basis for the methods of statistical inference described later in this chapter.

4.2 **Summarizing Sample Data**

Epidemiological data consist of measurements or observations on the **variables** (the disease status, risk factors, exposures, demographic characteristics, etc.) collected from the subjects selected. The choice of summary measures, graphical displays, and analyses depends on the type of variable.

There are two main types of variable: **quantitative** (or **measurable**) and **qualitative** (or **categorical**).

Quantitative variables

A **continuous** variable is measured on a continuous scale with an associated unit of measurement; it is recorded to a certain degree of accuracy. So, for example, height is a continuous variable but is often recorded to the nearest centimetre. A **discrete** variable is one that takes a list of values; in practice, it is often a **count**, for example the number of persons in a household.

Categorical variables

A characteristic of a patient may be described as belonging to one of several categories. If the categories are unordered, the variable is described as **nominal categorical**; for example the four blood groups A, B, AB, and O. When there are only two categories, the variable is usually described as **binary** or **dichotomous**; for example, the presence or absence of a factor. When the categories have a natural ordering, for example a variable representing some outcome with categories poor, satisfactory, good, the variable is described as **ordinal** or **ordered categorical**. Sex, social class (see Chapter 17), and smoking habit are examples of categorical variables: (smoking habit is grouped into categories such as never, ex-smoker, light (1–14 cigarettes per day), medium (15–24), and heavy (25+) smokers).

A quantitative variable can be converted into a binary variable or an ordered categorical variable by the application of suitable cut-points to the original variable. The cut-points may be calculated from the sample data, for example using the three sample quartiles (see Box 4.1) as cut-points divides the sample into four approximately equal-sized groups. Alternatively, cut-points that are in widespread use can be chosen, for example body mass index (BMI) in adults is categorized as underweight, normal weight, overweight, obese by the cut-points 20, 25, 30 kg/m² (see Chapter 8).

A large sample of observations on any type of variable can be summarized in a **frequency table**, which could include frequencies and relative frequencies (or percentages). In the case of a continuous variable or a discrete variable with many distinct values, suitable classes of equal width, usually between 10 and 20 in number, need to be defined before the calculation of the frequencies. For such variables the relative frequencies or the percentages of the classes can be displayed in a **histogram** (see Figures 4.1 and 4.2). For a categorical variable or a discrete variable with few distinct values, the frequencies can be displayed in a **bar chart**, which emphasizes the discrete nature of the variable (see Chapter 6, Figure 6.6).

In the case of a quantitative variable, more succinct summary measures are available: the appropriate measures depend on the distribution of the observations in the sample which can be inferred from the

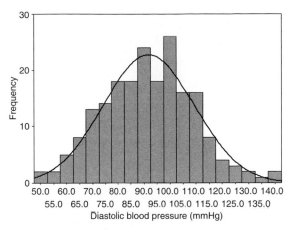

Fig. 4.1 Histogram of the diastolic blood pressures of a random sample of 200 males with fitted normal distribution curve.

shape of the histogram. If the histogram has a long tail to the right, as shown in Figure 4.2, the sample is **skewed to the right** or **positively skewed** (if **skewed to the left** then it is **negatively skewed**).

The following sample summary measures are described in Box 4.1. The most widely used measure of location of the 'centre' of a sample is the **mean**. However, it is inappropriate for highly skewed data, and the **median** or fiftieth percentile is then preferable. The **standard deviation** is a common measure of variation usually presented in conjunction with the sample mean. For a skewed sample, the dispersion is better described by a pair of percentiles, for example the twenty-fifth and seventy-fifth percentiles or by their difference, **interquartile range**. By its definition, this range contains half of the distribution. Finally, the **coefficient of variation** expresses the standard deviation as a percentage of the

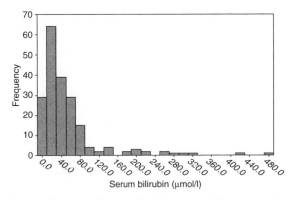

Fig. 4.2 Histogram of serum bilirubin values in 200 patients with cirrhosis.

BOX 4.1 **SAMPLE SUMMARY MEASURES**

Let $x_1, x_2, ..., x_n$ denote the observations on a quantitative variable in a sample of size n.

The **mean**, denoted by $\bar{x}$, is the arithmetic mean of the observations:

$$\bar{x} = (x_1 + x_2 + ... + x_n)/n = \sum x_i / n.$$

The **standard deviation**, denoted by **s**, is defined by

$$s = \sqrt{\sum (x_i - \bar{x})^2 / (n-1)},$$

that is, the square root of the approximate mean of the squares of the deviations, $(x_i - \bar{x})$, of the observations from the sample mean.

The **coefficient of variation**, denoted by **c**, is only defined for variables taking positive values:

$$c = \frac{s}{\bar{x}} \quad 100\%.$$

Percentiles are calculated by sorting the observations in order of magnitude. The percentiles divide the distribution of observations into 100 equal-sized parts.

The fiftieth percentile is the **median** or second quartile, Q_2; the twenty-fifth and seventy-fifth percentiles are the first and third quartiles, Q_1 and Q_3, and define the **inter-quartile range** $= Q_3 - Q_1$.

The mean and standard deviation are the most commonly used summary measures if the distribution of observations or results is roughly symmetric (Figure 4.1). However, the median and inter-quartile range are used for heavily skewed distributions (Figure 4.2).

---

mean and provides a measure of relative variation that is independent of the units of measurement and hence can be used to compare the variation of variables measured in different units. Coefficient of variation is therefore widely used for quantifying measurement error in laboratory work.

The relation between two categorical variables can be displayed in a two-way frequency table, also called a **contingency table** (see Chapter 5, Table 5.1) For two quantitative variables, or a quantitative variable and a categorical variable, a **scatter diagram** (see Chapter 17, Figure 17.4) indicates the form of any association; for quantitative variables any linear association can be summarized by a **correlation coefficient**, r, ranging from −1 (perfect inverse association) through 0 (no

linear association) to +1 (perfect direct association). See examples in Chapter 6.

It may be beneficial to transform a quantitative variable to another scale so that the assumptions for a statistical method are satisfied. How to choose an appropriate transformation is beyond the scope of this text but in medical studies the **logarithmic transformation** is very commonly used because many variables exhibit positive skewness. Having analysed the logarithmically transformed data, the results should be interpreted on the original scale. Another type of variable that is extensively used in comparison studies is the standardized version of a quantitative variable, often called a **z-score**:

z-score = (variable value – sample mean) / sample standard deviation.

An example is given in Chapter 13 (see Figure 13.3).

Finally, in some statistical methods (for example non-parametric), the ordered sample of n values of the variable is replaced by the set of **ranks** 1, 2, ..., n.

4.3 **Simple Methods of Statistical Inference**

Statistical inference is the process of drawing conclusions from sample data about the characteristics of the population or populations that have been sampled. Because the information available is incomplete, these conclusions are subject to uncertainties, which are expressed in terms of probabilities and probability distributions. Statistical methods require the assumption that the samples obtained are random samples drawn from the populations being studied in order that inferences are valid. The possibility of biased conclusions resulting from the use of non-random samples (as is often the case in practice) must be assessed by the researcher. Generally, statistical methods only take **sampling error** into account and do not quantify biases due to non-random sampling. The two forms of statistical inference are **estimation** and **hypothesis testing**.

Suppose a characteristic of a population (for example the 'average' value) is represented by a single quantity (for example the population mean). Such a quantity is called a **parameter** and is typically unknown. Given a sample from the population, a single value, often referred to as a **statistic**, is calculated as an **estimate** of the parameter. For example, the sample mean is an estimate of the population mean. The properties of the **statistic** or **estimate** are determined by its **sampling distribution**: the frequency distribution obtained by calculating the statistic for every possible sample (of the same size) from the population. When the sample size is large, the sampling distribution is often approximated by a **normal distribution** (see Figure 4.1 (distribution of diastolic blood pressure) and Box 4.2). The precision of a statistic is measured by its **standard error** (SE), the standard deviation of its sampling distribution, which can be reduced by increasing the sample size; standard errors are used in calculating confidence intervals and in hypothesis testing.

An alternative that provides more insight into the precision of a statistic is **confidence interval estimation**: for a chosen degree of confidence (usually 95%), an interval is calculated from the sample data and is said to include the unknown parameter with the specified degree of confidence. The **confidence limits** (the lower and upper values of the interval) are generally calculated

from knowledge of the sampling distribution of the statistic. For means, proportions, and their differences, approximate 95% confidence limits are given by

$$\text{statistic} \pm 1.96 \times \text{SE (statistic)}$$

when samples are large. For odds, odds ratios, and relative risks (see Chapter 3) similar calculations of confidence limits are performed on a logarithmic scale. In repeated samples (of the same size) and for the same degree of confidence, the confidence limits will change from sample to sample. However, for 95% confidence intervals, it is expected that 95% of these intervals will contain the unknown parameter. For a chosen degree of confidence, the narrower the confidence interval the better is the estimation process. Using a larger sample reduces the standard error and hence narrows the confidence interval. An example of the calculation of a confidence interval for a proportion is given in Box 4.2.

The second form of statistical inference is **hypothesis testing** (also called **significance testing**). The general

---

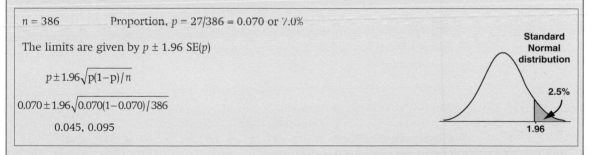

BOX 4.2 EXAMPLE OF CALCULATION OF A CONFIDENCE INTERVAL FOR A PROPORTION

To investigate the risk of irritable bowel syndrome after an episode of bacterial gastroenteritis, 386 patients were surveyed by questionnaire 6 months after bacterial gastroenteritis infection and it was found that 27 had developed irritable bowel syndrome. Assuming that these 386 patients represent a random sample from the population of all bacterial gastroenteritis patients, calculate 95% confidence limits for the proportion of the population who develop irritable bowel syndrome.

$n = 386$ Proportion, $p = 27/386 = 0.070$ or 7.0%

The limits are given by $p \pm 1.96\ \text{SE}(p)$

$$p \pm 1.96\sqrt{p(1-p)/n}$$

$$0.070 \pm 1.96\sqrt{0.070(1-0.070)/386}$$

$$0.045,\ 0.095$$

Standard Normal distribution

2.5%

1.96

The 95% confidence limits are 4.5 per cent and 9.5 per cent, while the 95% confidence interval is from 4.5 per cent to 9.5 per cent. Then 95% of intervals like this will include the actual proportion of the population of bacterial gastroenteritis patients who develop irritable bowel syndrome. A larger sample would give a narrower confidence interval.

Data from: Neal, K. R., Hebden, J. and Spiller, R. (1997). 'Prevalence of Gastrointestinal Symptoms Six Months after Bacterial Gastroenteritis and Risk Factors for Development of the Irritable Bowel Syndrome: Postal Survey of Patients'. *British Medical Journal*, **314**: 779–82.

aim of hypothesis testing is to investigate whether sample data are consistent with an assumption about the population (or populations) from which the samples were drawn (for example two population means are equal).

A hypothesis test can be considered as a series of six steps (see Box 4.4).

1 The study hypothesis is expressed in terms of two statistical hypotheses about the population distributions: the **null hypothesis**, usually representing the current state of knowledge, or expressing 'no difference' if two or more distributions are being compared; and the **alternative hypothesis**, which is often simply the negation of the null hypothesis. The null hypothesis is not rejected unless the sample evidence is strongly against it, in which case it is rejected in favour of the alternative hypothesis. In the worked example the alternative hypothesis is that the length of the neck of the femur has changed over the course of the twentieth century.

2 A suitable **test** is chosen. This choice depends on the number of groups, the type of variable, and the form of its distribution; Box 4.3 lists some widely used tests. Associated with the test is a **test statistic**, which is a function of the sample data and the nature of the hypotheses.

3 The **significance level** of the test is chosen, usually 0.05 (or 5 per cent), but smaller probabilities can be used. The choice of significance level depends upon the particular problem and how serious would be the consequences if a true null hypothesis were rejected.

4 The *P*-value is calculated using a statistical computer package: it is the probability of the observed value of the test statistic, with any other equally extreme or more extreme values that might have occurred, assuming that the null hypothesis is true. Whether a value is 'more extreme' is a statistical concept, and its biological relevance is generally more easily decided in practice.

5 The *P*-value is compared with the significance level, say 0.05. If $P \leq 0.05$, the **test is significant at the 5 per cent level**, the null hypothesis is rejected, and the alternative hypothesis is accepted; if $P > 0.05$, the test is not significant at the 5 per cent level and the null hypothesis is not rejected. In the worked example, the *P*-value is calculated as 0.0014 or 0.14 per cent, a low probability leading to rejection of the null hypothesis.

6 A statistically significant result must be interpreted with regard to the aims and size of the study;

BOX 4.3 GUIDE TO SELECTING THE APPROPRIATE STATISTICAL TEST FOR COMPARISONS BETWEEN SAMPLES

This table covers only the more commonly used methods for making simple comparisons between samples.

Type of variable	Two samples		R samples (R > 2)	
	Independent	Paired	Independent	Matched
Continuous (Normality assumptions satisfied)	Independent samples *t*-test*	Paired samples *t*-test*	One-way analysis of variance	Randomized block analysis of variance
Discrete, continuous (Normality assumptions **not** satisfied)	Mann–Whitney *U*-test *or* Wilcoxon rank sum test	Wilcoxon signed-rank test	Kruskal–Wallis analysis of variance	Friedman two-way analysis of variance
Categorical Two categories	χ^2 test for 2 × 2 table or Fisher's exact test	McNemar's test	χ^2 test for R × 2 table	Cochran's Q test
C categories (*C* > 2)	χ^2 test for 2 × C table	–	χ^2 test for R × C table	–

*Or equivalent large samples *z*-test.

BOX 4.4 HAS THE LENGTH OF THE NECK OF THE FEMUR CHANGED OVER THE COURSE OF THE TWENTIETH CENTURY IN SCOTLAND? A WORKED EXAMPLE OF A STATISTICAL HYPOTHESIS TEST

A study compared femoral neck lengths (in millimetres) in the anatomy collection of a Scottish University in 43 men who had died in the early twentieth century (1900–1920) with 22 men who had died in the late twentieth century (1980s).

$$n_{Early} = 43 \qquad\qquad n_{Late} = 22$$
$$\bar{x}_{Early} = 34.9 \text{ mm} \qquad\qquad \bar{x}_{Late} = 38.3 \text{ mm}$$
$$s_{Early} = 3.9 \text{ mm} \qquad\qquad s_{Late} = 3.8 \text{ mm}$$

Is there evidence of a change in femoral neck length between the two periods?

1 The means in these samples clearly differ by 3.4 mm, but does this provide evidence that the population means differ? The null hypothesis is that the mean femoral neck length in the male population of Scotland in the early twentieth century is the same as the mean in the late twentieth century. The alternative hypothesis is that there has been a change in length. It is assumed that each group of men is a random sample from the Scottish male population of the time.

2 Because femoral neck length is a continuous variable and is to be compared in two independent samples of men, reference to Box 4.3 shows that **the independent samples *t*-test** is appropriate. Femoral neck length must be assumed to follow a normal distribution, although this assumption can be relaxed in large samples.

3 The conventional 5 per cent significance level is chosen for this test, and consequently it must be accepted that there will be a 1 in 20 chance of making a type 1 error (that is, rejecting the null hypothesis when it is actually true).

4 From these two samples a *t*-statistic is calculated as 3.35 and used to derive from the *t* distribution with 63 degrees of freedom the *P*-value of 0.0014 (see inset). This represents the probability of seeing a difference in sample means as large as, or larger than, the difference actually observed in this study assuming that in reality there has been no change in femoral neck length.

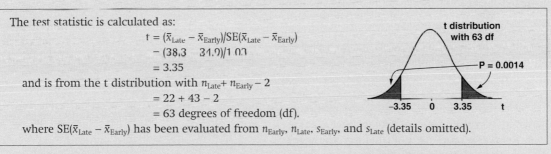

The test statistic is calculated as:
$$t = (\bar{x}_{Late} - \bar{x}_{Early})/SE(\bar{x}_{Late} - \bar{x}_{Early})$$
$$= (38.3 - 34.9)/1.03$$
$$= 3.35$$
and is from the t distribution with $n_{Late} + n_{Early} - 2$
$$= 22 + 43 - 2$$
$$= 63 \text{ degrees of freedom (df)}.$$
where $SE(\bar{x}_{Late} - \bar{x}_{Early})$ has been evaluated from n_{Early}, n_{Late}, s_{Early}, and s_{Late} (details omitted).

5 This *P*-value is less than the chosen significance level for the test, so the null hypothesis is rejected. A difference as large as that observed between the samples is not likely to arise often if the null hypothesis were true.

6 There is evidence of an increase in the femoral head diameter in Scottish men during the period. The risk of type 1 error is small (the null hypothesis would still have been rejected had we chosen to use a lower probability cut-off). However, some caution must be advised in interpreting these findings since men whose bodies were donated to the university may not necessarily have been representative of the male population of Scotland at the time.

Data from: Duthie, R. A., Bruce, M. F. and Hutchison, J. D. (1998). 'Changing Proximal Femoral Geometry in North East Scotland: An Osteometric Study'. *British Medical Journal*, **316**: 1498.

a statistically significant result need not necessarily be clinically or biologically important. In certain situations (as in the worked example) there were doubts about the representativeness of the sample, and this can also cast doubt on the conclusion of the test.

Statistical significance and power

A non-significant result does not imply that the null hypothesis is true but that, on the available evidence, the null hypothesis cannot be rejected. A significant result often, but not invariably, indicates that the alternative hypothesis is true. Hence errors may occur in this decision-making process. **A type I error occurs if the null hypothesis is rejected when in fact it is true**; it has a 1 in 20 chance of happening when the 5 per cent level of significance is chosen. Accordingly, testing of numerous hypotheses in a study may result in an increased chance of type 1 error (a 'false-positive' result). Adjustment for multiple testing is usually made by adopting a smaller probability cut off, for example a 1 per cent level of significance. **A type II error occurs if the null hypothesis is not rejected when in fact the alternative hypothesis is true**; the probability of this happening can be calculated for a specified alternative hypothesis. Box 4.5 displays the possible outcomes of a hypothesis test. The probability of not making a type II error is called the **power** of the test. The concept of power is important in designing a study to ensure that it is of adequate size to detect a clinically worthwhile difference; typically a power of at least 0.8 (80 per cent) is recommended. Many research studies are underpowered, and research protocols usually include an estimate of the necessary sample size to ensure a conclusive result.

Generally, a statistic together with its associated confidence interval is more useful than a hypothesis test, because a statistic gives information on the magnitude and direction of an effect, and the confidence interval provides a measure of the precision of the statistic. In many analyses, a confidence interval can also be used to test the null hypothesis (the null hypothesis is rejected only if the confidence interval does not include the value specified by the null hypothesis).

4.4 **Regression Modelling**

The methods of section 4.3 can be used to investigate the association between the disease state (represented by a quantitative or a categorical variable) and a single exposure or treatment variable (again either quantitative or categorical), except when they are both quantitative. In this latter case, **correlation analysis** or preferably **simple linear regression** (univariable model) may be appropriate procedures. However, where there are possibly several exposure variables and other available information about the subjects being studied, multivariable regression modelling is a suitable approach (see Chapter 6, Table 6.2).

The general aim of **regression modelling** is to explain the variation in a response or outcome variable, usually representing the disease state, in terms of explanatory or predictor variables which can be quantitative or categorical; specific objectives may be the testing of hypotheses of the effect of an explanatory variable (also termed by some the independent variable), estimation of effects, and the making of predictions. In epidemiological studies regression modelling is generally considered to be the best approach for estimating an exposure effect after controlling or adjusting for the effects of confounding variables. (A **confounding variable** is one that is associated with the outcome and the exposure; for example, smoking habit is associated with risk of heart attack and socioeconomic status so smoking habit could confound an analysis of the association between socioeconomic status and heart attack.) (See also Chapter 2.) When a third variable modifies the relation between an exposure and the outcome, **effect modification** or **interaction** occurs; this can also be investigated in regression analysis. In Table 6.3 (Chapter 6), age is an effect modifier of smoking habit for the risk of myocardial infarction, because the relative risk of smoking decreases steeply with increasing age. In this text, two forms of regression modelling are considered: multiple linear regression for a continuous outcome; and binary logistic regression for a binary outcome.

A fitted **multiple linear regression** model takes the form

$$Y = b_0 + b_1 X_1 + b_2 X_2 + \ldots + b_k X_k$$

where Y represents a continuous outcome, and the Xs represent the explanatory variables (or functions of these variables). The bs are estimated **regression coefficients**: an individual coefficient represents the change in the outcome variable associated with a unit change in the corresponding X variable, when the remaining X variables are kept fixed. The relative contributions that variables such as age, smoking habit, and physical activity make to the prediction of

BOX 4.5 **CLASSIFICATION OF ERRORS IN HYPOTHESIS TESTING**		
	Result of test	
True situation	Reject null hypothesis	Do not reject hypothesis
Null hypothesis true	Type I error	Correct decision
Alternative hypothesis true	Correct decision	Type II error

continuous variables such as weight or body mass index are typically assessed by such methods.

A fitted **binary logistic regression** model takes the form

$$\log_e\{p/(1 - p)\} = b_0 + b_1 X_1 + b_2 X_2 + \dots + b_k X_k$$

where p represents the probability or risk of the outcome occurring, $p/(1 - p)$ is the odds of the outcome occurring, and the Xs represent the explanatory variables (or functions of these variables). The function $\exp(b_i)$ is the **odds ratio** associated with the variable X_i, that is, comparing the two odds obtained by a unit change in X_i, when the remaining X variables are kept fixed. Many risk factors have been shown to be associated with risk of coronary heart disease and the relative contributions of each risk factor is typically estimated using this approach.

In both models the bs are estimated from the sample data using a suitable statistical computer package, for example SPSS, Stata, or SAS. Not all the explanatory variables may be required to obtain an adequate fit to the data: a variable may not be associated with the outcome as a variable may be highly correlated with one or more of the other explanatory variables. Most statistical computer packages contain routines to select a subset of the explanatory variables. **Forward selection** successively adds the most significant X variable until none of the remaining variables makes a further contribution according to a predetermined significance level. In contrast, **backward elimination** starts with all X variables in the model and successively removes the least important at each stage until any further elimination would result in a significant variable being removed. **Stepwise** selection is a combination of these approaches which has the benefit that a decision to add (in the case of forward selection), or to remove (in the case of backward elimination), may be changed at a later stage. It may also be used as a generic term for these automatic selection procedures. However, the selection of variables should primarily be based on the researcher's understanding of the data and the context of the study, particularly in choosing confounders to be controlled.

Biostatistics is a core discipline of epidemiology and preventive medicine; students are encouraged to read one or more of the texts listed below to develop their ability to evaluate the current research literature.

Further Reading

Altman, D. G. (1997). *Practical Statistics for Medical Research.* London: Chapman & Hall.

Armitage, P., Berry, G., and Matthews, J. N. (2000). *Statistical Methods in Medical Research* (4th edn). Oxford: Blackwell.

Bland, M. (2000). *An Introduction to Medical Statistics* (3rd edn). Oxford: Oxford University Press.

Campbell, M. J. and Machin, D. (1999). *Medical Statistics: A Commonsense Approach* (3rd edn). Chichester: Wiley.

Kirkwood, B. R. and Sterne, J. A. C. (2003). *Essential Medical Statistics* (2nd edn). Massachusetts, USA: Blackwell Science Ltd.

Pereira-Maxwell, F. (1998). *A–Z of Medical Statistics. A comparison for critical appraisal.* London: Arnold.

Woodward, M. (2004). *Epidemiology Study Design and Data Analysis* (2nd edn). Boca Raton, USA: Chapman & Hall.

References

References for this chapter can be found at www.oxfordtextbooks.co.uk/orc/yarnell. Where possible, these are presented as *active links* which direct you to an electronic version of the work. If you are a subscriber to that work (either individually or through an institution), and depending on your level of access, you may be able to peruse an abstract or the full article if available. ⌨

Screening for disease

This chapter introduces the topic of screening in public health and medical practice. The principles, purposes, and methods of screening are discussed, and concepts of validity, which are common to screening tests used in the general population and to those used for clinical diagnosis. Case studies are given for prostate cancer, neuroblastoma, and antenatal screening for Down syndrome.

Introduction

To 'screen' is used in the general sense to mean 'to sift or investigate' and can be applied at the population or individual level. **Screening** results in a classification of an individual as either 'diseased' (or 'at risk of a disease') or 'not diseased' (or 'not at risk'). Many of the concepts and cross-tabulations relating to risk, developed in Chapter 3 (section 3.3), also apply to screening tests. Borderline cases are likely to be re-tested but, essentially, individuals are classified dichotomously or qualitatively by tests that are often quantitative. These tests, therefore, are indicators either for the disease itself, for a risk factor or for a particular trait that could affect the health of the individual or others. Issues about the **validity** of the test will be discussed later, but it is firstly necessary to discuss *why* and *how* a particular test is applied.

5.1 Types and Principles of Screening

Mandatory screening is usually designed for the preservation of the health or safety of others, often as a condition of employment, or before blood donation. Doctors, airline pilots, and applicants to many other occupations must expect to undergo a screening examination formulated according to medico-legal guidelines. Among blood donors, unexpected results may cause distress to individuals testing positive for human immunodeficiency virus (HIV) or hepatitis B or C for example, and informed consent and counselling are part of the procedures used by the Blood Transfusion Service in the UK.

Prescriptive screening implies potential benefit for the individual and is usually a systematic screening programme, either delivered as an integrated component of routine practice, as in antenatal and neonatal care, or as a voluntary public health programme such as those for cervical and breast screening. Screening may be: **uniphasic**, where one screening test is used, for example a blood test for cholesterol; **multiphasic**, for example screening for colorectal cancer where a preliminary filter test, such as the faecal occult blood test, identifies a subgroup at higher risk, and for whom further screening (colonoscopy) is recommended. Multiphasic is also used to indicate multiple screening tests used on the same occasion.

Opportunistic screening is also prescriptive but involves screening for a risk factor or disease when an individual presents for another reason; one example is when the opportunity to screen for raised blood pressure is taken during a routine visit to the general practitioner.

Screening can be further categorized as **selective**, if confined to individuals at high risk of a particular disease, or **mass**, if offered to the general public.

A few examples of the wide range of screening tests used in preventive medical practice are shown in Box 5.1. Detailed discussion of screening services available in the USA is to be found elsewhere (US Preventive Services Taskforce 1996).

Principles

Screening can be introduced at any phase of the natural history of a disease. However, whether this is useful or not in interrupting the natural progression of the disease depends on the speed of progression and other important characteristics of the natural history. Figure 5.1 shows stages at which screening tests can be performed, which relate particularly to cancers, but are relevant for all diseases. Screening is a preventive activity,

---

BOX 5.1 SCREENING TESTS IN PREVENTIVE MEDICAL PRACTICE

Mandatory	Prescriptive	Opportunistic (often in primary care)
Cardiovascular and optical examination for heavy-goods vehicle (HGV) drivers, airline pilots, train drivers, etc.	**Antenatal care** Urinalysis: glucose, protein, blood, etc.	Blood pressure Blood cholesterol Blood glucose
Donor blood tested for hepatitis B, HIV, syphilis, etc.	Blood analysis: haemoglobin, full blood count (FBC), etc.	Body weight/height (body mass index)
Occupational health monitoring in workers exposed to asbestos, X-rays, lead, carcinogens, etc.	Infectious diseases: rubella, syphilis, HIV, hepatitis B	
	Blood pressure Foetal ultrasound **Postnatal care** Neonatal blood tests for phenylketonuria, hypothyroidism, etc. **Selective screening** Tonometry in relatives of glaucoma patients **Women's health** Cervical smear Mammography	

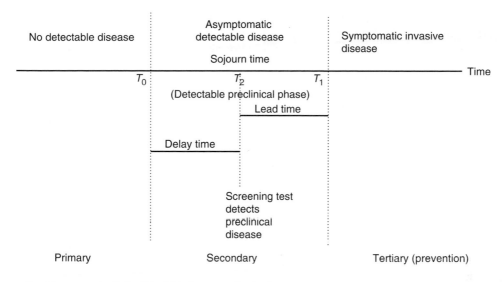

T_0 – Tumour potentially detectable by screening test
T_1 – Tumour detectable clinically
T_2 – Actual date of detection by screening test

Fig. 5.1 Principles and definitions in cancer screening
Source: Modified from Vainio, H. and Bianchini, F. (2002). *Breast Cancer Screening. IARC Handbook of Cancer Prevention* (vol. 7).
Lyon: IARC Press.

as illustrated previously in Chapter 1 (Figure 1.4), in which primary, secondary, and tertiary prevention were described. Screening activities can thus be categorized depending on whether or not the disease has been initiated (primary), become detectable by the screening test (secondary) or become clinically manifest (tertiary). In practice, screening tests usually aim either: to prevent the occurrence of detectable disease (as in the case of screening for risk factors for coronary heart disease, such as hypertension or high blood cholesterol); or to detect an asymptomatic disease or a tumour (as in the case of secondary prevention of the complications of diabetes, or of breast or cervical cancers). In practice, it can be difficult sometimes to distinguish adequately between primary and secondary prevention in screening tests, because the natural history of diseases offer a wide spectrum of possibilities.

5.2 **Evaluation**

Screening has considerable potential for the detection of pre-symptomatic disease but it was recognized early in medical screening that new screening tests should be fully evaluated before their general introduction.

For example, in the UK, chest X-rays were introduced in the 1950s to screen the general population for tuberculosis. This helped to reduce the considerable public health burden of the disease. The same programme was then adapted to screen for lung cancer but was found to be ineffective, as lung cancers were usually too advanced when detected (see Chapter 7). Wilson and Jugner (1968) proposed a set of criteria to be used when evaluating screening programmes, particularly prescriptive programmes, where there is implied benefit for an individual. These have been recently modified and updated by others (Box 5.2).

Most conditions or diseases that have important consequences for the individual or for the health of others can be viewed as eligible for consideration for preventive screening tests. As noted earlier, mandatory tests are designed to protect others and may not benefit the individual under test.

Difficulties have arisen for screening programmes for some diseases, such as prostate cancer, which demonstrates a wide range of invasiveness. It has an estimated prevalence of 55 per cent in men in their fifth decade of life and 64 per cent in the seventh; most of these malignancies remain localized and do not present clinically.

BOX 5.2 REQUIREMENTS FOR A SCREENING PROGRAME

The condition

- This should be an important health problem.

- The natural history of the disease including latent disease should be adequately understood and risk groups identified.

- There is a recognizable pre-disease or early symptomatic stage.

The test

- Should be safe, simple, effective, valid and acceptable.

- A suitable cut-point for the test value should be agreed in the target population.

The treatment

- Should be effective and lead to better outcome and improved survival with earlier intervention.

- Facilities exist for diagnosis and treatment.

The screening programme

- Evidence should be available from RCTs that the programme is effective in reducing mortality and morbidity.

- The benefit from the screening programme should outweigh the possible physical and psychological harm caused by the test, diagnostic procedures and treatment.

- The costs should be considered in the context of other demands for resources.

Modified from: UK National Screening Committee (2003), http://www.nsc.nhs.uk/.

The screening test should ideally be cheap, quick, and acceptable. It should be **reliable**, i.e. produce the same result if repeated. It should also be **valid**, i.e. good at discriminating those who have the disease from those who do not. Similar remarks also apply to tests used for clinical diagnosis (see section 5.3) except that, for clinical diagnostic tests, whereas diagnostic power is clearly important, the issue of cost and acceptability is less important than in mass screening in public health practice.

The choice of cut-off points for continuously distributed variables such as blood pressure, or intra-occular pressure, must be carefully considered, as all those screened must be categorized into either positive or negative for further investigation. If the cut-off is too low then too many subjects will be counted as positive and vice versa. This is critical to the issue of **sensitivity** and **specificity** in public health and clinical practice, and in laboratory medicine.

Validity, or the accuracy of a test, is measured using **sensitivity** and **specificity**. The **sensitivity** of a test is the measure of its ability to detect disease when present. A highly **sensitive** test has no or very few missed cases (**false negatives**). **Specificity** measures the ability to identify healthy people as such (non-diseased), and therefore there are few **false positives**. These definitions are shown in Box 5.3.

For serious diseases, screening tests should clearly have a high sensitivity, preferably close to 100 per cent, so that few cases are missed. However, the specificity, which reflects the percentage of false positives, will only be consequential if further procedures are indicated for a screenee; for example, in the case of positive mammography, needle biopsy will be necessary, which will create anxiety during the waiting period.

In the case of **quantitative variables**, such as **blood pressure**, **plasma cholesterol**, and **body mass index**, the choice of the cut-point to define **hypertension**, **high blood cholesterol**, and **overweight or obesity** will be critical in determining the 'sensitivity' and 'specificity' of the risk factor test for predicting future disease or non-disease (see Table 2.1 and Chapters 6 and 8). Risk factor cut-points can only be accurately determined from large-scale observational studies, reinforced, where possible, by randomized controlled trials (RCTs), because the diseases may take years to present clinically. Hypertension provides a recent example of this, as the World Health Organization and US, European, and UK medical societies recommended that the threshold for hypertension be lowered from at least 160/95 mmHg to 140/90 mmHg (see Chapter 6).

Two other measures are used to evaluate screening tests. These depend on the **prevalence** of the disease in the population and use the row values rather than the column values in Box 5.3: the **positive predictive value (PPV)** measures the ability of the test to correctly diagnose the disease; and the **negative predictive value (NPV)** the ability of the test to correctly identify absence of disease. Diseases with a high prevalence will have a higher chance of correctly testing positive than

BOX 5.3 INDICES USED TO EVALUATE ACCURACY OF A SCREENING OR DIAGNOSTIC TEST

Test result	Disease present	Disease absent
Positive	True positive (**TP**)	False positive (**FP**)
Negative	False negative (**FN**)	True negative (**TN**)

Sensitivity: percentage of positive results in those with disease = $\dfrac{TP}{TP+FN} \times 100\%$

Specificity: percentage of negative results in those without disease = $\dfrac{TN}{FP+TN} \times 100\%$

Positive predictive value: percentage of correct results in those with a positive test result = $\dfrac{TP}{TP+FP} \times 100\%$

Negative predictive value: percentage of true negative results in those with negative results = $\dfrac{TN}{TN+FN} \times 100\%$

those with a low prevalence for any given level of sensitivity and specificity (see Table 5.1).

Examination of the formulae in Box 5.3 and the examples in Tables 5.1 show that sensitivity and specificity are based on the test results only, whereas positive and negative predictive values are based on the numbers with disease. Predictive values of screening tests are more directly relevant to patients or screened subjects than are sensitivity and specificity, which are principally used by epidemiologists in their evaluation of screening tests.

Given a relatively high sensitivity and specificity for a particular test, PPV increases rapidly with a higher prevalence of disease. The PPV is also known as the **yield** for a particular test and, in clinical and public health practice, screening tests clearly provide a greater yield in 'high risk' groups, which have a higher initial prevalence of disease compared with that in the general population.

5.3 Clinical Epidemiology and Clinical Diagnosis

One simple definition of clinical epidemiology is '**epidemiology in patient populations rather than general populations**'. Fletcher *et al.* (1996) ▣ extended this definition to include all aspects of **clinical decision making** and have formulated the main clinical questions that fall within the remit of clinical epidemiology (see Box 5.4).

All these clinical questions could be equally applied to the general population; but in this chapter we will confine the discussion to that concerning the diagnosis of disease. Firstly, in the case of simple categorical tests (that is, disease present/absent) such as radiological detection of tumours or magnetic resonance imaging (MRI), opportunities exist for observer variation. If there are systematic differences in interpretation (inter-observer variation) this will result in **observer bias**,

| **TABLE 5.1** | Positive and Negative Predictive Values for Screening Tests in Diseases with a High and a Low Prevalence |

	Disease		Total
Low prevalence disease (1%)	Present	Absent	
Positive screening test	1.8 (TP)	39.6 (FP)	41.4
Negative screening test	0.2 (FN)	158.4 (TN)	158.6
Total	2	198	200

$$\text{Positive predictive value} = \frac{1.8}{41.4} \times 100\% = 4.3\%.$$

$$\text{Negative predictive value} = \frac{158.4}{158.6} \times 100\% = 99.9\%.$$

	Disease		Total
High prevalence disease (20%)	Present	Absent	
Positive screening test	36 (TP)	32 (FP)	68
Negative screening test	4 (FN)	128 (TN)	132
Total	40	160	200

$$\text{Positive predictive value} = \frac{36}{68} \times 100\% = 52.9\%.$$

$$\text{Negative predictive value} = \frac{128}{132} \times 100\% = 97.0\%.$$

(For both sets of results sensitivity of screening test = 90%; specificity = 80%.)

but even 'random' differences in interpretation will lead to lower levels of diagnostic certainty. 'Random' differences of re-categorization by individual observers is known as intra-observer variation. Fletcher *et al.* (1996) 💻 describe a study of MRI assessment of prolapsed inter-vertebral disease, which 'blinded' radiologists as to whether or not a subject had symptoms of back pain or was a healthy volunteer. Prolapsed or protruding discs were found in about two-thirds of asymptomatic subjects, a very similar proportion to that in symptomatic patients, indicating that MRI was unhelpful, at least in the initial clinical diagnosis.

For laboratory tests in immunology and biochemistry, the results are usually computed as quantitative variables. It is clearly important for new tests to establish a **'normal range' (mean ± two standard deviations)** in a large, unselected population encompassing healthy subjects from both genders, a wide range of social groups, and even different ethnic groups. 'Normal ranges' often differ by age, sex, and ethnic group and are often presented accordingly. It should be noted that laboratory tests often are not normally distributed (see Chapter 3)

and logarithmic or other transformations may be required to approximate 'normality'. Of critical importance is the choice of cut-point. Gerstman (1999) has provided an example from serological testing for exposure to HIV by using three different cut-points to define positive test (Figure 5.2).

When the cut-point is set at position A there are no false negatives and sensitivity is 100 per cent. In position B there are both false positives and false negatives (the usual situation in practice). In position C there are no false positives.

Receiver operator characteristic curves can be used to define a suitable cut-point by plotting the sensitivity (the true positive rate) against the false positive rate (1-specificity). These curves are particularly useful for comparing two different laboratory tests that both attempt to diagnose the same clinical entity. Figure 5.3 shows the level of diagnostic certainty for clinically confirmed congestive heart failure obtained using plasma levels of four different cardiac peptides (produced by cardiac endothelium in response to cardiac dilatation). The comparative standard for this test was heart size on radiography. Currently echocardiography would be more likely to provide a higher level of diagnostic certainty (see Chapter 6).

In this example the cardiac BNP performs better than other cardiac peptides in the prediction of a clinical diagnosis of congestive heart failure.

Both diagnostic testing and clinical interventions fall under the general remit of '**health technology assessment**'. This broad area of study can be considered an important component of evidence-based medicine (Chapter 20). The systematic quantitative use of external evidence using **Bayes's theorem** in health technology assessment is discussed in detail elsewhere (Spiegelhalter *et al.* 2000). 🖳 **Bayes's theorem** is particularly appropriate for this area of work, and for clinical decision making in general (see Chapter 21), as it incorporates the prevalence of the particular disease into the calculations of the predicted risk (odds) of

a true result: the higher the prevalence of the disease, the greater the probability that a positive test result will represent true disease.

5.4 Screening for Cancers

Many cancers carry a high case-fatality rate or a low five-year survival rate (see Chapter 15), and quality of life is often impaired. Early detection of tumours raises the possibility of intervention and cure, and new screening tests are being developed for this, which require full evaluation. Stages at which screening may be introduced into the natural history of cancer are shown in Figure 5.1.

Critical time points that are invariably approximate and variable between individuals are T_0, at which the screening test is capable of detecting asymptomatic disease, T_1, the average time of clinical presentation, and T_2, the time in practice when a screening test detects preclinical disease. Definitions that stem from these time points are shown in Figure 5.1.

Very small tumours are unlikely to be detected by conventional radiological techniques unless metabolites, which can be 'tagged', accumulate in the tumour. Biochemical tests for secretory products of tumours are often evaluated as potential markers (see Chapter 15). Mutations of certain genes, such as *p53*, *BRCA-1* and *BRCA-2*, are associated with a high risk of cancers (Chapter 15), but have a low prevalence in the general population, and effective non-surgical interventions are currently lacking. Prophylactic mastectomy is a surgical intervention occasionally used in women with *BRCA-1/2*. Another problem is a wide variation in the natural history and invasiveness of cancers with varying rates in malignant development or conversion of pre-cancerous cells, for example cervical and prostatic cancers.

Particular issues in the evaluation of screening tests for cancer are as follows.

Frequency of testing

If the period between tests (the screening interval) is too long, disease may develop between them. Such cancers are called **interval cancers**, and are made up of the following types of case:

- false negatives, i.e. the screening test failed to detect the cancer;
- cases in people who did not attend for follow-up investigation;
- true interval cases which appear 'de novo' and usually represent fast-growing tumours.

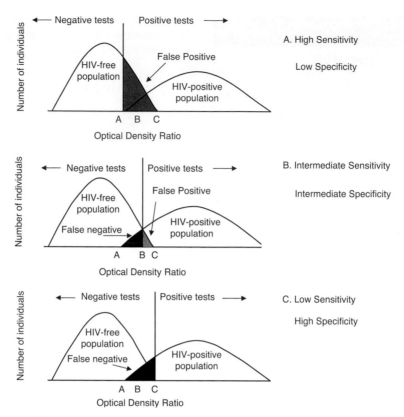

Fig. 5.2 The effect of setting different cut-points on the sensitivity and specificity of an enzyme-linked immunosorbent assay (ELISA) for HIV. Source: Modified after Gerstmann, B. B. (1999). *Epidemiology Kept Simple. An Introduction to Classic and Modern Epidemiology.* New York, NY: Wiley-Liss.

Screening frequency has to take account of the costs and benefits of more versus less screening. For example, screening every five years for cervical cancer will reduce the incidence of disease by 84 per cent, every three years by 91 per cent and annually by 93 per cent. Screening annually, as opposed to every three years, trebles the cost of the programme with only a 2 per cent reduction in disease (Eddy 1990).

Effective screening, by definition, leads to earlier diagnosis of disease, and consequently, a longer period between diagnosis and death, or longer survival. However, early diagnosis may not prolong the date of death, and it is important to consider this when comparing screened and non-screened groups for differences in outcome. **Lead time bias** cannot be measured directly except in RCTs and, therefore, adjustment for this bias is liable to error. The implication of this is that

it is not possible to distinguish between bias and real benefits of screening using observed case survival data only, such as those routinely obtained from cancer registries (see Chapters 2 and 15). The difficulty in evaluating observational data on prostate cancer in the USA, where testing for prostate-specific antigen (PSA) has been widely used for many years, has been reported elsewhere (Shaw *et al.* 2004). 🖥

Length bias

The screening test increases detection of low-risk tumours, which may never be detected otherwise, cause symptoms, or disease. It reflects the growth rate of the tumour and the detection by screening of slower-growing, less malignant tumours. These differences may be detected by histological grading of the tumour. In contrast, those cases presenting between screens

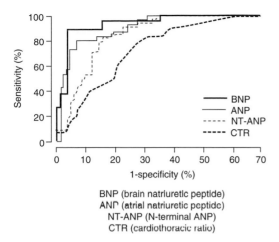

Fig. 5.3 Receiver-operating-characteristic curves for natriuretic peptides and cardiothoracic ratio in the prediction of clinically confirmed congestive heart failure.
Source: Cowie M. R., Struthers A. D., Wood D. A. *et al.* (1997). 'Value of Natriuretic Peptides in Assessment of Patients with Possible New Heart Failure in Primary Care'. *The Lancet*, **350**: 1347–51.

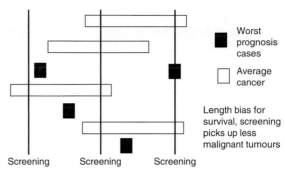

Four non-interval, slow growing cancers detected.
One interval, rapid growing cancer detected.

Fig. 5.4 Interval and non-interval cancer: relationship to screening examinations.

(**interval cancers**) tend to have a worse prognosis than those picked up at screening. Length bias, which is also influenced by the screening interval, is another major potential source of bias when examining survival rates in the context of screening (Figure 5.4).

Halving the screening interval would have detected one more interval cancer, but still fails to detect two interval cancers.

Selection bias

Case–control studies of screening have problems with selection bias. In a practical example, invitations to a screening programme may result in a 70 per cent acceptance, but those who accept have a lower underlying risk than the general population, perhaps 0.8. The 30 per cent refusers have a higher underlying risk at 1.5. The refusers therefore will contribute 45 per cent (30 per cent × 1.5) of the cases, and the acceptors will contribute 55 per cent (0.8 × 70 per cent) of the cases. An evaluation may find that there is a reduction in disease among those who attend for screening but would fail to detect the effect of the 45 per cent of cases who were not screened.

Will Rogers phenomenon

The importance of the role of changing diagnostic tools in screening is illustrated by the 'Will Rogers effect'. Will Rogers is reported to have said, 'When the Okies left Oklahoma and moved to California they raised the average intelligence level in both states.' The Will Rogers effect raises issues of reliability of stage-adjusted survival over time, and it is important to consider this in view of ongoing technological advances. In a disease with four defined stages, for example lung cancer, patients are allocated into these four categories using chest X-ray, stage 4 being the worst disease. If a newer and better diagnostic tool is discovered, for example scanning with computerized tomography (CT), it is likely that some of the stage 1 cases will be discovered to have more widespread disease than was previously thought, and they will be moved from stage 1 to stage 2. This will result in an improved survival of stage 1 as they lose their worst cases to stage 2. Stage 2 will get some less severe cases previously categorized as stage 1, and the worst stage 2 cases will become stage 3 on CT scan, so the prognosis for stage 2 cases will improve. The same happens with stage 3, whereas stage 4 gets some of the old stage 3, which had a better prognosis. Thus each stage has improved survival but the overall survival is the same (Feinstein *et al.* 1985).

The problems encountered in evaluating the effectiveness of treatments from routinely collected cancer registration and survival data are summarized in Box 5.5.

Negative aspects of screening

Routine screening tests can also have some negative consequences as well as potential benefits. Some of these can be predicted from the list of requirements in Box 5.2. Mandatory tests may not benefit an individual; indeed, they are designed to protect others and may prevent an individual taking up a particular occupation,

BOX 5.5 PROBLEMS IN THE INTERPRETATION OF TRENDS IN CANCER SURVIVAL

Observed improvements in survival may come about for the following reasons:

- There is early detection and better cure rates reflected by changes in stage.
- It may be the result of lead time bias, length bias and/or selection bias.
- It may be the effect of improvements in treatment or a change in the disease.
- It may reflect a change in the available information, for example, new diagnostic methods.

or continuing to work in it, or from donating blood. There may be no suitable treatment, and for this reason screening for several mature-onset genetic conditions, such as Huntington's disease, is not recommended.

For prescriptive screening, problems for screenees can arise if they are tested as false-positives and have to undergo further testing and unnecessary anxiety. Test specificity is the issue here; and for some common tests, such as mammography, it is sufficiently low as to create a sizeable proportion of false-positives. For some large screening programmes, testing false-positive has been shown to affect participation in subsequent routine testing in future years.

For screening tests with continuous distributions there is the problem of the choice of cut-point. This will determine the specificity and sensitivity of a particular test and, for risk factors such as hypertension or cholesterol which are classified as 'borderline raised' on testing, such results can create a group of 'worried well' individuals. Adequate communication about the level of risk, and the significance of the results to a screenee by health professionals should reduce the possibility of this outcome, which has been investigated only to a limited extent in research studies.

In the following worked examples we have used the framework provided in Box 5.2 to evaluate screening proposals. First, we examine the case for prostate cancer, for which screening has been introduced, particularly in the USA, without evidence of benefit from RCTs. Secondly, we discuss a trial of screening for neuroblastoma, the second commonest tumour in childhood. And thirdly, we examine the case for screening for Down syndrome during the antenatal period, when the mother has the option of termination of pregnancy.

CASE STUDIES

1. Should we screen for prostate cancer?

Is the disease an important health problem?

Yes, prostate cancer causes 18 per cent of male cancer deaths in the UK. It is a disease primarily of older men: 50 per cent of the cases are aged over 74 years at diagnosis. There is an increasing detection of cases, and death rates are rising. It is a disease that will assume increasing significance as the population ages.

Is the natural history known?

Latent prostate cancer is found in up to 40 per cent of males aged 60 years, rising further with age (Whitmore 1994). Most of these cancers will not become life threatening, but some evolve into invasive tumours.

Is there a recognizable latent early symptomatic stage?

Many cases of prostate cancer are clinically silent, the likelihood of a tumour progressing or metastasizing is highly variable, and the disease outcome is uncertain. There are two main tests for detecting prostate cancer: digital rectal examination, which is prone to inter-examiner variability, and the prostate-specific antigen (PSA) blood test, which may also be raised in benign hypertrophy, prostate inflammation, and after prostate surgery. For the PSA test there is no uniform standard so results between laboratories and countries are not comparable. It is recognized that these tests involve the risk of treating benign tumours (Cancer Research Campaign 2002). Table 5.2 compares the validity measures of the two available screening tests for prostate cancer.

These data suggest that the sensitivity, specificity, and 'yield' (PPV) of digital rectal examination as a

TABLE 5.2 Evaluation of the Digital Rectal Examination for Prostate Cancer (Verified By Biopsy) at Two Ranges Of Prostate-Specific Antigen (PSA)

PSA cut-point	Sensitivity (%)	Specificity (%)	PPV (%)	NPV (%)
<3.0 ng/ml	62	42	0.9	55
<4.0 ng/ml	50	54	16	86

Adapted from: Postma, R. and Schröder, F. H. (2005). 'Screening for Prostate Cancer'. *European Journal of Cancer*, **41**: 825–33.

screening test are low at PSA levels under 4.0 ng/ml. In this study up to 65 per cent of 'cancers' were missed by digital rectal examination and ultrasonography at PSA levels between 2.0 and 4.0 ng/ml, but these 'cancers' may have a more favourable prognosis than those in subjects with higher PSA levels.

Is there an effective treatment?

Treatments for prostate cancer are 'watchful waiting' with regular reviews of PSA levels, radiotherapy, surgery and palliative hormonal therapy. These last interventions are not without side effects; for example, several studies report that impotence is still present in 15–51 per cent of surgical patients, and some degree of incontinence is found in 4–72 per cent of patients at 18 months of follow-up (Selley *et al.* 1997; Jonler *et al.* 1994). There is a 14 per cent relapse rate for early tumours seven years after surgical treatment or radiotherapy. After 15 years follow-up, neither stage nor treatment was found to be predictive of outcome, perhaps because patients are generally old at time of diagnosis (50 per cent of cases are 70 years or over when diagnosed) (Selly *et al.* 1997).

Does early diagnosis improve survival?

Survival from prostate cancer is strongly related to the stage of disease at diagnosis. The five-year relative survival for clinically detected cancer confined to the prostate is 70 per cent without systematic screening in the UK. If the disease is widespread, with bony metastases, five-year relative survival is about 20 per cent (Cancer Research Campaign 2002).

The UK National Screening Committee does not recommend screening for prostate cancer but many doctors use PSA testing as a screening tool (Melia *et al.* 2005). Population-based trials of screening for prostate cancer are currently ongoing; the screening trial of the National Cancer Institute in the USA needed to recruit 74 000 men to be followed over

10 years to achieve sufficient statistical power for a clear result. It is due to report in 2008, together with a large European trial (Postma and Schroder 2005).

2. Screening for neuroblastoma

This is one of the most common childhood malignancies, which arises anywhere in the neuronal network of the autonomic nervous system (most commonly in the adrenal medulla), but the number of cases is small (fewer than 100 per year in the UK). At present more than 50 per cent of tumours have spread from the original site at time of diagnosis, and for such tumours there has been little improvement in survival in the past 20 years. There is a validated screening test available, which measures catecholamines and its metabolites in the urine. The prognosis in the disease depends on the age and stage of disease at diagnosis; the earlier the detection, the better the prognosis.

Currently there is no neuroblastoma screening programme in the UK, but a national programme has been established in Japan. It is known that neuroblastomata may undergo spontaneous regression and there is a possibility of over-diagnosis with screening.

Q1 How would you set up a study to investigate the value of neuroblastoma screening?

Q2 How would you evaluate such a study?

Neuroblastoma screening in Germany

A case–control study of neuroblastoma screening using catecholamines was established in Germany between 1995 and 2000, with 2.6 million children in the screening area. There were 1634 false positives, 150 neuroblastomas detected by screening, and 68 false negatives, giving a total of 218 neuroblastomas in the screening area. The outcome from the neuroblastoma screening was an increase in cases, 7.7 excess cases per 100 000 screened. The results are summarized in Table 5.3.

Q3 What could have caused this increase?

The conclusions from this study about neuroblastoma screening were:

- the study does not support mass screening for neuroblastoma at one year of age;
- mass screening leads to unnecessary treatment;
- the policy of neuroblastoma screening in Japan should be reconsidered.

TABLE 5.3 Neuroblastoma: Estimate of Cases Detected Early and Excess Cases not Explained by Early Detection[a]

Cases per 100 000 births*	Control cohort (births 1994–1999)	Study cohort participants (births 1994–1999)	Difference
Diagnosis-by-screening age 12–24 months	3.3 [2.5,4.1][b]	11.0 [9.3,12.7]	Excess in screening cohort 7.7 [5.8,9.6]
Diagnosis above screening age 24–60months	4.6 [3.7,5.5]	3.6 [2.6,4.6]	Cases detected early 1.0 [−0.4,2.3]
Sum 12–60 months	7.9 [6.7,9.1]	14.5 [12.6,16.5]	Overdiagnosis 6.7 [4.4,9.0] Excess not explained by early detection.

[a]Apparent discrepancies are due to the rounding of the presented figures.

*Cases registered by 30 June 2002.

[b]Approximate 95% confidence intervals.

Source: Schilling, F. H., Spix, C., Berthold, F. *et al.* (2003). 'Children May Not Benefit from Neuroblastoma Screening at 1 Year of Age. Updated Results of the Population Based Controlled Trial in Germany'. *Cancer Letters*, **197**: 19–28.

3. Screening for Down syndrome

Down syndrome (DS) is caused by an extra chromosome 21 in 90 per cent of cases, hence the name trisomy 21. The extra chromosome is usually of maternal origin. DS is characterized by learning disability, developmental delay, characteristic facial features, and is often associated with cardiac anomalies and duodenal atresia.

The risk of having a baby with DS increases with maternal age. For mothers under 30 years of age, the total prevalence (see Chapter 14 for a definition of total prevalence of congenital anomalies) is approximately 0.7 per 1000 births. At 30–34 years, the average risk increases to 1.5 per 1000 births, and above the age of 35 years the average risk is around six per 1000, although the risk increases sharply with each single year of age within this age group. Thus at age 44 years the risk is approximately 34 per 1000, but it seems risk does not continue to increase in older mothers (Morris *et al.* 2003).

Because of the high risk associated with high maternal age, prenatal screening started as the offer of prenatal diagnostic (rather than screening) tests to all mothers over an age threshold (35 years in some countries, 36 or 38 years in others). Chorionic villus sampling (first trimester) and amniocentesis (second trimester) can be used to look for the extra chromosome in a foetal sample. These are invasive methods with a small risk of miscarriage. Unusually given the principles of screening, there is no effective treatment, and the main option offered is termination of pregnancy.

Q4a. Why is the proportion of DS cases with older maternal age in Table 5.4 much greater than the proportion of all births with older maternal age?

Q4b. What is the maximum proportion of cases that would be prenatally diagnosed if invasive tests were offered to all mothers of 35 years or over in the five regions shown in Table 5.4?

Q4c. Which of the columns in Table 5.4 is approximately equivalent to an attributable fraction for older maternal age?

Because a large proportion of DS cases are born to mothers younger than 35 years (Table 5.4), biochemical

TABLE 5.4 Proportion of Births and Proportion of Down Syndrome Cases[1] to Mothers of 35 Years of Age and Over, Five European Regions, 1995–99

Region	Births	Down Syndrome cases
	Per cent in mothers 35+ years	Percent to mothers 35+ years
Wales (UK)	14.9	44.7
Tuscany (Italy)	18.0	47.4
Dublin (Ireland)	18.7	51.4
Basque Country (Spain)	23.8	54.3
Paris (France)	23.9	60.9

[1]Includes livebirths, stillbirths and terminations of pregnancy.

Source: EUROCAT Working Group (2002), *EUROCAT Report No. 8: Surveillance of Congenital Anomalies in Europe 1980–99*, University of Ulster, Belfast. http://www.eurocat.ulster.ac.uk/pubdata/report8

screening methods have been developed to identify high-risk mothers, whatever their age, to whom amniocentesis could be offered. These methods use a combination of maternal age and the levels of serum markers such as alphafetoprotein (AFP) and human chorionic gonadotrophin (hCG) to estimate risk in second trimester screening. Using multiple markers gives higher specificity and sensitivity for the screening test as a whole, hence the triple and quadruple tests now in common use. Ultrasound-soft markers (nuchal translucency) at the end of the first trimester have been added to biochemical markers in some centres (providing combined or integrated tests), and have replaced biochemical markers in others. The best screening strategy is as always one that detects the highest number of confirmed cases (sensitivity) with the least number of invasive diagnostic tests being performed (high specificity); potential harm as a result of a false positive result (both psychological and from risk of miscarriage after invasive testing) should be balanced against the perceived benefit. As noted earlier, the yield (based on the positive predictive value) is likely to be greater in a high-risk population.

In 2004 the National Institute of Clinical Excellence (NICE) recommended that all pregnant women should be offered a test that provides a detection rate over 60 per cent, and a false-positive rate lower than 5 per cent (NICE 2004). Nevertheless, there are major issues about prenatal screening of this kind, including: the 'medicalization of pregnancy'; the anxiety experienced by mothers receiving the inevitable false positive test results; and staff training for prenatal genetic counselling when offering tests or communicating test results. Recently, more rapid (1–3 day) limited karyotype analysis has become available which detects trisomy 21 and a few other major chromosomal anomalies. This test does not detect the full range of rarer chromosomal anomalies, but has the advantage of not raising the ethical and counselling dilemma of detecting chromosomal anomalies that are of unknown significance, or are compatible with a normal life (often otherwise going undetected). Research is ongoing to find a non-invasive way of determining the foetal karyotype (Kumar and O'Brien 2004); 🖳 clearly screening methods that cause minimal harm to both mother and foetus are required.

Screening tests are likely to feature strongly in future preventive efforts in medicine both at a primary and a secondary level of disease progression. The future of **genetic testing** is particularly controversial since many ethical issues arise as a result of its increasing availability. These occur largely because of multiple testing for many disorders at the same occasion, many of which do not fulfil many of the disease criteria for a screening test beneficial to an individual listed in Box 5.2. Genetic testing is further discussed in Chapter 18.

Evaluation of the efficacy and effectiveness of all public health screening programmes increasingly include consideration of their cost-effectiveness, which is discussed in Chapter 21.

Further Reading

Bhopal, R. (2002). *Concepts of Epidemiology – An Integrated Introduction to the Ideas, Theories, Principles and Methods of Epidemiology*. Oxford: Oxford University Press.

Fletcher, R. H., Fletcher, S. W. and Wagner, E. H. (1996). *Clinical Epidemiology. The Essentials* (3rd edn). Philadelphia, PA: Lippincott, Williams and Wilkins.

Gerstmann, B. B. (1999). *Epidemiology Kept Simple. An Introduction to Classic and Modern Epidemiology*. New York, NY: Wiley-Liss.

US Preventive Services Taskforce (1996). *Guide to Clinical Preventive Services* (2nd edn). Baltimore, MD: Williams & Wilkins.

Web Addresses

Cancer Research Campaign (2002), *Cancer Statistics: Prostate Cancer UK*, http://www.crc.org.uk.

EUROCAT Working Group (2002), *EUROCAT Report No. 8: Surveillance of Congenital Anomalies in Europe 1980–99*, University of Ulster, Belfast. http://www.eurocat.ulster.ac.uk/pubdata/report8.html.

National Institute for Clinical Excellence (2004), http://www.nice.org.uk/.

UK National Screening Committee (2003), http://www.nsc.nhs.uk/.

References

References for this chapter can be found at www.oxfordtextbooks.co.uk/orc/yarnell. Where possible, these are presented as *active links* which direct you to an electronic version of the work. If you are a subscriber to that work (either individually or through an institution), and depending on your level of access, you may be able to peruse an abstract or the full article if available. 🖳

Model answers

Q1

- Cases detected in a screened population would be compared with those found clinically in an unscreened population. The populations would be monitored during a fixed time period and would be of sufficient size to detect a significant difference in the detection rate between the two populations.

- Define the age group to be studied in each population.

- Ethical approval and parental consent would be required.

- Ensure that there are adequate resources for the test, follow-up investigation, treatment and clinical outcomes.

- Provide public information about the study, training of research and involved health professionals, and a pilot study.

- Ensure that population data are available to enable the calculation of mortality from neuroblastoma in the two study areas.

Q2 By assessing the following items:

- The practical process and cost of screening.

- The numbers accepting screening, age group etc.

- The calculation of sensitivity, specificity, PPV and NPV.

- The numbers being treated.

- Calculation of the rates of spontaneous regression.

- Clinical outcomes such as disability and death.

- Five-year survival rates in screenees and non-responders in population screened and in control population.

Q3

These could be due to lead time bias and possible over-diagnosis (this may be distinguished by examining the age at diagnosis). Lesions detected early were calculated at one per 100 000 and over-diagnosis at 6.7 per 100 000. There were three deaths, all related to treatment, in children with early disease.

Q4a

This would be expected as the occurrence of DS is much more common in births to older mothers.

Q4b

60.9 per cent (the estimate for Paris).

Q4c

The second column.

Systems-Based Epidemiology

Circulatory diseases

This chapter deals with the circulatory diseases, which are the leading cause of death in developed countries and are rapidly increasing in incidence in most developing countries. The major cardiovascular disorders are: coronary heart disease, stroke, congestive heart failure, and peripheral vascular disease. Examples of epidemiological studies, which have been used extensively in examining the causes of cardiovascular diseases, are given as follows: ecological (monitoring and surveillance of coronary heart disease and stroke), case–control (smoking habit of hospitalized heart attack patients), and cohort (cholesterol level and risk of heart disease and stroke in Shanghai).

Introduction

In developed countries of the world, circulatory diseases are the leading cause of death. In developing countries they are usually of lesser importance than malnutrition and infectious diseases, but are becoming more so. For example, even in some of the poorest countries in Africa hypertension is relatively common, particularly in urban areas, leading to stroke and congestive heart failure as important causes of hospital admission or death in adults.

The major circulatory diseases (sometimes known as cardiovascular diseases) are those of the arterial blood vessel system and involve a pathological process known as atherosclerosis. This involves lipid deposition in the arterial wall, initially known as fatty streaks, but potentially developing into raised plaque encapsulating liquid lipid material, atheroma (Greek: gruel or porridge), which can endanger the integrity of the arterial wall, and, in the smaller arteries can create a significant obstacle to normal blood flow. Some organs, known as end-organs, are particularly vulnerable to anoxia caused by this reduction in blood flow (**ischaemia**) both acutely and chronically. The heart, brain, and lower limbs are especially liable to the anoxic consequences of atherosclerosis. Acute obstruction of the coronary arteries appears to be often associated with rupture of a vulnerable plaque. This releases atheromatous material, which is highly thrombogenic, promoting a local cellular inflammatory/thrombotic response. Figure 6.1 shows the main components of a ruptured plaque.

Both platelet and plasma factors control the extent of this response, which can produce large, aggregated platelet emboli; these proceed in the coronary circulation to block smaller vessels. In the larger and middle-range coronary and cerebral arteries, acute obstruction will result in acute anoxia and subsequent death of heart muscle or brain cells over a substantial region, giving rise to myocardial or cerebral **infarction**. These acute events are associated with the typical clinical symptoms of **heart attack** or **stroke**; smaller emboli that may be a result of extensive plaque formation, irregularity, and erosion of the arterial endothelium often lead to blockage of minor blood vessels and chronic anoxia. In heart muscle, chronic anoxia results in the slow death of muscle and its replacement by fibrous tissue (**ischaemic heart disease, IHD**).

Diseases of the venous blood system represent only a small proportion of the total burden of circulatory disease, but **deep vein thrombosis** (DVT) and **pulmonary**

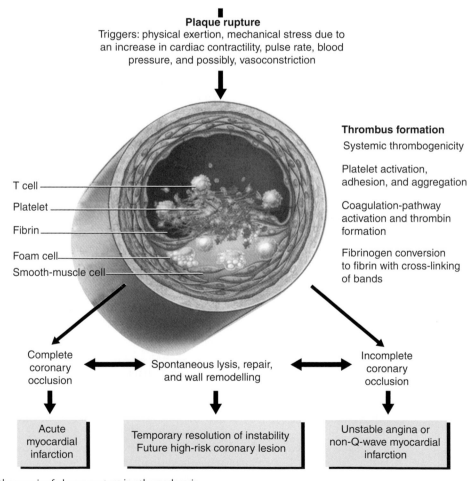

Fig. 6.1 Pathogenesis of plaque rupture in atherosclerosis.
Source: Yeghiazarians, Y., Braunstein, J. B., Askari, A., and Stone P. H. (2000). 'Unstable Angina Pectoris'. *New England Journal of Medicine*, **342**: 101–14.

embolism are of clinical importance. These diseases are thrombotic and embolic in nature and largely occur in the chronically ill or those undergoing major orthopaedic surgery (for which anticoagulant prophylaxis is usually given). Recent interest has focussed on DVT and pulmonary embolism as a complication of long-haul air flights, and preventive measures have been introduced by most airlines, although risk is low.

The major circulatory diseases are shown in Box 6.1.

6.1 **Coronary Heart Disease**

As shown in Box 6.1 coronary heart disease (synonym: ischaemic heart disease) (CHD or IHD) has a variety of clinical manifestations. Acutely these are now often termed **acute coronary syndromes** by clinicians and include **ventricular fibrillation**, **acute myocardial infarction** and **unstable angina**. In turn, acute myocardial infarction can be extensive enough to cause pump failure, usually of the left side of the heart, resulting in acute **congestive heart failure**; in the elderly, myocardial infarction is frequently free of significant chest pain and often presents with congestive heart failure. The bundle of His and other electrical conducting fibres of the heart are particularly vulnerable to sudden ischaemia; if the blood supply to these conducting tissues is restricted then arrhythmias, which can originate at the higher level of the atria or at the lower level of the ventricles, may develop. Atrial arrhythmias such as **atrial fibrillation** result in irregular ventricular contractions but are of near-normal rate, which are not usually life threatening, and are a common feature of chronic ischaemia. At the **ventricular** level, arrhythmias such as **fibrillation**, which are common in acute

coronary obstruction, effectively result in stasis of the arterial blood supply to the brain, and imminent death, but the heart can be restored to **sino-atrial** (**sinus**) rhythm by prompt electrical defibrillation. **Asystole**, when there is no residual electrical activity detectable in the heart tissue, will not respond to defibrillation attempts, but cardio-pulmonary resuscitation, using ventilation of the lungs with regular compression of the ventricles (usually externally), can maintain blood supply and oxygenation of vital organs such as the brain in the short term (30–60 minutes). In the absence of this, brain death will occur in approximately four minutes. Acute obstruction of the blood supply to a significant area of the myocardium will result in the death of the muscle in this region within a matter of minutes. Typically, this will result in 'crushing' chest pain often radiating down the left arm owing to the anatomical innervation of the pericardium and is often associated with sweating. Death or ischaemia of the ventricular myocardium is usually detectable as a particular abnormality of normal electrical conductance as depolarization of the avascular area of myocardium will not occur. Typical abnormalities of particular segments of electrocardiographs (ECGs), which record the electrical activity associated with each cardiac cycle, can be detected or read according to a standard protocol by experienced clinicians. Although computerized programmes do exist for the classification of these abnormalities, they still require refinement before being used routinely on their own. Important confirmatory evidence of myocardial damage is obtained by measurement of cardiac enzymes such as lactic dehydrogenase (LDH) or creatinine kinase (CK), which are released from dying myocardial muscle. Until recently a level of twice the upper limit of the normal range of LDH was considered pathognomic (diagnostic) of acute myocardial infarction. Currently, however, the increasing use for diagnostic purposes of troponins, which are released at very low levels of tissue damage, have blurred the distinction between myocardial infarction and **unstable angina** in which there is only minor tissue death. This is likely to lead to significant problems in case definitions for epidemiologists interested in monitoring trends in incidence of CHD over time. Clearly, the **acute coronary syndromes** constitute a broad spectrum of clinical disorders ranging from acute myocardial infarction, with or without chest pain, and with or without acute congestive heart failure, to unstable angina in which chest pain may be severe due to ischaemia, but where this ischaemia is insufficient to result in significant myocardial damage.

BOX 6.1 **CARDIOVASCULAR DISEASES**	
Major causes of mortality	**Major causes of morbidity**
Acute myocardial infarction	Angina: (stable) (unstable)
Ventricular fibrillation	
Chronic ischaemic heart disease	Congestive heart failure
Congestive heart failure	
Stroke (cerebrovascular disease)	Chronic cerebrovascular disease
Aortic aneurysm	Peripheral vascular disease

Chronic ischaemic heart disease constitutes another broad spectrum of diseases ranging from **stable angina** (formerly termed angina pectoris), through the various conduction defects (for example atrial fibrillation) and valvular disorders due to localized ischaemia, to **chronic congestive heart failure**, in which there is the gradual onset of pump failure of the heart. Usually this is of the left ventricle but sometimes of the right in **cor pulmonale** in which progressive inflammatory change to lung tissue (predominantly caused by smoking but sometimes exacerbated by occupational lung disease or chronic asthma) has resulted in chronic failure of the right ventricle.

Atrial fibrillation is found in only 0.5 per cent of the general population but in over 10 per cent of men and women aged more than 75 years of age. Increasingly it is due to chronic IHD but in past generations was strongly associated with mitral valve disease caused by rheumatic fever. Recently a review of epidemiological and clinical studies found the risk of embolic stroke to be increased in subjects with atrial fibrillation, and a prophylactic anticoagulant (for example warfarin) is recommended.

Epidemiology and risk factors for acute and chronic coronary heart disease

As noted in Chapter 1, CHD is not a new disease but it began to be increasingly prominent during the twentieth century. Clinicians in the USA and in some European countries, particularly the UK and Finland, noticed increasing numbers of patients with heart attack admitted to their hospitals; these patients, who were often men, could be relatively young, perhaps only in their thirties or forties. Many such patients never reached hospital, dying relatively suddenly at home or at work due to the rapid onset of myocardial ischaemia, often resulting in ventricular fibrillation or asystole. An early report from Northern Ireland showed that 60 per cent of patients died before reaching hospital (McNeilly and Pemberton 1968). 🖳 Post mortems tended to show thrombosis in the coronary vessels. Epidemiologists noted a rapid rise in deaths from these diseases, which were given a number of names by clinicians and pathologists, for example myocardial degeneration, coronary thrombosis, coronary occlusive heart disease, myocardial infarction, etc. Some large-scale cohort studies were established in the 1950s and 1960s to examine possible causes of the coronary epidemic. In the USA the National Institutes of Health funded a cohort study based on the inhabitants of a small town in Massachusetts called **Framingham**, and Ancel Keys established cohorts in **Seven Countries** with contrasting death rates from coronary disease. In Britain, the Department of Health funded a study of male civil servants (**Whitehall Study**); many of the epidemiological methods required for standardization and validation of clinical diagnoses were developed by cardiologists who had become epidemiologists, such as Geoffrey Rose, on behalf of the World Health Organization (WHO). This body had begun to take an interest in **chronic** non-communicable disease rather than **infectious** or communicable disease, which had tended to dominate its work previously.

Defining the disease

A rapidly increasing trend in mortality due to coronary or ischaemic heart disease was observed in the 1950s and 1960s in industrialized wealthy countries such as the USA, Britain, and other Western European countries. This was followed by a slow decline beginning in the 1970s in the USA and somewhat later elsewhere. However, there were great variations in the mortality rates in different countries. The MONICA Project (Multi-national MONItoring of trends and determinants of CArdiovascular disease) was established in the early 1980s to determine whether these differences were real or due to differences in diagnostic habits of doctors in different countries. Because incidence is made up of fatal and non-fatal events it is clearly also important to examine whether there are differences in mortality between centres due to differences in survival; that is, differences in case-fatality rates. As noted in Chapter 2, the coding scheme used for the International Classification of Diseases tends to rename common diseases according to the scientific fashion among clinicians. The bridge-coding exercise, performed in many countries, allows adjustment of official mortality data to take account of these changes in nomenclature.

In the MONICA project, in each participating country or study population a case register of non-fatal and fatal cardiac episodes was established and a strict set of diagnostic criteria used to define *definite* and *probable* cases of acute myocardial infarction. Geographic areas comprising populations of several hundred thousand persons of all ages were used to limit the boundary of each case register for 37 populations in 21 countries, and registration was restricted to those aged 25–64 years. Registration of potential and, after validation, of included cases, was made for a minimum of 10 years. A notification network was established in each centre to investigate all potential coronary deaths, both in the community and in hospital, and all potential non-fatal coronary events either, remaining at home and seen by a doctor, or admitted to hospital. Table 6.1 shows coronary incidence data from selected population registers collected from 1985–87.

> **Q1(a)** What clinical criteria do you think were used to establish the case definitions of coronary events used in all centres?
>
> **Q1(b)** Why do you think the investigators in defining case fatality chose 28 days as the cut-point for fatal events following the onset of symptoms?
>
> **Q1(c)** If you were told that Tarnobrzeg is a large, rural area in southern Poland, would this help to explain the high case-fatality rates in this region?

Trends in coronary risk factors, which included plasma cholesterol, blood pressure, and smoking habit, were monitored in two or more cross-sectional surveys among random samples of the general population in each centre during the period of coronary event registration. Trends in coronary incidence in the whole geographic region from the coronary events register were compared and correlated with the changes in risk factors in the samples from the general population (Kuulasmaa *et al.* 2000). 🖳

> **Q2** What is the overall study design of the WHO MONICA study (see Chapter 3)?

The search for causes of the coronary heart disease epidemic

In a series of metabolic experiments in human volunteers, Ancel Keys and others established in the 1950s that plasma cholesterol levels could be influenced by the proportion of saturated (mainly from dairy and meat products) and polyunsaturated fatty acids (mainly from vegetable products) in the diet. The more saturated fat, the higher the cholesterol; and the more polyunsaturated fats, the lower the cholesterol. Convinced of the need for population studies, he moved from hospital-based studies into international epidemiological studies, having noted that countries with high consumption of saturated fats tended to have high mortality from coronary disease. Countries such as Finland, the USA, and the UK had the highest rates in the world

TABLE 6.1 Coronary incidence in selected populations in the WHO MONICA Project from 1985–87

Population	Men		Women	
	Incidence per 100 000 (95% CI)	Case fatality at 28 days (%) (95% CI)	Incidence per 100 000 (95% CI)	Case fatality at 28 days (%) (95% CI)
Finland: North Karelia	915 (±62)	48 (±3)	165 (±25)	44 (±8)
UK: Glasgow	823 (±39)	49 (±2)	256 (±20)	49 (±4)
UK: Belfast	781 (±36)	40 (±2)	197 (±17)	44 (±4)
Canada: Halifax	605 (±43)	38 (±3)	138 (±20)	31 (±6)
Denmark: Glostrup	529 (±34)	52 (±3)	141 (±17)	57 (±6)
Czech Republic	495 (±24)	48 (±2)	89 (±10)	51 (±5)
Poland: Tarnobrzeg	465 (±26)	81 (±2)	110 (±12)	91 (±3)
Germany: Augsburg (urban)	353 (±32)	52 (±4)	70 (±13)	66 (±9)
Italy: Friuli	270 (±14)	49 (±2)	50 (±6)	50 (±6)
France: Toulouse	240 (±15)	45 (±3)	37 (±5)	65 (±7)
Spain: Catalonia	187 (±12)	41 (±3)	30 (±4)	46 (±8)
China: Beijing	76 (±9)	53 (±6)	37 (±6)	69 (±8)

Source: Tunstall-Pedoe, H., Kuulasmaa, K., Amouyel, P., Arveiler, D., Rajakangas, A.-M. and Pajak, A. for the WHO MONICA Project (1994). 'Myocardial Infarction and Coronary Deaths in the World Health Organization MONICA Project: Registration Procedures, Event Rates, And Case-Fatality Rates in 38 Populations from 21 Countries in Four Continents'. *Circulation*, **90**: 583–612.

whereas Mediterranean countries like Spain, Italy, and Greece had much lower rates, but not as low as those in countries such as Japan and China.

Ancel Keys pioneered the first major international epidemiological study of coronary heart disease by conducting cardiovascular examinations in population or occupational groups of men in seven countries with a range of coronary mortality. Several potential risk factors were examined at the baseline examination, and men were followed over several years to determine which risk factors predicted future coronary events. The Seven Countries study and other cohort studies conducted in single populations, such as Framingham and Whitehall, helped establish the major classic risk factors of coronary disease: high plasma cholesterol, hypertension, and cigarette smoking (Luepker *et al.* 2004). ⌨ Official mortality data also show that there is a strongly increasing relation with age (exponential) in both sexes; mortality rates are much lower in middle-aged women than in men, but are almost equal in men and women over 85 years of age. With the possible exception of age, none of these risk factors is in itself *sufficient* to predict CHD, although hypercholesterolaemia may be a *necessary* factor in that, in countries where the average population levels of plasma cholesterol are low, CHD is relatively uncommon. An example of a large prospective study conducted in such a country is shown in Table 6.2. However, all these risk factors predict future risk of CHD in individuals rather poorly and, because CHD is still such a major cause of premature death, there has been an intensive search for additional risk factors. Over 200 'new' risk factors have been investigated. Most of these have been investigated in **longitudinal** studies. These may have a **cohort** design in which all the population exposed and unexposed

to the risk factor are followed up for subsequent fatal or non-fatal CHD, or a **nested case–control** design in which stored biological samples taken at baseline are tested for the risk factor after a certain period of follow-up, for example 10 years.

All the classic risk factors show a graded relation (**dose–response**) with risk of subsequent CHD. Such a relation is important in indicating a **causal** link with the disease in question, but a link established in an intervention study is considered to be the highest level or 'gold standard' of evidence. Within the past decade large, multicentre trials have established the **efficacy** of statins, which are powerful lipid-lowering drugs, in reducing the incidence of CHD. Similarly, large-scale, multicentre studies have demonstrated the efficacy of anti-hypertensive treatments against cardiovascular disease, but practical and ethical difficulties have limited the possibility of randomized intervention studies on smoking. However, the weight of evidence from observational studies and animal experiments linking smoking with cardiovascular risk, risk of respiratory diseases, and many cancers is so strong as to render this unnecessary for public health and clinical practice.

As part of an investigation into risk of heart attack and the strength of cigarettes normally smoked (low-tar versus medium and high-tar cigarettes), Parish *et al.* (1995) ⌨ collected data shown in Table 6.3. A multicentre study of 14 000 men and women admitted to hospital with a final diagnosis of myocardial infarction were asked by questionnaire about their current smoking habits. For each case of myocardial infarction two or more of their relatives were given the same questionnaire. Table 6.3 shows the distribution of cases and controls according to their reported smoking habit and by their age group.

TABLE 6.2   Number of deaths from coronary heart disease and from stroke during 8–13 years of follow-up in 9021 men and women aged 35–64 years from Shanghai according to their initial cholesterol level

| | Number of deaths (relative risk*) | | | | | |
| | Cholesterol level (mmol/l) | | | | | |
Deaths from:	≤3.53	3.54–4.10	4.11–4.62	≥4.63	**All subjects**	**χ^2 for trend**
Coronary heart disease	4 (0.38)	9 (0.88)	12 (1.07)	18 (1.63)	43 (1.00)	8.35**
Stroke	34 (1.01)	35 (1.00)	34 (0.87)	43 (1.11)	146 (1.00)	

*Relative risk adjusted for age, sex (and cohort).

**$p < 0.01$.

Source: Chen, Z. M., Peto, R., Collins, R., MacMahon, S., Lu, J. R. and Li, W. X. (1991). 'Serum-Cholesterol Concentration and Coronary Heart Disease in a Population with Low Cholesterol Concentrations'. *British Medical Journal*, **303**, 276–82, reproduced with permission from the BMJ Publishing Group.

6.2 Stroke

Stroke (synonym: cerebrovascular accident) is a sudden neurological deficit or malfunction from a vascular cause which could range from loss of consciousness to partial loss of motor or sensory function. To be classified as stroke, these symptoms must persist for 24 hours or more; shorter periods of deficit are termed **transient ischaemic attack**. However, improved diagnostic techniques have shown that a proportion of these result in focal areas of brain infarction and would be better termed **mini-strokes**. Clinical examination cannot always distinguish between stroke due to **ischaemia** or that due to rupture of a blood vessel (**haemorrhagic** stroke), but neurological examination can often point to the particular part of the brain affected. **Subarachnoid haemorrhage** is clinically and epidemiologically distinct, as the blood vessels are those of the subarachnoid space surrounding the brain; cerebrospinal fluid tapped from a lumbar puncture needle at the level of L-4/5 inter-vertebral space is blood stained, which is diagnostic.

For clinical and epidemiological purposes, it is useful to distinguish ischaemic from haemorragic stroke. Haemorrhagic strokes should be referred for neuro-surgical opinion, and antiplatelet or thrombolytic drugs should be withheld. Haemorrhagic strokes may have different epidemiological risk factors to those for ischaemic stroke. Ischaemic stroke can be due to local occlusion of an artery of the brain (the bifurcation of the internal carotid is a common site for atherothrombosis) but **thrombi** can also originate either from the left atrium in atrial fibrillation or from the left ventricle in acute myocardial infarction or congestive heart failure. Haemorrhagic strokes, particularly subarachnoid haemorrhage, are frequently associated with aneurysm (berry aneurysm), which need to be fully investigated for possible surgical repair.

In advanced industrialized countries, computerized tomography (CT), which produces radiological, cross-sectional images sequentially of the whole brain, is frequently used to distinguish haemorrhagic from ischaemic stroke. However, in the developing world these expensive diagnostic facilities are not available. In Figure 6.2 the principal results of a survey done in urban and rural Tanzania are compared with data from England and Wales. Regular censuses and prospective monitoring of all deaths in three defined populations

TABLE 6.3	Smoking habit in cases of myocardial infarction admitted to hospital and in controls				
	Current smoker of manufactured cigarettes only		**Non-smoker with no regular cigarette use in past 10 years**		**Ratio of smoking rates* in cases compared with that in controls**
Age (years)	Cases (*n*)	Controls (*n*)	Cases (*n*)	Controls (*n*)	Risk ratio (95% CI)
30–39	78	1784	35	4873	6.33 (4.22–9.51)
40–49	293	1497	190	4306	4.66 (3.82–5.69)
50–59	435	861	508	2701	3.10 (2.64–3.65)
60–69	416	653	707	2299	2.54 (2.16–2.98)
70–79	111	163	369	942	1.92 (1.45–2.54)

*Smoker v non-smoker rates standardized for age and sex.

Source: Parish, S., Collins, R., Peto, R. *et al.* (1995). 'Cigarette Smoking, Tar Yields, and Non-Fatal Myocardial Infarction: 14000 cases and 32000 Controls in the United Kingdom'. *British Medical Journal*, **311**, 471–7, reproduced with permission from the BMJ Publishing Group.

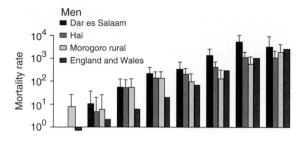

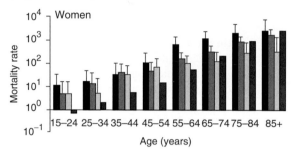

Fig. 6.2 Number and yearly rate per 100 000 with 95% CI of deaths from stroke in 10-year age-bands in adult men and women in Dar es Salaam, Hai district, Morogoro rural district, and England and Wales (1993).
Source: Walker, R. W., McLarty, D. G., Kitange, H. M. *et al.* (2000). 'Stroke Mortality in Urban and Rural Tanzania'. *Lancet*, **355**: 1684–7.

in Tanzania were performed between 1992 and 1995. **Verbal autopsies** (witness statements of the symptoms and signs preceding death) were obtained from relatives or carers of those who died. Mortality in men and women in three areas of Tanzania and in England and Wales are shown in Figure 6.2.

The scale used for the mortality rate is logarithmic; the results indicate that the stroke death rates rise exponentially with age. The mortality from stroke is highest in the urban area of Dar es Salaam (the largest city and commercial capital), intermediate in Hai (a well-developed rural area) and lower in Morogoro (a poorly developed rural area), but lowest of all in England and Wales (except in men and women aged 75 or more years). Death rates from most other causes were, of course, much higher in Tanzania than in England and Wales. The authors noted that atheroma was rare in Africa and ischaemic strokes may have been mainly due to cardiac emboli, possibly from **rheumatic heart disease**; haemorrhagic strokes probably contributed disproportionately to the total as other studies indicate that this group contributes 28–33 per cent of the total burden of stroke in Africa (Walker *et al.* 2000). 🖳 The

high level of stroke mortality in Tanzania was attributed to untreated hypertension (Walker *et al.* 2000). 🖳

Risk factors

As noted above, the mortality from stroke (and the incidence) rises exponentially with age. Subarachnoid haemorrhage is the most common category in men and women under 45 years of age in Western countries but rises only linearly with age. Most studies on stroke epidemiology treat subarachnoid haemorrhage separately, although the major risk factors – hypertension and smoking habit – are shared with both ischaemic and haemorrhagic stroke. In Western countries the proportion of strokes that are haemorrhagic is relatively low (6–14 per cent) (Wolfe *et al.* 2000). 🖳

Compared with CHD, the epidemiology of stroke is in its infancy. A major review for the Stroke Council of the American Heart Association (Goldstein *et al.* 2001) 🖳 concluded that potentially modifiable risk factors were; hypertension, smoking, diabetes mellitus, carotid stenosis, hyperlipidaemia, and atrial fibrillation. Although other risk factors have been established in observational studies (such as obesity, sedentary lifestyle, alcohol consumption, hyperhomocysteinaemia, hypercoagulability, hormone replacement therapy, and inflammatory markers), the evidence that modification of these factors was beneficial or achievable was less convincing. Most public-health strategies, however, should include reduction of obesity, increasing physical activity, and reduction of heavy alcohol consumption in preventive strategies to reduce the incidence of stroke (Goldstein *et al.* 2001). 🖳 Smoking is a major risk factor for both ischaemic and haemorrhagic stroke, but is a particularly strong risk factor for subarachnoid haemorrhage, whose epidemiology is less well explored (as the population incidence is low compared with that of other types of stroke).

Figure 6.3 shows the major impact of blood pressure on the risk of stroke taken from a meta-analysis of 61 observational studies among one million men and women with a combined total of 12.7 million person-years at risk.

Prevention of cardiovascular disease

Observational epidemiological studies have clearly shown the major roles of hypertension and smoking as risk factors for CHD and stroke. Raised cholesterol is a major risk factor for CHD, and international comparisons of the incidence in Western and Eastern countries suggest that it may be a **necessary** factor for CHD.

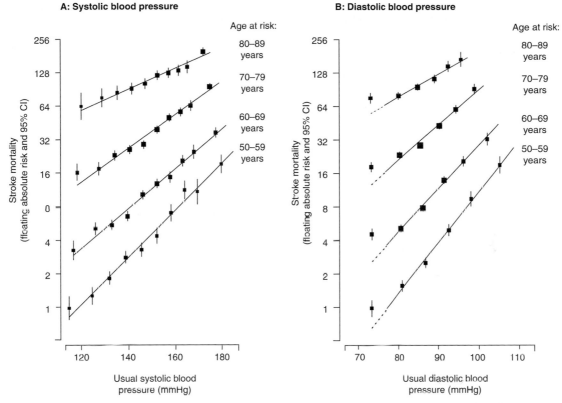

Fig. 6.3 Stroke mortality rate in each decade of age versus usual blood pressure at start of that decade (meta-analysis of cohort studies). Source: Prospective Studies Collaboration (2002). 'Age-Specific Relevance of Usual Blood Pressure to Vascular Mortality: A Meta-Analysis of Individual Data for One Million Adults in 61 Prospective Studies'. *The Lancet*, **360**: 1903–13.

But the role of cholesterol as a risk factor for stroke is less clear.

A meta-analysis of cohort studies indicates strongly reduced risk of death after myocardial infarction in patients who quit smoking (Wilson *et al.* 2000); 🖳 and a large cohort study shows clearly reduced risk of stroke in subjects who have quit smoking (Wannamethee *et al.* 1995). 🖳 Experimental evidence from large, multi-centre clinical trials has shown convincing benefit of antihypertensive treatment particularly for stroke (Blood Pressure Lowering Treatment Trialists' Collaboration 2000). Within the past 10–15 years, major multicentre trials have shown clear benefit in treatment of hypertension in the elderly whose blood pressure tends to be high (blood pressure increases with age in the general population) and who are at high risk of stroke. Until these trials published their results in the late 1980s, blood pressure in the elderly was rarely treated. Now the weight of observational and experimental

evidence has resulted in the recommendation that 140/90 mmHg in all age groups should be used as the new threshold for initiation of preventive treatment (both non-pharmacological and pharmacological), replacing the previous threshold of 160/95 mmHg (Guidelines Subcommittee 1999). 🖳 The Health Survey for England (Primatesta *et al.* 2001) 🖳 estimated that with this threshold 38 per cent of the general population will require investigation and treatment using the diastolic cut-point of at least 90 mmHg. Full implementation of the strategy would bring considerable health gain, but the costs to the health service would also be large. Generic (off-patent) anti-hypertensive drugs are relatively inexpensive compared with effective antilipaemic drugs such as statins, which were more recently introduced. Most statins and more recent cardiovascular drugs remain expensive, however, and cost implications to the National Health Service are considerable (Marshall 2003). 🖳

Patients who are discharged from hospital after a myocardial infarction tend to be prescribed several different cardiovascular drugs. A recent paper suggested that similar drugs should be combined in a 'polypill' in the primary prevention of cardiovascular disease without necessarily screening for risk factors (Wald and Law 2003). ⬛ Commentators questioned the likely effectiveness of this polypharmacy and raised the question of possible side effects. Others have suggested that dietary intervention (the Polymeal) could reduce cardiovascular disease by a similar amount (75 per cent) (Franco *et al.* 2004). ⬛

Non-pharmacological treatments and preventive strategies for the general population to lower the 'population mean' of a particular risk factor remain the public-health strategy of choice but require major cultural and policy changes that may be difficult to achieve in practice (see also Figure 1.3 and Chapters 8 and 21).

6.3   Congestive Heart Failure

A steady and perhaps unexpectedly sustained decline in mortality due to CHD (and also to stroke) in Western countries has been witnessed during the past 25–35 years, with an increase in adult life expectancy. This is believed to be due largely to a decline in the population prevalence of risk factors but also in part to improvements in treatment (Unal *et al.* 2004). ⬛ In mirror image to the decline in coronary mortality, hospitalization rates for congestive heart failure have increased. This has not been reflected in an increase in official mortality statistics from congestive heart failure as coding regulations by the International Classification of Diseases require the coding of the underlying cause of death, which as noted below, is most frequently attributed to CHD.

Congestive heart failure is the result of pump failure of the heart. This may be acute, after acute myocardial infarction, or chronic, usually in Western societies owing to chronic ischaemia and fibrosis of the heart muscle; but in developing countries hypertrophic cardiomyopathy is a major cause of failure, usually because of untreated hypertension. When pump failure of the left side of the heart occurs there is back-pressure in the pulmonary venous system, and, when the osmotic (oncotic) pressure of the blood in the pulmonary capillaries exceeds that in the interstitial space, fluid moves into the pulmonary alveoli, resulting in breathlessness and increased respiration. Clinical diagnosis may be particularly difficult in the elderly owing to co-morbidity. Cardiologists prefer to use **echocardiography** (ultrasound) in the diagnosis but suitable equipment may not be readily available in all centres, and may not be available to outpatients. Measurement of one of the cardiac peptides produced as a response to pressure stress of the ventricular and atrial walls shows considerable promise as a possible simple screening test for cardiac failure (Maisel *et al.* 2002) ⬛ (see also Chapter 5, Figure 5.3). Echocardiography can be used to distinguish systolic and diastolic (pre-symptomatic) congestive heart failure (Vasan and Levy 2000) ⬛ but this has been questioned by others (Caruana *et al.* 2000). ⬛

Population prevention

Congestive heart failure in hospitalized patients carries a one-year mortality of 50 per cent (Cleland 1998). ⬛ As Cleland notes, in population terms prevention may not be achievable, but 'it may be possible to slow the increasing morbidity associated with heart failure'. Clinical trials of ACE inhibitors and β-blockers provide some optimism in this respect (Cowie and Zaphiron 2002). ⬛

6.4   Peripheral Vascular Disease

Peripheral vascular disease is defined as atherosclerosis of the major vessels supplying the lower limbs, resulting in ischaemia which can produce the symptoms of calf pain on exertion (claudication) or in more severe cases chronic anoxia to the lower limbs resulting in gangrene. Cigarette smoking is a strong risk factor for this disease and coexistence with other manifestations of atherosclerotic disease is common. As with congestive heart failure, trends in the prevalence of peripheral vascular disease are likely to increase owing to an ageing population and delay in the onset of cardiovascular disease; but there have been relatively few epidemiological studies for this condition. Recent reviews of the epidemiology and treatment are to be found elsewhere (Hiatt 2001). ⬛

Aortic aneurysm is presumptively atherosclerotic in nature, with a strong genetic element, and is a potentially preventable cause of death, particularly when confined to the abdominal aorta. The prevalence is 5 per cent in men aged 60 years or more and 1–2 per cent in women. Screening for this condition has been suggested because elective surgical repair carries a 5–8 per cent 30 day mortality compared with 50 per cent mortality for ruptured aneurysm; a trial of screening conducted in the south of England has shown encouraging results (The Multicentre Aneurysm Screening Study Group 2002). ⬛

References

References for this chapter can be found at www.oxfordtextbooks.co.uk/orc/yarnell. Where possible, these are presented as *active links* which direct you to an electronic version of the work. If you are a subscriber to that work (either individually or through an institution), and depending on your level of access, you may be able to peruse an abstract or the full article if available. 🖳

Model answers

Q1(a) The WHO established three separate clinical criteria, two of which had to be fulfilled before a case could be classified as definite myocardial infarction. These criteria were: severe chest pain lasting 30 minutes or more; certain ECG changes classified according to the Minnesota coding scheme (this had to be done by specially trained technicians); two or more-fold elevation of cardiac enzymes signifying myocardial necrosis. Currently troponins provide a sensitive marker of myocardial necrosis, but international standards for these markers have not been agreed.

Q1(b) Risk of death from complications of acute myocardial infarction, and of further infarction, are highest in the first few days after the initial infarction, but decline gradually over the next four weeks.

Q1(c) Case-fatality rates may have been high in this region because of significant delays in patients receiving medical care. There may have also been delays in the recognition and significance of symptoms by patients and their relatives.

Q2 The overall study design in MONICA is ecological, as individual data on risk factors and on coronary incidence obtained from registrations are not directly linked.

Q3(a) This is an unmatched case–control study. Because the information on exposure and disease status is collected cross-sectionally, it could also be classified as a cross-sectional case–control study.

Q3(b) The researchers probably chose relatives as a control population for ease of access and possibly also to achieve a higher response rate than may have been possible from unrelated subjects.

Q3(c) Smoking habits tend to cluster within families and close relatives may have been more likely to have been smokers if the hospitalized case patient also smoked. This may have reduced the possibility of finding an association between smoking habit and myocardial infarction.

Q3(d) Smoking habit is significantly associated with increased risk of myocardial infarction at all ages. Young cases of myocardial infarction are more likely to be smokers than older cases.

Q3(e) The rate ratio or relative risk.

Respiratory system

This chapter describes the role of respiratory infection as a leading worldwide cause of death in infancy and a major cause of death in the elderly. Many lung diseases are closely linked to cigarette smoking: for example 90 per cent of cases of lung cancer (the commonest cancer in men and the second commonest in women) and most chronic obstructive airways disease. Cigarette smoking is also an important factor in reducing resistance to respiratory infections, which can lead to life-threatening respiratory diseases such as bronchopneumonia and tuberculosis. The effects of air pollution and occupational exposures are also reviewed.

Introduction

The delicate ciliated epithelial lining of the bronchial airways is vulnerable to pathological damage throughout life but is most vulnerable during infancy. At birth there are around 64 000 terminal bronchioles and 20 million alveoli, which increase to about 300 million during the first year of life although the lungs do not reach complete development until the age of 7 or 8 years. The surface area of the lungs is exposed in adults to an average of 7000 litres of air a day. The bronchial epithelium has several highly efficient defence mechanisms against particulate and microbiological invasion but is particularly vulnerable in infancy when the airways are at their earliest stage of development. Respiratory infections are therefore an important cause of **infant mortality (deaths during the first year of life)**, particularly in the **post-neonatal period (after 28 days)**; and this mortality occurs more frequently in developing countries, often with tropical climates, than in industrialized, well-developed countries. There is often a problem with host resistance or immunological competence, which can be due to malnutrition (or at least sub-optimal nutrition: see Chapter 8). Measles is a common killer in developing countries, often paving the way for bacterial pneumonia as the mode of death. Similarly, in old age **hypostatic pneumonia** is often the mode of death in a body incapacitated by other major diseases such as cancer or stroke. As noted in Chapter 2, death certificates should provide information on the underlying cause of death rather than the mode of death. Variability in the completeness of death certification can lead to over-representation of pneumonia as a 'true' cause of death; ICD10 has attempted to reduce this possibility.

Besides being vulnerable to micro-organisms, lungs are prone to damage from exposure to inhaled chemical or physical agents such as tobacco smoke and atmospheric and workplace pollutants. Another important group of respiratory diseases are believed to have a mainly allergic basis. These include **asthma**, which is showing a rising prevalence and **occupational asthma**, which is highly prevalent in certain industrial environments.

Box 7.1 shows the respiratory diseases that are responsible for major mortality and morbidity in the UK.

Pneumonia is the consequence of a sustained infection of the lower (or distal) part of the respiratory tract. Alveoli are party filled with fluid, and gas exchange is severely restricted. The generic term **bronchopneumonia** tends to be used for non-specific pneumonias but can be made more specific, for example **hypostatic** pneumonia, **lobar** pneumonia, **aspiration** pneumonia, etc.

The terms **chronic bronchitis**, **emphysema**, and **chronic obstructive airways (or pulmonary) disease (COAD or COPD)** are terms that reflect different aspects of the same disease: chronic bronchitis describes the inflammatory nature of the disease, (productive cough for at least 3 months per year); emphysema the result of overinflation of the alveoli (destruction of their structure and functional capacity); and COPD, which describes the overall condition. **Pneumoconioses** are a group of diseases of the lung which are the result of occupational exposure to dusts such as silica (silicosis), beryllium (beryllosis), asbestos (asbestosis), and fungi such as *Aspergillus* (aspergillosis: farmer's lung). Finally, **pulmonary tuberculosis** is the most important cause of mortality in adults in many parts of the developing regions of the world. Antibiotic resistance and malnutrition are closely associated with the high mortality in many areas.

Acute upper respiratory tract infections (infections above the level of the bronchi) are circulating in populations continuously and cause significant symptoms in children and adults usually several times a year. They are the leading cause of sickness absence but are usually self-limiting. In susceptible subjects they can precede the development of lower respiratory infections and bacterial pneumonias. **Influenza** is epidemic in nature and new strains of influenza virus can be charted across the globe. **Asthma** is a major wheezing disorder of children and adults whose prevalence appears to be climbing steadily with other **atopic** diseases such as hay fever.

7.1 Acute Upper and Lower Respiratory Infections, Influenza, and Pneumonia

Upper respiratory tract infections

These are the commonest presenting illness in primary care. Table 7.1 provides an estimate of mortality and service use for the major respiratory diseases in the UK.

BOX 7.1 MAJOR CAUSES OF RESPIRATORY MORTALITY AND MORBIDITY

Mortality	Morbidity
Bronchopneumonia	Acute upper respiratory tract infections
Lung cancer	Acute bronchitis (middle respiratory tract infections)
	Influenza
Chronic bronchitis	Asthma
Emphysema	Hay fever (allergic rhinitis)
Chronic obstructive pulmonary disease	
Pneumoconioses	
Tuberculosis (developing countries)	

TABLE 7.1 Expected mortality and service use in district with population of 500 000 in the UK per year (1998–99)

	Deaths	Hospital bed-days	GP consultations
Upper respiratory infections	2	1310	106 550
Acute bronchitis and bronchiolitis	5	863	35 950
Pneumonia	562	17 012	1450
Influenza	6	227	10 250
Chronic bronchitis, emphysema, and COPD	242	9084	5650
Asthma	13	10 914	21 250
Lung cancer	280	5211	400

Adapted from: Walters, S. and Ward, D. J. (2004). 'Lower Respiratory Disease', in A. Stevens, J. Raftery, J. Mant (eds.). *Health Care Needs Assessment, The Epidemiologically Based Needs Assessment Reviews.* Oxford and New York: Radcliffe Medical Press, 245–371.

A large range of viruses are responsible for upper respiratory tract infections (URTIs) including influenza A and B, parainfluenza, rhinovirus, adenovirus, enterovirus, and respiratory syncytial virus (RSV). Viruses particularly associated with bronchiolitis in children are the RSV and parainfluenza 3, and several viruses predispose to pneumonia (influenza, chickenpox, RSV, parainfluenza, measles, and adenoviruses). Many patients seek treatment from their general practitioner, but a systematic review suggests that antibiotic therapy is usually unnecessary except for some bacterial infections, for example haemolytic streptococcal infection of throat with local complications (Fahey *et al.* 1998). 🖥 Vaccines are unavailable for most URTIs, but a review of cohort studies and trials suggests that influenza vaccination significantly reduces the risk of death associated with the complications of influenza in the elderly (Gross *et al.* 1995); 🖥 this has been adopted as public health policy for those older than 65, in key public sector workers, and in patients with chronic disease with reduced immune function, including those who have had a splenectomy.

Pneumonia is most simply classified into two distinct epidemiological types: **community-acquired** and **hospital-acquired** (or **nosocomial**; Greek: hospital). In infancy and childhood, acute respiratory infections such as bronchitis and bronchiolitis can develop into pneumonia and are a common cause of hospital admission in developed countries, but mortality is low.

In developing countries, however, the situation is completely different, and mortality from respiratory infections is second only to 'perinatal causes' as the leading cause of death in infancy and childhood (see Chapter 14). **Community-acquired pneumonia** is a disease of the middle-aged and elderly and causes over one million hospital admissions per year in the UK. In middle-aged adults, cigarette smoking is a major risk factor, and alcohol and corticosteroid therapy can also impair ciliary and immune function. In the elderly, general debility, recent influenza, other URTIs or major co-morbidities predispose to pneumonia. It has been estimated that 40 per cent of hospitalized patients with pneumonia do not receive a microbiological diagnosis. Both bacterial and viral diagnoses include; streptococcus pneumoniae (30 per cent +), chlamydia pneumoniae (10 per cent), myoplasma pneumoniae (9 per cent), legionella pneumoniae (5 per cent), influenza, parainfluenza, measles, RSV, and chicken pox, all of which have distinct clinical and epidemiological characteristics. Studies in the USA show a similar pattern (Ruiz *et al.* 1999). 🖥

Hospital-acquired pneumonia is defined as a pneumonia that develops a minimum of 48 hours after admission to hospital. It may result as a direct result of surgery (post-operative and aspiration pneumonia) but is more often a result of major co-morbidity, for example COPD or general debility in the elderly. Some 2–5 per cent of hospital admissions are complicated by the development of this condition. The spectrum of micro-organisms responsible for hospital-acquired pneumonia are different to those found in the disease acquired in the community. Gram-negative organisms predominate: *Escherichia coli*, pseudomonas and *Klebsiella*. Methicillin-resistant *Staphylococcus aureus* (MRSA), widely found in hospitals, may also cause this condition (see Chapter 16).

Until the introduction of the tenth revision of the International Classification of Diseases (ICD), **bronchopneumonia** tended to be used as main cause of death in the elderly even when it was a complication of 'old age' or a major co-morbidity. With the introduction of ICD-10, deaths due to bronchopneumonia have fallen substantially within the UK (see Chapter 2).

7.2 Chronic Lower Respiratory Disease

COPD, which includes chronic bronchitis and emphysema, dominate this group of diseases, which occur mainly in the middle aged and elderly. **Occupational lung diseases** form a separate, relatively small but largely preventable group. Their epidemiological characteristics are described after the following section.

In developed countries, COPD is the second most important respiratory cause of death in men (fourth most important cause of death overall) after lung cancer. In developing countries it is second to tuberculosis in men but is the leading cause of respiratory death in women. COPD is characterized by **dyspnoea**; chronic cough is often insidious in onset but often leads to a protracted long-term illness, premature mortality, and dependency on domiciliary oxygen. It is unsurprising, therefore, that in the developed world COPD is the leading cause of **disability-adjusted life years (DALYs)** lost, but in the developing world this ranking is surpassed only by tuberculosis (World Health Organization 2003).

Cigarette smoking is the major cause of COPD, although it is estimated that only 15 per cent of lifetime smokers develop the condition (Croxton *et al.* 2003). In developed countries Ezzati and Lopez (2003) estimated that 84 per cent of COPD in men and 62 per cent in women under 70 years of age can be attributed to cigarette smoking. In those older than 70 the figures are 77 per cent and 61 per cent, respectively. In developing countries, widespread smoking among men began only in the past few decades, and just less than 50 per cent of COPD can be attributed to smoking in men and only 20 per cent in women. A recent National Heart, Lung and Blood Institute (USA) review of clinical research in COPD provides an excellent overview of the epidemiology of the condition and a list of research questions for the future (Croxton *et al.* 2003). 🖥

7.3   **Cancers of the Respiratory Tract**

Although this group of cancers includes those of the upper respiratory tract – lip, mouth, and oropharynx – the group is dominated by lung cancer, which is the commonest non-skin cancer worldwide. In European countries it is the leading cause of cancer deaths in men and a rising cause of cancer death in women (see Tyczynski *et al.* 2003). 🖥 There are four major histological types: squamous cell (35 per cent), adenocarcinoma (30 per cent), small-cell (20 per cent), and large-cell (15 per cent), which have different epidemiological characteristics and respond differently to treatment. However, difficulties in obtaining samples (from bronchoscopy) preclude a histological diagnosis in up to a third of cases.

Epidemiology and risk factors for respiratory cancers

At the beginning of the twentieth century lung cancer was rare, accounting for less than 1 per cent of cancer deaths, but by the end of the century it had emerged in the developed world to be the leading cause of cancer deaths in men and, in most of these countries, either the first or second cause of cancer deaths in women. By the midpoint of the twentieth century the scale of the lung cancer epidemic was recognized by physicians and epidemiologists. The search for causes launched the first major epidemiological investigations into non-infectious or chronic diseases and stimulated a major debate among medical scientists. Undoubtedly this paved the way for improved methodological rigour in epidemiology, and the link between smoking and lung cancer provides a model for the 'causal criteria' proposed by Bradford Hill (see Chapter 1, Box 1.3). The strong association between cigarette smoking and the risk of respiratory cancer was tested in many longitudinal epidemiological studies. One of the best-known British studies is summarized in Table 7.2 (see also Doll *et al.* 2004). 🖥

Although randomized trials of smoking cessation have been attempted (Rose and Colwell 1992), 🖥 most epidemiological evidence on risk reduction after smoking cessation comes from observational studies. Table 7.3 illustrates data available from two case–control studies from Britain conducted in 1950 and 1990.

In developed countries over 90 per cent of lung cancers can be attributed to cigarette smoking in men (Ezzati and Lopez 2003) 🖥 whereas there is less epidemiological certainty in the estimates for women (approximately 71 per cent). Similarly, in developing countries other factors may also be important as 65 per cent of lung cancer in men under 70 years of age can be attributed to smoking, and in women the figure is only 26 per cent (Ezzati and Lopez 2003). 🖥 Unfortunately this pattern is likely to change to the pattern in developed countries unless global action on smoking cessation and tobacco consumption is initiated effectively in the developing world (see Chapter 17, section 17.1).

The pattern of histological tumour types appears to be changing over time with an increasing prevalence of adenocarcinomas in Western countries (Tyczynski *et al.* 2003). 🖥 This seems to be due to the introduction of low-tar and low-nicotine cigarettes, which may be inhaled more deeply and more often than cigarettes with higher nicotine levels, resulting in the distribution of carcinogens to the peripheral regions of the lungs which predisposes this tissue to adenocarcinoma.

TABLE 7.2   Mortality by smoking habits from respiratory disease by 40 years of follow-up in British doctors

Type of disease (number of deaths, 1951–91)	Non-smokers (never smoked regularly)	Former cigarette smokers	Current cigarette smokers Number per day			Relative risk ≥25 daily versus non-smokers
			1–14	15–24	≥25	
Pulmonary tuberculosis (66)	4	8	7	9	20	5.0
Chronic obstructive lung disease (542)	10	57	86	112	225	2.3
Pneumonia (864)	71	90	113	154	169	2.4
Asthma (70)	4	11	6	8	6	1.5
Other respiratory disease (216)	19	28	26	31	33	1.7
All respiratory disease	107	192	237	310	471	4.4
(Number of deaths 1758)	(131)	(455)	(161)	(170)	(159)	
Cancers						
Upper respiratory sites (98)	1	3	12	18	48	48.0
Lung (893)	14	58	105	208	355	25.4

Source: Doll, R., Peto, R., Wheatley, K., Gray, R. and Sutherland, I. (1994). 'Mortality in Relation to Smoking: 40 years' Observations on Male British Doctors'. *British Medical Journal*, **309**: 901–11, reproduced with permission from the BMJ Publishing Group.

TABLE 7.3   Smoking status versus cumulative risk of death from lung cancer by age 75, from 1950 and 1990 studies

	Men				Women			
	Percentage of cases/controls		Cumulative risk (%)*		Percentage of cases/controls		Cumulative risk (%)*	
Smoking Status	1950	1990	1950	1990	1950	1990	1950	1990
Lifelong non-smoker	0.5/4.5	0.5/19.0	~0.4	~0.4	37.0/54.6	7.6/50.3	~0.4	~0.4
Former smokers	5.2/9.1	42.7/52.5	2.9	5.5	9.3/7.4	29.8/29.4	0.9	2.6
Current pipe or cigar only	3.9/7.2	8.5†/7.1	2.8	8.1†	0/0	0.6/0.1	—	—
Current cigarette smokers	90.4/79.2	48.3/21.5	5.9	15.9	53.7/38.0	61.9/20.1	1.0	9.5
Amount smoked (% of smokers)								
<5/day	3.6/7.0	6.2/9.5	2.8	10.4	20.6/36.7	4.1/10.1	0.6	3.4
5–14/day	38.2/47.5	33.5/39.7	4.4	12.8	44.1/44.9	32.3/37.8	1.0	7.7
15–24/day	33.0/31.5	39.1/37.3	5.7	16.7	35.3/18.4	44.1/42.4	2.0	10.4
≥25/day	25.2/14.0	21.1/13.5	9.8	24.4		19.5/9.7		18.5
Total	100/100	100/100			100/100	100/100		
Number of cases	1357/1357	667/2108	—	—	108/108	315/1077	—	—

*Calculated from published relative risk estimates.

†In 1990 88 per cent of these subjects were also former cigarette smokers.

Modified from: Peto, R., Darby, S., Deo, H. *et al.* (2000). 'Smoking, Smoking Cessation, and Lung Cancer in the UK Since 1950: Combination of National Statistics with Two Case–Control Studies'. *British Medical Journal*, **321**: 323–9, reproduced with permission from the BMJ Publishing Group.

Other risk factors for lung cancer include occupational causes such as exposure to asbestos, metals (for example nickel, arsenic, and cadmium), ionizing radiation, radon gas (which may be found either in the workplace or in the domestic environment in association with regions of natural granite formation), and passive smoking of the cigarette smoke of others (see section 7.5).

Prevention of respiratory cancers

The scientific case for primary prevention of lung cancer and other respiratory cancers by the elimination of tobacco smoking is overwhelming, but commercial interests have effectively limited public health initiatives since the 1960s (see below and Chapter 17). In view of the high-case fatality associated with lung cancer, screening programmes have been introduced to detect early cancers. Several major trials of radiological screening for the early detection of lung cancers have indicated no overall benefit despite improved survival for asymptomatic tumours. The usual epidemiological problems associated with the evaluation of cancer-screening initiatives impede the complete evaluation of these programmes (lead-time bias, length bias, and overdiagnosis) (Henschke *et al.* 1999) ▢ (see also Chapter 5).

7.4 **Asthma**

Asthma (Greek: panting) is characterized by reversible airflow obstruction due to bronchospasm or constriction of the musculature of the bronchi and bronchioles and with chronic inflammation of the airways. Untreated severe cases cause hypoxia, cyanosis, and can lead to respiratory failure and death. Fortunately, most asthma attacks can be limited in their severity by the judicious use of beta-2 agonists which act with **adrenaline** in the dilatation of bronchial smooth muscle. But this treatment is sometimes not without its problems; increased mortality among teenagers and young adults in the 1960s and 1970s in Westernized countries was attributed to inappropriate or excessive use of early beta-2 agonists, which have largely been replaced by safer drugs.

As shown in Table 7.1, asthma is a common cause of consultation in general practice and is the most common chronic disease of childhood. Recent epidemiological surveys of asthma prevalence have focused on the issue of standardizing questionnaires which elicit asthma symptoms. One such study used a standardized questionnaire worldwide often with the assistance of clinical videos showing symptoms (International Study of Asthma and Atopy in Childhood: ISAAC) and

found a prevalence of asthma symptoms (wheeze) ranging from 32 per cent in the UK, to 22 per cent in the USA, 14 per cent in France and Germany, and 2 per cent in Indonesia in school-children aged 13 and 14 years (The ISAAC Steering Committee 1998). ▢ The questionnaire that elicited the symptoms is shown in Box 7.2.

Peak expiratory flow before and after exercise has been used by some investigators to define asthma in epidemiological surveys, particularly in children (see Burr *et al.* 1994). ▢ A more invasive approach is the use of bronchial challenge testing. Although this has been used in surveys, its invasiveness and the necessity to have trained staff on hand in case of anaphylaxis has limited its use in the general population. It has been used in young adults with asthma symptoms drawn from the general population in the European Community Respiratory Health Survey (Janson *et al.* 2001). ▢

Prevalence, time trends, and risk factors

Surveys performed using the ISAAC protocol in the UK and Ireland indicate a prevalence of diagnosed asthma and treated wheeze of 22 per cent in schoolchildren aged 13–14 years and of 25 per cent in 5- to 8-year-olds. Time trends in asthma using standardized questionnaires of asthma symptoms have strongly suggested a steep increase in prevalence of the disorder in many Western countries. The 'hygiene hypothesis', which suggests that the lack of antigenic stimulation in our modern, relatively sterile environment is responsible for the development of an inappropriate chronic, allergenic, inflammatory response in many individuals, has been developed to account for this increase, and there is some epidemiological evidence to support this (Matricardi *et al.* 2000). ▢

Table 7.4 shows the results of the study by Matricardi *et al.* in which past exposure to infectious agents was investigated in 240 atopic and 240 non-atopic Italian military cadets.

Significantly fewer atopic cadets had evidence of past exposure to *Toxoplasma gondii* and to hepatitis A virus than had non-atopic cadets.

Q1 What additional analyses would strengthen the case of the investigators that past exposure to orofaecal and food-borne infections protects against the development of atopy?

Q2 The investigators also measured immunoglobulin E (IgE) levels in their sample. What additional biological measurements might be useful to establish the causal mechanisms in asthma?

BOX 7.2 SECTION A: BREATHING

1 Has your child ever had wheezing or whistling in the chest <u>at any</u>   Yes .....   No .....
   <u>time</u> in the past?
   If you have answered "No" please skip to question 11

2 Has your child had wheezing or whistling in the chest <u>in the last 12 months</u>?   Yes .....   No .....
   If you have answered "No" please skip to question 11

3 How many attacks of wheezing has your child had <u>in the last 12 months</u>?
   ..... None   ..... 1 to 3   ..... 4 to 12   ..... More than 12

4 <u>In the last 12 months</u>, how often, on average, has your child's sleep
   been disturbed due to wheezing?
   ..... Never woken with wheezing   ..... Less than one night per week
   ..... One or more nights per week

5 <u>In the last 12 months</u>, has wheezing ever been severe enough to limit your   Yes .....   No .....
   child's speech to only one or two words at a time between breaths?

6 <u>In the last 12 months</u>, how much did this wheezing interfere with
   your child's daily activities?
   ..... Not at all   ..... A little   ..... A moderate amount   ..... A lot

7 <u>In the last 12 months</u>, has your child's chest sounded wheezy during   Yes .....   No .....
   or after exercise?

8 <u>In the last 12 months</u>, has your child's chest sounded wheezy when he/she   Yes .....   No .....
   HAD NOT recently taken exercise?
   Colds

9 <u>In the last 12 months</u>, has your child had a wheezing or whistling in   Yes .....   No .....
   the chest when he/she **HAD** a cold or flu?

10 <u>In the last 12 months</u>, has your child had a wheezing or whistling in   Yes .....   No .....
    the chest when he/she **DID NOT** have a cold or flu?

11 Has your child <u>ever</u> had asthma?   Yes .....   No .....

12 <u>In the last 12 months</u>, has your child taken any treatment (medicines, tablets,   Yes .....   No .....
    inhalers) for wheezing or asthma?
    If YES, what?

    Inhaler/Nebulizer?   Yes   No   (Please circle)

    If Yes, Name(s) (or describe)   1. ....

    2. ....   3. ....

    Medicine/Tablets?   Yes   No   (Please circle)

    If Yes, Name(s) (or describe)   1. ....

    2. ....   3. ....

Atopy is a well-established risk factor for asthma, although a systematic review of population-based studies indicated that fewer than 40 per cent of asthma cases can be attributed to atopy. Both asthma and atopy are believed to be polygenic disorders and clearly interact with environmental factors such as biological allergens, tobacco smoke, atmospheric pollution, and domestic atmospheric pollutants. A recent report from the European Community Respiratory Health Survey suggests that sensitization to mould spores and to house-dust mite, among other allergens, is an important risk factor for severe asthma in young adults (Zureik *et al.* 2002). Similar findings have been reported from the city of Bombay, India, in a study using an identical protocol.

TABLE 7.4 Prevalence of antibodies against selected infectious agents in 240 atopic and 240 non-atopic Italian military cadets. Values are numbers (percentages) of participants unless stated otherwise

Infectious agent	Non-atopic group	Atopic group	Crude odds ratio (95% CI)
Orofecal and foodborne infections			
Toxoplasma gondii	63(26)	42(18)*	0.60(0.38–0.93)
Helicobacter pylori	44(18)	35(15)	0.76(0.47–1.24)
Hepatitis A virus	73(30)	39(16)†	0.44(0.29–0.69)
Infections transmitted by other routes			
Measles	233(97)	231(96)	0.77(0.28–2.11)
Mumps	92(38)	112(47)	1.41(0.98–2.03)
Rubella	211(88)	198(83)	0.65(0.39–1.08)
Chickenpox	157(65)	157(65)	1.00(0.69–1.46)
Cytomegalovirus	112(47)	132(55)	1.40(0.97–2.00)
Herpes simplex virus type 1	181(75)	168(70)	0.76(0.51–1.14)

*$p = 0.027$.

†$p = 0.004$.

Source: Matricardi, P. M., Rosmini, F., Riondino, S. *et al.* (2000). 'Exposure to Foodborne and Orofecal Microbes versus Airborne Viruses in Relation to Atopy and Allergic Asthma: Epidemiological Study'. *British Medical Journal*, **320**: 412–17, reproduced with permission from the BMJ Publishing Group.

7.5 Environmental Factors in Respiratory Disease

Environmental tobacco smoke

This smoke comes both from exhaled tobacco smoke and directly from the burning end of the cigarette in which the concentration of some carcinogens is higher than in smoke inhaled by the smoker. The US Department of Health, Education and Welfare (1986) 🖳 and the US Environmental Protection Agency (1992) 🖳 produced the first major reviews of the effects of environmental tobacco smoke on the health of adults and children in contact with it. More recently, Hackshaw *et al.* (1997) 🖳 reviewed 37 studies with a pooled relative risk of lung cancer of 1.24 (95% CI 1.13, 1.36). Evidence from many cross-sectional and short-term longitudinal studies supports the view that environmental tobacco smoke is hazardous to the respiratory health of children. A World Health Organization (WHO) consultation in 1999 concluded that environmental tobacco smoke (largely parental) caused pneumonia and bronchitis, middle ear disease, and worsening of respiratory symptoms and asthma (relative risk of maternal smoking for lower respiratory tract infection in infancy 1.7

(95% CI 1.6, 1.9)). The weight of scientific evidence linking passive smoking with impairment of respiratory health in others fully supports public health and WHO initiatives to limit public and occupational exposure to the tobacco smoke of smokers and parental education on household smoking (see also Chapter 17).

Air pollution

In the UK, public health concern was raised when a notable London smog was associated with about three times the number of deaths normally expected in one week in the winter of 1952; many of the deaths were attributed to bronchitis and pneumonia, and also to ischaemic heart disease (IHD). Smog was caused largely by carbon particles suspended in a moist atmosphere and associated with high levels of sulphur dioxide. Regional research in a longitudinal study of children born in 1946 found that heavily polluted areas were associated with a higher incidence of childhood bronchitis and pneumonia (Douglas and Waller 1966). 🖳 Accumulated evidence suggested that most of the elements producing smog were caused by domestic coal consumption; the Clean Air Act 1956 required the use of smokeless coal in British cities. Since then smogs caused by coal have declined but have been partly replaced by pollution due to vehicle exhaust gases. The main pollutants are shown in Box 7.3. Most pollutants are more highly concentrated in winter months; ozone is produced by sunlight, however, and significant health effects can occur in dry, hot conditions in association with vehicle pollution. In many developing countries pollution levels are similar or worse than in European cities when domestic coal was used but with additional pollutants from vehicle exhaust gases (McMichael and Smith 1999). 🖳

The London smog episode is an example of a **'natural experiment'** and many subsequent epidemiological studies have investigated seasonal effects on respiratory and cardiovascular mortality and admissions to hospital of adults and children with acute respiratory disease including asthma. Estimates on attributable mortality from the best available data from three European countries have been published (Künzli *et al.* 2000) 🖳 (Table 7.5).

Some attempts have been made by epidemiologists to monitor the contribution of air pollution to mortality during a longer period of time. In one such study in the US, Dockery *et al.* (1993) 🖳 followed a cohort of 8000 adults in six cities with a range of pollution levels.

BOX 7.3 HEALTH EFFECTS OF ATMOSPHERIC (MAINLY VEHICLE) POLLUTION

Pollutant	Source	Health effect
Nitrogen dioxide (NO_2)	Vehicle exhaust.	May exacerbate asthma and possibly increase susceptibility to infections.
Particulates PM10 Total suspended particulates, black smoke	Those less than 10 pm in diameter (PM10) penetrate the lung fairly efficiently and are most hazardous. Diesel produces more particulates than petrol.	Associated with respiratory symptoms. Long-term exposure is associated with death from heart and lung disease. Particulates can carry carcinogenic materials into the lungs.
Acid aerosols	Airborne acid formed from common pollutants including sulphur and nitrogen oxides.	May exacerbate asthma and increase susceptibility to respiratory infection. May reduce lung function in asthma.
Carbon monoxide (CO)	Comes mainly from petrol car exhausts.	Lethal at high doses. At low doses can impair concentration. May present a risk to the foetus.
Ozone (O_3)	Secondary pollutant produced from nitrogen oxides and volatile organic compounds in the air.	Irritates the eyes and air passages. Exacerbates asthma. May increase susceptibility to infection.
Lead	Compound present in leaded petrol to help the engine run smoothly.	Impairs brain development of children.
Volatile organic compounds (VOCs)	A group of chemical solvents from petrol fuel. Also present in vehicle exhaust.	Benzene has given cause for concern in this group of chemicals. It is a cancer causing agent and can cause leukaemia at high doses.
Polycyclic aromatic hydrocarbons (PAHs)	Produced by incomplete combustion of fuel. PAHs become attached to particulates.	Includes a range of chemicals and carcinogens. PAHs in traffic exhaust poses a low cancer risk to the general population.
Asbestos	May be present in brake pads and clutch linings especially in heavy duty vehicles. Asbestos fibres and dust are released into the atmosphere when vehicles brake.	Asbestos can cause lung cancer and mesothelioma. The consequences of low exposure from braking vehicles are not known.

TABLE 7.5 Health outcomes and those attributable to effects of atmospheric pollution in three European countries

Health outcome	Effect estimate relative risk (95% CI)	Health outcome frequency per million inhabitants per year			Attributable number of cases per 10µg/m³PM$_{10}$ per 1 000 000 inhabitants (95% CI)		
		Austria	France	Switzerland	Austria	France	Switzerland
Total mortality (adults >30 years, excluding violent death)	1.043 (1.026–1.061)	9330	8390	8260	370 (230–520)	340 (210–480)	340 (200–470)
Respiratory hospital admission (all ages)	1.013 (1.001–1.025)	17 830	11 550	10 300	230 (20–430)	150 (20–280)	130 (10–250)
Cardiovascular hospital admission (all ages)	1.013 (1.007–1.019)	36 790	17 270	24 640	450 (230–670)	210 (110–320)	300 (160–450)
Chronic bronchitis incidence (adults ≥25 years)	1.098 (1.009–1.194)	4990	4660	5010	410 (40–820)	390 (40–780)	430 (40–860)
Bronchitis episodes (children <15 years)	1.306 (1.135–1.502)	16 370	23 530	21 550	3200 (1410–5770)	4830 (2130–8730)	4620 (2040–8350)
Restricted activity days (adults ≥20 years)*	1.094 (1.079–1.502)	2 597 300	3 221 200	3 373 000	208 400 (175 400–241 800)	263 700 (222 000–306 000)	281 000 (236 500–326 000)
Asthma attacks (children <15 years)†	1.039 (1.019–1.059)	173 400	169 500	172 900	6280 (3060–9560)	6190 (3020–9430)	6370 (3100–9700)

*Total person-days per year. †Total person-days per year with asthma attacks.

Source: Künzli et al. (2000).

Künzli, N, Kaiser, R, Medina, S. et al. (2000) 'Public-Health Impact of Outdoor and Traffic-Related Air Pollution: A European Assessment'. The Lancet, **356**: 795–801.

After adjustment for confounding factors such as smoking, occupational exposure, etc., the excess mortality associated with air pollution was 26 per cent. Future studies such as these would appear to be essential in monitoring the health effects of atmospheric pollutants. A recent report from the American Heart Association provides a review of cohort studies, which show a consistent increase in risk of cardiovascular mortality associated with air pollution (Brook *et al.* 2004). 💻 Future monitoring systems also have to consider pollution in the upper atmosphere and issues of global warning, which are likely to have major health effects. These effects include thermal stress (which already claimed 15 000 excess deaths in France in 2003), floods and droughts, increased air pollution, and the spread of tropical diseases to temperate countries (Haines and Patz 2004). 💻

Housing environment

Attempts have been made to investigate housing factors and health in observational studies, but problems of confounding render the interpretation of such studies problematic. One study, designed after an extensive pilot study, conducted in Edinburgh, Glasgow, and London, showed that damp and mould growth were associated with a higher prevalence of reported respiratory symptoms, particularly in children, unexplained by confounding factors and study design (Platt *et al.* 1989). 💻 Although many aspects of the housing environment such as overcrowding, inadequate and contaminated water suppliers, damp, and ambient pollution clearly have had important effects in the UK and other developed countries in the past, these problems are particularly relevant today in developing countries owing to rapid, poorly controlled urbanization. For the reasons given above, these specific environmental effects can be difficult to quantify directly, but are likely to be a major factor in determining sub-optimal health status in the developing world.

7.6 Occupational Exposures

The workplace environment is often associated with both acute and chronic respiratory disease. This may be the office environment, for example 'sick-building syndrome', legionnaire's disease, etc., or more often the industrial environment where well-documented effects range from upper respiratory tract disease, middle respiratory tract disease (bronchitis, bronchiolitis), asthma, COPD, lung cancer, fibrotic diseases (for example asbestosis, silicosis), granulomatous diseases, and

inhalation fever. In the developed world, the pattern of disease has changed markedly over the past 100 years. In the first half of the twentieth century, heavy manufacturing industries and agriculture predominated. Fibrotic lung diseases, such as silicosis, asbestosis, and coal miner's pneumoconiosis were important causes of morbidity. During the same industrial period, COPD also contributed to poor health among workers. In the developing world, these occupational diseases persist because of poor environmental control of working conditions.

It is estimated that occupational exposures account for about 5 per cent of lung cancers. Neoplasms of the lung may be associated with specific industries. Smelters working with nickel, coke oven workers engaged in steel production, and insulation workers in the shipbuilding and construction industries working with asbestos, all have a higher incidence of bronchial carcinoma. The decline of these industries and the improvement of controls have led to a switch in emphasis to public-health issues such as air pollution or passive smoking. However, one important occupational neoplasm has had an increasing incidence. Mesothelioma is a malignant tumour of the pleura. It has a long latent period of 35–40 years. It is associated with asbestos exposure, in particular blue asbestos or crocidolite. Although blue asbestos was banned at the beginning of the 1970s, the incidence of mesothelioma in the UK is still increasing, and is likely to do so for several more years. The importance of early regulatory action based on good epidemiological evidence is demonstrated by a different experience in the USA, where the incidence of mesothelioma is now falling (Treasure *et al.* 2004). 💻 Industrial diseases are notified to the coroner's office in the UK to facilitate epidemiological monitoring and legal redress for workers when environmental controls have been poorly implemented.

The progressive shift from heavy manufacturing industry to service and high-tech manufacturing has been matched by a change in the pattern of occupational lung disease. In a recent surveillance study of occupational lung disease, asthma is now the most frequently reported cause (Ross 1999). 💻 Chemicals such as isocyanates, which are used in paint spraying, and soldering flux (used in the electronics industry), are important examples of respiratory sensitizers; biological agents are also important: for example, laboratory technicians may become allergic to inhaled animal proteins (such as rabbit fur) and bakers to flour.

Biological agents can produce other adverse immunological responses; for example, extrinsic allergic alveolitis, which may also result in fibrosis. This is a granulomatous inflammatory reaction that occurs in response to inhaled organic dusts. Examples are mouldy hay causing farmer's lung and bird excreta causing bird fancier's lung. The pattern of occupationally acquired respiratory infections has also changed. Diseases such as anthrax, in wool sorters, are now very rare. Tuberculosis (TB) has always been an important occupational disease, particularly among health-care workers. With a falling prevalence and the availability of treatment, it became less prominent in developed countries. However, in the UK, notifications of cases of TB have not fallen since the 1980s. The increasing mobility of workers worldwide, HIV infection, and the emergence of multi-drug resistance strains of TB have, however, caused new concern and interest in this old disease. The changing working environment has led to the emergence of new potential occupational infections, such as legionnaire's disease. Old and new viral illnesses such as influenza and severe acute respiratory syndrome (SARS), which can evolve in working environments, present continuing challenges (see also Chapter 16).

Further Reading

US Department of Health and Human Services (1986). The health consequences of involuntary smoking. A report of the Surgeon General. US DHHS, Public Health Services, Office of the Assistant Secretary for Health, Office of Smoking and Health, Washington, DC. DHHS Pub. No. (PHS) 87-8398.

US Environmental Protection Agency (1992). Respiratory health effects of passive smoking: lung cancer and other disorders. Office of Research and Development, Office of Health and Environmental Assessment, Washington, DC. SAB Review Draft. EPA/600/6-90-006B.

References

References for this chapter can be found at www.oxfordtextbooks.co.uk/orc/yarnell. Where possible, these are presented as *active links* which direct you to an electronic version of the work. If you are a subscriber to that work (either individually or through an institution), and depending on your level of access, you may be able to peruse an abstract or the full article if available. 🖳

Model answers

Q1 In Table 7.4 only data for the crude (unadjusted) odds ratio for each of the infectious agents are presented. It would be helpful to know whether the cases and controls had been adequately matched for potential confounding factors. If this was not the case then some attempt should be made to adjust for possible confounders in subsequent analyses.

Q2 Investigators may also measure genetic polymorphisms which may predispose to asthma in subjects with and without atopy.

CHAPTER 8

Nutritional, endocrine, and metabolic diseases

Chapter contents

This chapter deals with the major nutritionally related diseases that are of public-health importance internationally. In the developing world, malnutrition and suboptimal nutrition are endemic, whereas an epidemic of overweight and obesity has occurred in the developed world. Three examples of epidemiological studies are given: a major cohort study on mortality in American nurses according to the amount of body fat; a landmark multicentre clinical trial on the prevention of complications of insulin-dependent diabetes; and a community-based trial of iodine supplementation to fertile women in Papua New Guinea to reduce the likelihood of cretinism in their offspring.

Introduction

Several nutritionally related diseases are of major public-health importance and include both diseases of **deficiency** and of **excess**. Deficiency of calories or food energy, tragically experienced to some degree by well over half of the world's population, is **malnutrition**; the diseases of calorie excess have led to an epidemic of **overweight** and **obesity**, even paradoxically among low-income groups in affluent countries. The epidemics of coronary heart disease preceded those of overweight and obesity in such countries and have been closely linked with high consumption of foods containing saturated fatty acids (particularly dairy and meat products) which raise blood cholesterol levels (see Chapter 6). There is also much epidemiological evidence linking diet with many cancers on a worldwide basis (see Chapter 15).

Former micronutrient deficiency diseases such as **beriberi** (thiamine deficiency), **pellagra** (niacin deficiency), and **scurvy** (vitamin C deficiency) lie beyond the scope of this book but are important for a more complete understanding of the development of nutritional epidemiology (see Truswell 1999). 🖥 **Vitamin A deficiency** remains a major preventable cause of blindness in developing countries, and is often associated with protein–calorie malnutrition. **Rickets and osteomalacia** (vitamin D deficiency), once a major blight on children's skeletal development in large, industrialized cities, can still be problematic in Asian communities in the UK for whom vitamin D supplementation in childhood is recommended. **Maternal folate deficiency**, which has been closely associated with risk of neural tube defects (spina bifida) and for which pre-conceptual supplementary folate is advocated in the UK, is discussed in more detail in Chapter 14. Truswell notes that half of the vitamins are required in daily amounts of 1 mg or less (Truswell 1999), and with a balanced varied diet supplementation should be rarely necessary. Furthermore, in pregnant women excess levels of vitamin A have been linked with developmental abnormalities, and multivitamins containing vitamin A are not recommended in early pregnancy.

The term **metabolic disease** is used rather loosely in medical practice. Hormones play an essential role in many metabolic processes and endocrine diseases are essentially metabolic in nature. **Maturity-onset diabetes mellitus** is characterized by increasing resistance to the effects of insulin and a marked increase in insulin requirements. A rising trend in the incidence of this disorder is closely linked with the rising trend in overweight and obesity. **Iodine** is an essential micronutrient for normal thyroid function, and maternal iodine deficiency remains an important public-health problem worldwide, as a cause of **endemic cretinism**; it may also cause a major proportion of cases of mental retardation in the developing world. However, the major public health and sociopolitical problems that require remedies are the problems of deficiency of food energy, protein, and micronutrients in the developing world, and of excess elsewhere.

8.1 Malnutrition

Malnutrition was common in both urban and rural populations in Europe during the nineteenth and early twentieth century, particularly in children. Specific deficiency diseases such as rickets were very common, particularly in urban environments, and rickets was known as 'a disease of poverty and darkness'. Dairy products (milk, butter, eggs, etc.) were not generally available to the poor, and up to 75 per cent of poorer children showed some evidence of the disease in some large European cities. Nutritional science blossomed at the beginning of the twentieth century with the demonstration of the almost total absorbtion and energy balance of the primary nutrients (protein, carbohydrate, and fats) in humans by Atwater (1902), 🖥 and the gradual discovery of the vitamins, originally recognized by Hopkins (1912) 🖥 as 'accessory food factors'. This new knowledge led to new initiatives in public health and **nutritional surveillance** to monitor the changes in the level of attainment of full, healthy growth potential in childhood, as it was increasingly recognized that inadequate growth in children was related to susceptibility to frequently fatal infectious diseases such as tuberculosis, diphtheria, whooping cough, measles, and influenzal or bacterial pneumonia, which accounted for much of infant and childhood mortality at that time. **Growth standards** in childhood were developed; in Glasgow the average height of 13-year-old Glasgow schoolchildren increased by 4.5 inches (11.43 cm) between 1915 and 1959 and a further 8–10 cm by the early 1990s. Nutrition in childhood in Europe and in industrialized countries in general has become adequate for almost all, but unfortunately excessive for some, partly because of an increasing cultural tendency towards sedentary activities such as watching television or playing computer games, and also to widespread availability of high-calorie fast foods. It is instructive to inquire of our grandparents their daily way of life, now termed **lifestyle**, to discover how radically this has changed during the past 50 years.

For large parts of the less affluent world, malnutrition is a crippling reality and a major drain on human development. **Marasmus** (Greek: wasting) is hard to misdiagnose but milder forms of **protein–calorie malnutrition** can have major developmental and health consequences in children. **Kwashiorkor** (originally a local name in Ghana), another form of protein–calorie malnutrition, presents without gross wasting when carbohydrate intakes are sufficient to maintain insulin secretion (averting the need for gluconeogenesis from body protein), but is also life-threatening if untreated. Several **reference standards** have been devised for children, which relate to **achieved weight or height for a given age**, although some indices have standardized for height, which is done for adults. In children, skeletal vertical growth varies at different ages; periods of accelerated growth, even in younger children, and the problem of stunting (reduced height but normal body shape) make a universal index difficult

---

BOX 8.1 ASSESSMENT OF MALNUTRITION: COMMONLY USED INDICES

	Per cent reference[1] population	No oedema	Oedema
Weight for age[2]	60–79	Under-nourished	Kwashiorkor
	<60	Marasmus	Marasmic kwashiorkor
Mid-upper arm circumference[3] (cm)	>14	Normal	
	12.5–14.0	Suboptimal nutrition	
	<12.5	Definite malnutrition	

[1]National Child Health Surveys (USA) are preferred reference population (National Centre for Health Statistics 1987).
[2]Height for age and weight for height have also been used as common indices.
[3]Constant between ages of 1–5 years, but can also be used on older age groups of children against reference standards.
Sources: Truswell (1999); Golden and Golden (2000).
Truswell, A. S. (1999). *ABC of Nutrition* (3rd edn). London: BMJ Books.
Golden, M. H. N. and Golden, B. E. (2000). 'Severe Malnutrition', in J. S. Garrow, W. P. T. James and A. Ralph (eds.), *Human Nutrition and Dietetics* (10th edn). Edinburgh: Churchill Livingstone.

---

to achieve; however, Box 8.1 shows two commonly used childhood indices to assess significant malnutrition.

Mid-arm circumference is particularly simple to use under field and famine conditions in young children as no scales are needed, and it is normally constant (greater than 13.5 cm) between one and five years of age. This has the advantage that simple tape-measures marked appropriately in colour can be produced in bulk and are easy to use by front-line staff. Adults can also be malnourished and here **Quetelet's index** (weight (kg) ÷ height[2] (m)) has become universally used as a standard index for assessing under- and overweight in both men and women. Unless otherwise stated, the term '**body mass index**' (BMI) usually refers to this definition, although other indices have also been used by some investigators (see Box 8.2).

In 1992 the United Nations World Declaration on Nutrition reported 20 per cent of the population of developing countries were malnourished in terms of energy and growth requirements, and 2000 million people (about 60 per cent of the developing population), mainly children and women, had deficiencies in one or more micronutrients. These levels of malnutrition have been recently reported to have declined only slightly, and a World Health Organization (WHO) Global Database on child growth and malnutrition has now been established (de Onis and Blossner 2003). ⌨ These statistics relate to **endemic malnutrition** rather than epidemic malnutrition induced by famine conditions, often precipitated by

social disruption such as civil war. Endemic malnutrition is associated with reduced immune response and resistance to infection, particularly in infants and young children; countries in which endemic malnutrition is common experience high infant and child mortality, particularly from respiratory and gastro-intestinal infections. Malnutrition particularly affects the cellular immune system, T-cell counts can be reduced and phagocytosis is impaired. Nevertheless, immunization programmes in developing countries, supported by the WHO, have had a major impact on the infant and childhood mortality, and should be developed in parallel with programmes designed to improve the nutritional status of infants and children.

8.2 Eating Disorders

Anorexia nervosa is a behavioural disorder mainly of teenage girls and young women in affluent societies, usually in better-off families with a prevalence of about 0.7 per cent. In anorexia there is usually a disturbance of the body image (the patient believes she looks fat), the body mass index is maintained at less than 17.5 kg/m[2] (normal 20–25), and commonly there is amenorrhoea and inadequate intake of protein and micronutrients.

Bulimia nervosa is a related condition in which there are recurrent episodes of binge eating, often in private, weight fluctuations, and frequently self-induced vomiting and purging. Usually there is the psychological problem of denial of the condition or the pattern of eating. The combined prevalence of bulimia and anorexia nervosa is about 2–3 per cent in women aged 15–35 years. The natural history and prognosis of the conditions imply that many patients eventually improve, although established anorexia is reported to have a relatively high risk of eventual death due to medical complications or suicide. A review of outcome studies based on clinic attenders for anorexia nervosa among a total patient population of 5334 indicated that 5 per cent died, 47 per cent recovered, 34 per cent improved, and 21 per cent remained chronically ill. In community studies, standardized questionnaires such as the Eating Attitude Test (EAT) and (SCOFF: Sick, Control, One (stone), Fat, Food) have been examined as potential screening tools. A series of case–control community studies has investigated risk factors for anorexia nervosa and bulimia nervosa (Fairburn and Harrison 2003), 💻 but population-based cohort studies are lacking. A summary of the descriptive epidemiology of eating disorders is shown below (Table 8.1).

8.3 Overweight and Obesity

In some ancient cultures being fat carried with it the mark of wealth and high social status, but in most modern cultures the converse is the case; in addition overweight and obesity carry a considerable health burden. As noted by Garrow (2000), 💻 obesity is the most important 'nutritional' disease in industrialized countries and in many parts of the developing world; it is a major risk factor for cardiovascular disease, maturity-onset diabetes mellitus (also known as non-insulin-dependent diabetes mellitus (NIDDM) or type 2

diabetes), some cancers, and several other major chronic diseases. As noted earlier, Quetelet's index (weight/height^2 (kg/m^2)) has been almost universally adopted as a standard measure of relative weight for men, women, and more recently for children. This provides a proxy measure of the amount of body fat. Technically precise, accurate methods, 'gold' standards, have been used to validate this simple measurement, and these and other proxy indices are shown in Box 8.2.

Assessment

As in the case of all continuously distributed variables, the cut-point at which the balance shifts to a significant future health risk in an individual has to be defined with a degree of precision from epidemiological studies; typically these are prospective studies with health outcome data. Such studies have placed at least 30 kg/m^2 as a suitable cut-point for a definition of **obesity** at which there is clearly increased health risk to an individual, if not currently, then in the short- to middle term (5–20 years), and in the longer term in young adults (20 years +) (Fontaine *et al.* 2003). 💻 The WHO has also adopted the standard definition of overweight as 25–29 kg/m^2 in adults, although the level of evidence is not as substantial as that for obesity. And, although there is a positive linear relation between body mass index and cardiovascular mortality in prospective studies, the relation is U-shaped for all-cause mortality (see Figure 8.1).

The Nurses Health Study report was based on over 100 000 mainly white American nurses aged 30–55 years followed for 16 years. Most studies examining the relation between body mass and mortality show this pattern.

TABLE 8.1	Epidemiology of eating disorders	
	Anorexia nervosa	**Bulimia nervosa**
Worldwide distribution	Predominantly Western societies	Predominantly Western societies
Ethnic origin	Mainly White people	Mainly White people
Sex	Most female (about 90%)	Most female (uncertain proportion)
Age	Adolescents (some young adults)	Young adults (some adolescents)
Social class	Possible excess in higher social class	Even distribution
Prevalence	0.7% (in teenage girls)	1–2% (in 16–35 year old females)
Incidence (per 100 000 per year)	19 in females, 2 in males	29 in females, 1 in males
Secular change	Possible increase	Likely increase

Source: Fairburn, C. G. and Harrison, P. J. 'Eating Disorders'. *The Lancet*, **361**: 407–16.

BOX 8.2 MEASUREMENT OF BODY FAT

Gold standards	Comment
Measurement of total body water, total potassium and body density using underwater weighing and isotopic measures	Technically demanding, used for research purposes only in specialized laboratories
Proxy measures	
Overall body fat	
Quetelet's index (weight/height^2) (kg/m^2)	Best overall index for men and women
Ponderal index (weight/height^3) (kg/m^3)	Differs for men and women
Weight/height (kg/m)	Estimates better for women
Skinfold thickness at various sites (mm)	Requires careful standardization and training
Bioimpedence (electrical conductance through body tissues)	Widely used but lacking universal standardization
Central obesity	
Waist/hip ratio	Differs for men and women
Waist circumference (cm)	Little epidemiological information
Abdominal/subscapular skinfold (mm)	As above (overall body fat)

Source: Garrow, J. S. (2000) 'Composition of the Body' in J. S. Garrow, W. P. T. James and A. Ralph (eds.), *Human Nutrition and Dietetics* (10th edn). Edinburgh: Churchill Livingstone.

Q1(a) What is the most likely explanation for the pattern of risk shown in Fig. 8.1?

Q1(b) How could you check this explanation?

Q1(c) Why is the relation different in non-smokers?

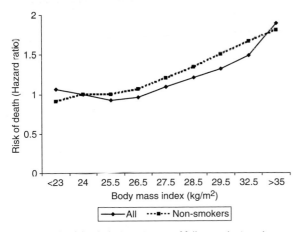

Fig. 8.1 Risk of death during 16 years of follow-up in American nurses by category of body mass (relative to lowest risk category). Source: Data from Allison, D. B., Fontaine, K. R., Manson, J. E., Stevens, J. and VanItallie, T. B. (1999). 'Annual Deaths Attributable to Obesity in the United States'. *Journal of the American Medical Association,* **282:** 1530–8.

Accurate measurement and assessment in populations is particularly important to monitor the steep rise in the prevalence of overweight and obesity. This has been described as pandemic in the USA, where two out of three adults are overweight or obese compared with one in four in the 1960s (Manson and Bassuk 2003). 🖥 These authors also suggest that obesity will soon overtake smoking as the primary preventable cause of death should the current rise in obesity continue. European countries show similar trends, but with slightly lower levels of overweight and obesity. In a recent Department of Health survey for England (2002), 🖥 the prevalence of overweight and obesity was: 68 per cent in men and 57 per cent in women; for obesity alone it was 24 per cent in women and 21 per cent in men.

Assessment and trends in children

In childhood, because vertical growth is accelerated at intervals, a fixed cut-point suitable for all ages cannot be used. Cole *et al.* (2000) 🖥 have proposed international standards that correspond to the cut-points of overweight and obesity in adulthood for children of a specific age to the nearest 6 month interval. As for most population standards, these are gender-specific (Figure 8.2).

Until recently, suitable standards were unavailable to reliably monitor trends in childhood obesity, but

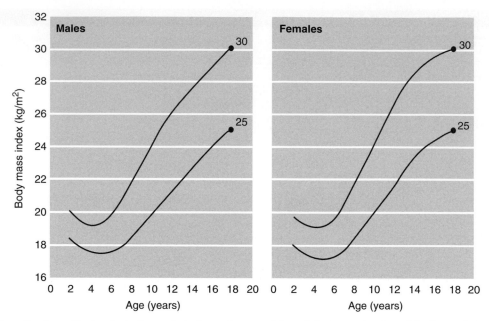

Fig. 8.2 International cut-off points for body mass index by sex for overweight and obesity, passing through body mass index 25 and 30 kg/m² (data from Brazil, Britain, Hong Kong, The Netherlands, Singapore, and USA).
Source: Cole, T. J., Bellizzi, M. C., Flegal, K. M., Dietz, W. H. (2000). 'Establishing a Standard Definition for Child Overweight and Obesity Worldwide: International Survey'. *British Medical Journal*, **320**: 1240–3, reproduced with permission from the BMJ Publishing Group.

available data suggest that this has doubled or tripled over 25 years in North America, Europe, and in developing countries such as Egypt (Ebbeling *et al.* 2002). 💻 Type 2 diabetes ('maturity onset' diabetes), one of the most significant complications of obesity, which is discussed in the following section, now accounts for 50 per cent of new cases of diabetes in adolescents in parts of North America, compared with almost no cases a generation previously. Although not all overweight or obese children **track** this into adulthood most do, which contributes further to the adult epidemic.

What are the complications of overweight and obesity?

Health consequences are related to the degree of excess weight, and this has been clearly demonstrated in epidemiological studies to be associated with the risk of hypertension, diabetes mellitus, and an overall increased risk of cardiovascular disease in general. These data are largely from observational studies, but a recent meta-analysis of intervention studies indicate that systolic blood pressure can be reduced by 10 mmHg for every 10 kg of weight loss irrespective of the initial body mass index (Neter *et al.* 2003). 💻 Perhaps underestimated, except by overweight or obese individuals, are the social consequences of obesity, which frequently result in prejudice in others, even in their family doctor, and may provide a psychological basis for the adolescent obsessions with body image in bulimia and anorexia nervosa. Many other clinical consequences of overweight and obesity are well established and are listed in Box 8.3.

What are the main causes of overweight and obesity, and are these preventable?

In the early 1900s Atwater showed that humans absorb, metabolize, and store over 90 per cent of food energy nutrients: protein, carbohydrate, fat, and alcohol. The law of conservation of energy applies, and 1 g protein and carbohydrate each contribute four calories of food energy, 1 g alcohol contributes seven calories, and 1 g of fat contributes nine calories. Animals and humans can survive without carbohydrate and alcohol in their diet (non-essential nutrients) but protein, fat, and a very long list of micronutrients are essential to life. Recommended nutrient intakes (RNIs) have been

BOX 8.3 COMPLICATIONS OF OVERWEIGHT AND OBESITY

Mortality	Life expectancy
Overweight	Reduced 3.1 years in men/ 3.3 years in women
Obese	Reduced 6.7 years in men/ 7.1 years in women

Morbidity	
Cardiovascular diseases	(Coronary disease, stroke, congestive heart failure, hypertension)
Metabolic diseases	Type 2 diabetes, 'insulin resistance syndrome'
Cancers	Colorectal, endometrial, post-menopausal breast cancer
Reproductive health	In women: infertility, menstrual disorders, gestational diabetes, birth problems
Mental health	Depression, social isolation

BOX 8.4 ENERGY REQUIREMENTS/ EXPENDITURE BY OCCUPATION AND IN DIFFERENT LEISURE ACTIVITIES

Men	MJ/day[1]	Range	
		Min	Max
Occupation[2]			
Elderly retired	9.7	7.3	11.8
Office workers	10.5	7.6	13.7
University students	12.3	9.4	18.5
Forestry workers	15.4	12.0	19.2
Activity	MJ/hour		
Sleeping	0.25		
Brisk walking	0.57		
Badminton	1.00		
Squash	1.71		

Women		Range	
		Min	Max
Occupation[2]			
Elderly retired	8.3	6.5	10.1
Laboratory technician	8.9	5.6	10.6
University students	9.6	5.8	10.5
Bakery workers	10.5	8.2	14.2
Activity	MJ/hour		
Sleeping	0.22		
Brisk walking	0.50		
Badminton	0.88		
Squash	1.50		

[1]1 Megajoule = 239 kcal.
[2]Occupational activity assessed 1950–65.
Source: Davidson, S., Passmore, R., Brock, J. F. and Truswell, A. S. (1979). *Human Nutrition and Dietetics* (7th edn). Edinburgh: Churchill Livingstone.

published for these micronutrients. Surveys conducted in the UK suggest that most of the population, both adults and children, have an adequate intake of essential micronutrients. In affluent countries and among the better-off in developing countries, a wide choice of foods is available, including **energy-dense foods** high in calories. Conversely the need for physical activity and energy expenditure has declined rapidly in industrialized and urbanized societies. A recent cohort study conducted in US children over a 10 year period reported that the decline in physical activity during adolescence was more closely associated with the development of overweight and obesity than were changes in energy intake (Kimm *et al.* 2005). ▢ Typical energy intakes and expenditures at different levels of physical activity, nowadays mainly during leisure, and in different occupations are shown in Box 8.4. Labourers in poorer countries, however, work long hours and have high energy expenditure. In times of civil disturbance or war, negative energy balance is common.

Environmental causes of overweight and obesity have been reviewed by Ebbeling *et al.* (2002) ▢ who note that many factors conspire to promote energy intake and limit physical activity, particularly in children. They estimate that excess calorie consumption of only 120 kcal per day (one sugar-sweetened soft drink) would produce a 50 kg increase in body weight over 10 years. A double cheeseburger, French fries, soft drink, and dessert may contain 2200 kcal and is unlikely to be the only meal of the day. Foods with a high proportion of refined carbohydrate – breads, many breakfast cereals, potatoes, soft drinks, cakes, and biscuits – cause a large post-prandial insulin response. Foods such as those with a high 'glycaemic index' (the level of insulin response) have been linked with the development of type 2 diabetes in prospective studies.

Psychosocial and family factors clearly play a role in childhood and adult obesity. Television viewing and solitary playing of computer games are linked with inappropriate snacking and parental neglect; these and other adversities are associated with the risk of early overweight (Ebbeling *et al.* 2002). 🖳 In adults, a recent report from the Nurses' Health Study (50 000 nurses, non-obese and non-diabetic at baseline followed up for six years) indicated that a sedentary lifestyle and high television viewing hours were closely related to the development of both obesity and diabetes mellitus. They estimated that 30 per cent (95% CI, 24–36 per cent) of new cases of obesity and 43 per cent (95% CI, 32–52 per cent) cases of diabetes could be prevented by the adoption of a relatively active lifestyle (less than 10 hours per week television watching and at least 30 minutes of brisk walking per day). This cohort study was observational rather than interventional, but interventional studies in children (largely school-based), which have used single or multiple interventions on physical activity or on diet have shown some positive results. Twin studies suggest that obesity is partly genetic in origin but, with the exception of very rare genetic disorders, the usual mode of inheritance appears to be polygenic (see Chapter 18).

Prevention or limiting the size of the epidemic of overweight and obesity has become an international concern of the WHO, which has established the International Obesity Task Force to devise strategies for public-health programmes. Implementation of these programmes may take considerable international effort and political will, such as that finally being attempted in tobacco control, some 40 years on from establishing the link between cigarette smoking and major chronic diseases (see Chapter 7).

8.4 Diabetes Mellitus

This disorder is the result of failure of insulin to regulate blood glucose levels after meals and, particularly in its acute form, is characterized by excess urine production (polyuria) and the presence of glucose in the urine (glycosuria). Hyperglycaemia (high blood glucose) is diagnostic of diabetes mellitus and this metabolic defect appears to be the main factor in producing the serious **microvascular**, and possibly also the **macrovascular**, complications of diabetes. There are two distinct types: **insulin-dependent diabetes mellitus** (IDDM) or **type I** in which there is failure of production of insulin owing to progressive destruction of the β-cells of the islets of Langerhans in the pancreas. This is considered by many to be an autoimmune inflammatory disorder, and islet cell antibodies can be detected in blood. In **non-insulin-dependent diabetes mellitus** (NIDDM) or **type 2** there is progressive

metabolic resistance to the effects of insulin which can also progress to insulin deficiency, but without islet cell antibodies. Type I commonly occurs in childhood, but can occur at any age although there is no increase in incidence with age in adults. Type 2 accounts for most (about 75 per cent) cases of diabetes, shows a steeply rising trend with age, and is closely associated with obesity. Owing to the rapid rise in the prevalence of obesity in some populations, particularly in North America, type 2 diabetes now accounts for about half of the newly diagnosed cases of diabetes in children and adolescents.

Insulin-dependent diabetes mellitus

The epidemiology of IDDM is most accurately studied in countries with advanced health-care systems and specially created disease registers for children. Data for adults are less widely available as type 2 diabetics may also progress to insulin dependence; prevalence and incidence data are therefore likely to be more accurate in childhood registries. It has been estimated that 10–15 per cent of childhood cases present as diabetic ketoacidotic coma, although fewer than 1 per cent die at the time of diagnosis.

IDDM is a relatively common major chronic disease of childhood with an overall prevalence of 0.25 per cent (one case per 400 children aged 0–14 years), and in UK registries a standardized incidence rate of 16.4 new cases per 100 000 person years (95% CI, 15.6–17.3) has been reported. In Europe the standardized incidence rate varies 10-fold between countries and is rising in most of these at the rate of 3.2 per cent per annum (95% CI, 2.7–3.7 per cent) (Green and Patterson 2001). 🖳 Reasons for the major differences in incidence between countries and the north–south gradient within Europe are poorly understood. There is a seasonal pattern coinciding with an increase in autumn and winter infections in children, but studies on viral aetiology have proved inconclusive. About 90 per cent of cases occur in children from families without a family history of IDDM, and studies investigating risk markers such as lack of breast feeding and socioeconomic conditions have proved inconclusive to date. Although the obscure aetiology does not currently provide opportunities for primary prevention, secondary prevention and, at the least, delay in the appearance of complications, appears to be achievable in many cases by maintenance of tight glycaemic control.

Non-insulin-dependent diabetes mellitus

This type of diabetes mellitus is more insidious in onset than IDDM and frequently presents asymptomatically on routine urine or blood testing. Blood sugar levels, taken after an overnight fast, of 7.8 mmol/l and above were formerly used by the WHO as an internationally agreed cut-point for the diagnosis of NIDDM, but the American Diabetic Association recently proposed a cut-point of 7.0 mmol/l (Expert Committee on the Diagnosis and Classification of Diabetes Mellitus 1997). 🖳 This cut-point has not been formally agreed in Europe, although prospective studies support the American proposal. Such problems contribute to the difficulty of accurately defining the prevalence of this disorder, which results in similar microvascular and macrovascular disease to that arising from IDDM.

Since the disease is defined by asymptomatic glycaemia it may be present for some years in many individuals before detection; such individuals are therefore at high risk of early development of complications. Thus there is a strong case for screening for diabetes, particularly in high-risk individuals, which is frequently done opportunistically in the UK using a paper strip dipped in urine (glycosuria test). Screening tests were recently discussed by the American Diabetes Association, which recommends fasting plasma glucose as a first-line screening test used opportunistically, based on the current level of evidence from screening intervention studies (American Diabetes Association 2004) 🖳 (see also Chapter 5).

Prevalence and incidence

The overall prevalence in the British population is about 5 per cent in men and 7 per cent in women. There is a steep rise with age (about 1 per cent in 20–44 year olds rising to up to 20 per cent in 65–74 year olds), which probably accounts for the higher overall prevalence in women who form a greater part of the elderly population. The incidence among middle-aged men is about 2 per 1000 person–years (Perry *et al.* 1995), 🖳 but in this cohort study the incidence was increased 11-fold in the top fifth of the distribution of body mass index. Clearly the pandemic of overweight and obesity in both the advanced industrialized countries and in some developing countries is set to cause a major increase in the worldwide prevalence of NIDDM (an estimated doubling in prevalence from 1994 to 2010) (Zimmet *et al.* 2001). 🖳 A pre-diabetic state categorized as the **metabolic** or **insulin resistance syndrome** has been proposed by the WHO and other bodies, but its clinical and epidemiological validity seem questionable.

In the UK, ethnic Indians from the Indian subcontinent show a large excess prevalence of NIDDM not accounted for by overweight or obesity alone; and in North America the prevalence of diabetes in Pima Indians is about 40 per cent in adults. Twin studies indicate a significant genetic contribution. Similar findings in minority populations in other parts of the world are likely to be due to the combined effects of a genetic predisposition and change in the diet and lifestyle of such populations (gene–environment interaction), although the rapidly increasing trend in incidence of both types of diabetes points to environmental causes as the major factor.

Prevention and control of complications of diabetes

The complications of diabetes are broadly classified into **microvascular** and **macrovascular**. Microvascular changes are at the capillary level and can cause significant renal damage and failure (**nephropathy**), retinal damage and blindness (**retinopathy**), and sensory impairment, particularly to the lower limbs (**peripheral neuropathy**) The latter is closely associated with vascular impairment and diabetic gangrene. Macrovascular complications are those of increased risk of cardiovascular diseases, which can be explained only in part by elevations in well-established risk factors. Both IDDM and NIDDM are associated with premature mortality and risk of complications in the medium to long term.

Two recent major trials demonstrated the importance of careful control of hyperglycaemia (the major risk factor for microvascular complications) by randomizing diabetics to intensive and normal control regimes. The development of complications was significantly reduced in those patients randomized to the intensive treatment group. These results have major implications for the treatment of both IDDM and NIDDM. The trial in patients with IDDM is illustrated below.

One thousand four hundred and forty-one patients (mean age 27 years) with IDDM, 726 with no retinopathy at baseline (primary prevention cohort), and 715 with mild retinopathy (secondary prevention cohort) were randomly assigned to intensive therapy (insulin pump or three or more daily insulin injections) or conventional therapy with one or two daily insulin injections. Patients were followed for an average of 6.5 years, and the appearance and progression of retinopathy and other complications of diabetes were assessed at intervals by 'blinded' observers. Results were calculated per 100 person-years of follow-up but are summarized graphically in Figure 8.3 as the percentage of patients developing significant complications: retinopathy (left panel) and nephropathy (right panel) according to the mode of treatment.

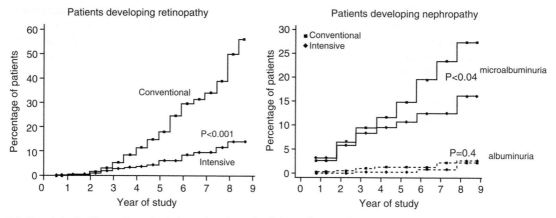

Fig. 8.3 Cumulative incidence of sustained change in retinopathy (left panel) assessed by six-monthly fundus photography and of nephropathy (right panel) defined by development of albuminuria or microalbuminuria in patients with type 1 diabetes receiving intensive or conventional therapy for diabetes mellitus.
Source: Data from Diabetes Control and Complications Trial Research Group (1993). 'The Effect of Intensive Treatment of Diabetes on the Development and Progression of Long-Term Complications in Insulin-Dependent Diabetes Mellitus'. *New England Journal of Medicine*, **329**: 977–86.

Q2(a) The results indicate significant reductions in the development of complications in young diabetics for intensive insulin treatment rather than conventional treatment. What is likely to be the main side effect of intensive insulin treatment and how would you evaluate its impact?

Q2(b) Why would it be important to 'blind' the observers who examined patients for complications of diabetes to the treatment regime?

Q2(c) In a multi-centre trial what pre-requisites are required for clinical and quantitative outcome measures?

Q2(d) Why might the comparison of albuminuria rates between treatments not have attained significance although the comparison of microalbuminuria rates did attain significance?

Q2(e) What other parameters should be evaluated following the results of this major trial?

Such studies have led to the development in the UK of National (Health) Service Frameworks for the prevention and treatment of major chronic diseases such as diabetes, which provide guidance and clinical standards to specialist physicians, primary care trusts, and other health-care workers involved in the prevention and treatment of these conditions. National Service Frameworks for coronary heart disease (CHD), the elderly, and for diabetes have been produced so far (see also Chapter 20). However, for the primary prevention of NIDDM, intervention studies combining weight loss with increased exercise have shown encouraging results (Tuomilehto *et al.* 2001).

8.5 Endocrine Disorders

Numerous endocrine disorders have been described clinically and are usually manifested by over-production or under-production of specific hormones. Examples are: hyperpituitarism, which includes Cushing's syndrome (overproduction of adrenocorticotropic hormone (ACTH)) and acromegaly (overproduction of growth hormone); diabetes insipidus (deficiency of antidiuretic hormone (ADH)); and thyrotoxicosis (overproduction of thyroid hormone). None of these is as common worldwide, or as readily preventable, as deficiency of thyroid hormone, most commonly caused by lack of dietary iodine.

Iodine deficiency

Iodine is an essential constituent of the thyroid hormones thyroxine (T4) and tri-iodothyroine (T3). Iodine deficiency commonly causes enlargement of the thyroid gland (goitre), particularly in adolescent girls and in women. The consequences of maternal iodine deficiency can be severe for the foetus, leading to mental retardation and cretinism. Iodine deficiency is believed to be the most common preventable cause of mental defect at the world level, with some 1000 million people (20 per cent of the world's population) living in iodine-deficient regions. Many of these are in the developing world, but in many European countries iodine is added to salt as a preventive measure. In the UK, iodine may also get into the diet as a bi-product of the disinfection process in milk production.

Hypothyroidism is routinely screened at birth in most affluent countries, and occurs in approximately 1:10 000 births. However, it is usually due to an intrinsic hormonal deficit rather than to iodine deficiency.

Goitre is a sign of dietary iodine deficiency (or less commonly of the presence of goitrogens in the diet, which interfere with iodine absorbtion). In the 1990s some 200 million people worldwide were estimated to have goitre, which the WHO has classified into grade 1 (palpable goitre only) and grade 2 (visible goitre) to standardize definitions used in epidemiological surveys. Confirmation of iodine deficiency can also be made in field surveys by measuring urinary iodine. This is conserved by the kidneys in iodine-deficient areas with the result that little iodine is excreted in the urine. In such populations, which are often remote, most mothers have goitre and 1–5 per cent of babies are born with cretinism.

Cretinism is a syndrome with a variable presentation. It comprises two or more of the following conditions: mental deficiency, deaf-mutism, ataxia, squint, dwarfism, and spasticity. In epidemiological surveys, deaf-mutism is the most readily measured disorder, and this is likely to apply also to routine birth registers in advanced industrialized countries.

Prevention and control

It was in Switzerland in the late nineteenth century that the link between endemic goitre and cretinism was first made in extensive epidemiological surveys.

Switzerland had a major problem with both, and several trials were done in schoolchildren, which demonstrated that iodized salt or milk effectively shrunk goitres to a normal size. In 1922 the Swiss Goitre Commission recommended the use of salt with added potassium iodide on a voluntary basis and the distribution of additional weekly iodine tablets to schoolchildren. The public-health situation was monitored closely during the next 40 years, and the prevalence of goitre and cretinism was reduced 10-fold.

In the 1990s a campaign to promote iodized salt in developing countries at risk of iodine deficiency was made by the WHO with UNICEF. It was estimated that the number of children born with cretinism has been halved in less than a decade since the programme began (Truswell 1999).

In more remote areas, iodinated oil in depot injections or iodine tablets are used. A double-blind controlled trial in fertile young women was performed by Pharoah *et al.* between 1966 and 1972 in the remote Jimi valley of the Papua New Guinea highlands. Endemic cretinism was known to be high in this region. In collaboration with the local administrators, a census of families in the district was made; alternate families were given either i.m. (intramuscular) iodized oil or saline. Women of child-bearing age were asked if they were pregnant. Follow-up surveys were done until children of mothers enrolled into this community study were between 10 and 16 years of age. The study results are shown in Figure 8.4. A follow-up of children born to these women was completed by 1982 (Pharoah and Connolly 1987).

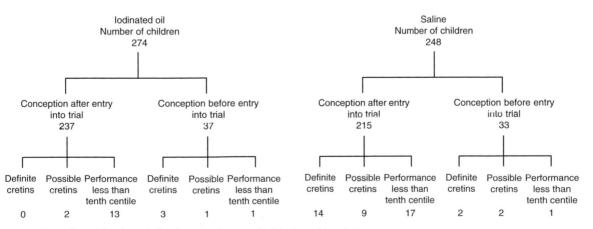

Fig. 8.4 Controlled trial of depot iodine injection (versus saline) in Papua New Guinea.
Source: Pharoah, P. O. D., and Connolly, K. J. (1987). 'A Controlled Trial of Iodinated Oil for the Prevention of Endemic Cretinism: A Long-Term Follow-Up'. *International Journal of Epidemiology*, **16**: 68–73.

Q3(a) Why was a double-blinded controlled trial the ideal choice of study design?

Q3(b) What other data would be helpful to provide an overall assessment of the effectiveness of this procedure?

Q3(c) This trial was performed in 1966 when few trials of this type had been carried out. Under what circumstances would it be ethical to perform similar trials to extend this work?

Model answers

Q1(a) On average, people who are ill, particularly those with terminal illness, tend to be lighter than average and hence experience a higher mortality than those who are not relatively undernourished.

Q1(b) It is usual to exclude deaths within the first 1–5 years of a follow-up study to reduce the possibility that the seriously ill individuals may be responsible for this or similar phenomena.

Q1(c) Tobacco smoking is associated with reduced appetite and smokers tend to be substantially lighter in weight than their non-smoking counterparts. Smokers are more likely to suffer from premature mortality and may contribute to the U-shape of the curve by causing increased mortality among lighter individuals. Smoking and body mass index are therefore set to interact with each other in their association with mortality. However, in non-smokers a dose–response relation is evident between increasing body mass index and mortality.

Q2(a) Intensive insulin treatment should produce a stabilization of the high glucose peaks likely to be experienced after food in conventionally treated young diabetics. The main side effect is hypoglycaemia, which can lead to disorientation and unconsciousness. The frequency of these episodes should be compared in those intensively treated and those treated under the conventional regimes.

Q2(b) Foreknowledge of the treatment given to the patient under examination may influence the observer's assessment of the clinical sign that is being observed.

Q2(c) Outcome measures should be carefully standardized to reduce the possibility of observer variation and to be as accurate and reproducible as possible to reduce random variation.

Q2(d) Albuminuria is much less frequent than microalbuminuria, which is a more sensitive test of renal function. Consequently, the power of the statistical analysis comparing the albuminuria end-point between treatments is lower. Possibly the test of the albuminuria end-point has produced a type II error (section 4.3), and in reality there is also a difference in the albuminuria end-point between treatments, but a much larger trial would be required to detect it.

Q2(e) An attempt should be made to measure peripheral neuropathy, which is the other main complication of diabetes. Significant episodes of hypoglycaemia should also be evaluated, hospital admissions, and in the longer term, mortality.

Q3(a) Rendering both the mother and the observer unaware of the treatment allocation should ensure an objective assessment of each infant's clinical status.

Q3(b) Mortality experience in the first year of life would also be a useful measure of the overall effectiveness of this procedure.

Q3(c) Because this trial provides good evidence that depot iodine considerably reduces the likelihood of cretinism provided that the iodine is given pre-conceptually, then it is unethical to repeat the experiment using a placebo. However, different doses of iodine or different modes of delivery could be tested in randomized controlled trials (RCTs) (a new treatment or mode of delivery is compared with the standard treatment).

Further Reading

Ferguson, A. and Griffin, G. E. (2000). 'Nutrition and the Immune System', in J. S. Garrow, W. P. T. James and A. Ralph (eds.), *Human Nutrition and Dietetics* (10th edn). Edinburgh: Churchill Livingstone.

Golden, M. H. N. and Golden, B. E. (2000). 'Severe Malnutrition', in J. S. Garrow, W. P. T. James and A. Ralph (eds.), *Human Nutrition and Dietetics* (10th edn). Edinburgh: Churchill Livingstone.

Krauss, R. M., Eckel, R. H., Howard, B. *et al.* (2000). 'AHA Dietary Guidelines. Revision 2000. A Statement for Healthcare Professionals from the Nutrition Committee of the American Heart Association'. *Circulation*, 102: 2284–99.

Truswell, A. S. (1999). *ABC of Nutrition* (3rd edn). London: BMJ Books.

Willett, W. (1998). *Nutritional Epidemiology* (2nd edn). New York, NY: Oxford University Press.

WHO Technical Report Series, No. 916 (2003). 'Diet, Nutrition and the Prevention of Chronic Diseases. Report of a Joint WHO/FAO Expert Consultation'. Geneva, Switzerland. http://www.who.int/hpr/NPH/docs/who_fao_expert_report.pdf.

Web Addresses

International Obesity Task Force, www.iotf.org.
Food Standards Agency, www.foodstandards.gov.uk.

References

References for this chapter can be found at www.oxfordtextbooks.co.uk/orc/yarnell/. 🖳

Digestive system

This chapter discusses the epidemiology of dyspepsia, which is one of the commonest gastro-intestinal problems presenting in primary care, the diseases associated with *Helicobacter pylori* infection, and the epidemiology of colorectal cancer, inflammatory bowel disease, and cirrhosis of the liver.

Introduction

It is beyond the scope of this textbook to discuss the epidemiology of all chronic gastro-intestinal diseases. Instead, several important topics have been chosen, which include dyspepsia, because of the substantial health costs associated with this group of symptoms and *Helicobacter pylori*. This is the most common bacterial infection known to man, and its association with diseases has only recently become known through epidemiological and clinical studies. The epidemiology of colorectal cancer, as the major alimentary cancer, soon to be incorporated into routine screening examinations in the UK, will be reviewed. The inflammatory bowel diseases ulcerative colitis and Crohn's disease are discussed as examples of disorders that are pathologically distinct, but sometimes difficult to distinguish clinically, and whose causes are largely unknown. Basic immunological, epidemiological, and genetic research will be required for progress to be made in the understanding, treatment, and prevention of these disorders. Finally, because of the medical and social importance of alcohol abuse, and of other causes of cirrhosis of the liver, its epidemiology is reviewed here.

9.1 Dyspepsia

The term 'dyspepsia' covers a variety of symptoms affecting the upper gastro-intestinal tract, which include

---

BOX 9.1 THE ROME I CLASSIFICATION OF DYSPEPSIA

Pain or discomfort centred in the upper abdomen. Discomfort may be characterized by postprandial fullness, early satiety, nausea, retching, vomiting, upper abdominal bloating. Patients with symptoms of heartburn and acid regurgitation are considered to be distinct from patients with dyspepsia.

Adapted from: Westbrook, J. L. *et al.* (2000). 'The Impact of Dyspepsia Definition on Prevalence Estimates: Considerations for Future Researchers'. *Scandinavian Journal of Gastroenterology*, **3**: 227–33.

BOX 9.2 UPPER GI SYMPTOMS INVESTIGATED IN DIGEST

Postprandial fullness, early satiety, localized epigastric pain, diffuse epigastric pain, heartburn, regurgitation, belching, nocturnal/fasting pain, abdominal distension.

Source: Stanghellini, V. (1999). 'Three-Month Prevalence Rates of Gastrointestinal Symptoms and the Influence of Demographic Factors: Results from the Domestic/International Gastroenterology Surveillance Study (DIGEST)'. *Scandinavian Journal of Gastroenterology, Supplement*, **231**: 20–8.

---

epigastric pain or discomfort, heartburn, acid regurgitation, excessive burping or belching, a feeling of slow digestion, early satiety, nausea, and bloating. Standardization of the definition of dyspepsia has proven very difficult, and although consensus definitions of dyspepsia are available, for example the Rome I criteria (Box 9.1), they have not been widely used in epidemiological studies.

Prevalence

A recent systematic review of population-based studies of dyspepsia in developed countries showed substantial variation in the reported prevalence of dyspeptic symptoms, ranging from 8 per cent to 54 per cent (Heading 1999). 🖳 This could reflect major differences in the occurrence of these symptoms, but probably results from the use of different definitions of dyspepsia, and the evaluation of the symptoms in differing age-groups or time periods. The utility of these data is therefore questionable, highlighting the importance in epidemiological research of using standardized, internationally agreed definitions of diseases, syndromes, or symptom complexes (see Chapter 2). The Domestic/International Gastroenterology Surveillance Study (DIGEST) (Stanghellini 1999) 🖳 examined the 3 month prevalence of upper gastro-intestinal symptoms (Box 9.2) in random population samples from 10 countries using, as far as possible, the same methods. Symptoms were considered clinically significant if they were moderate in intensity and occurred at least once a week. This study confirmed a high overall prevalence of these symptoms: 28.1 per cent of the subjects studied reported having symptoms in the 3 months before interview. However, symptom prevalence differed between the countries, ranging from 9.4 per cent in Japan to 41.8 per cent in the USA (see Figure 9.1) (Stanghellini 1999). 🖳 These country-specific differences in the prevalence of

dyspepsia are less likely to be artefactual than estimates from previous studies, although slight differences in methodology and response rates between countries may contribute to part of the differences seen. The incidence of dyspepsia is more difficult to assess as symptoms are relapsing and remittent in most subjects.

Risk factors

Women are approximately 50 per cent more likely to report dyspeptic symptoms than men, and dyspepsia prevalence increases slightly with age until 65 years. Smokers are more likely to have dyspeptic symptoms, especially heartburn and regurgitation, but alcohol consumption in moderate amounts does not appear to be a risk factor. Psychological factors play an important

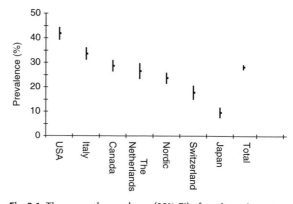

Fig. 9.1 Three month prevalence (95% CI) of moderate/severe upper GI symptoms among 5581 DIGEST respondents, by country or region.
Source: Stanghellini, V. (1999). 'Three-Month Prevalence Rates of Gastrointestinal Symptoms and The Influence of Demographic Factors: Results from the Domestic/International Gastroenterology Surveillance Study (DIGEST)'. *Scandinavian Journal of Gastroenterology, Supplement*, **231**: 20–8.

role both in reporting dyspeptic symptoms and seeking medical attention for these symptoms. Obese people are approximately three times more likely to suffer from heartburn and regurgitation (Murray *et al.* 2003) 🖳 but being overweight is less clearly related to other dyspeptic symptoms. A recent meta-analysis of randomized controlled trials has confirmed that users of non-steroidal anti-inflammatory drugs (NSAIDs) are three times more likely to experience dyspepsia than non-users. This risk is limited to the use of high doses of any NSAIDs or to any dose of indomethacin, meclofenamate, and piroxicam. The relation between infection with *H. pylori* and dyspepsia is discussed later in this chapter.

Time trends

The interpretation of trends in dyspepsia is difficult for reasons related to the problems of definition, and because of a paucity of population-based studies before the 1980s. It is clear though, that dyspeptic symptoms have been very common for many years in people living in developed countries. Indeed, Milk of Magnesia was invented as a treatment for dyspepsia by Sir James Murray in Belfast in 1812. However, it is unclear whether dyspeptic symptoms in general, or subgroups of symptoms, have become more common. The incidence of oesophageal adenocarcinoma has increased markedly in developed countries since the 1970s (Devesa *et al.* 1998). 🖳 Gastro oesophageal reflux is a risk factor for this cancer, and gastro-oesophageal reflux disease has been increasingly diagnosed in recent decades. Greater use of endoscopy has contributed to the trend in diagnosis of reflux oesophagitis, and data are not available to confirm whether this reflects an increase in heartburn and regurgitation in the general population.

Functional dyspepsia

The most common underlying conditions in patients presenting with dyspeptic symptoms in primary care are oesophagitis (15 per cent), gastric (4 per cent) or duodenal (9 per cent) ulceration, gallstone disease (2 per cent), and malignancy (2 per cent). However, more than 50 per cent of patients have no underlying pathology and are considered to have functional dyspepsia. This proportion may vary between countries, and increase over time as the incidence of pathology associated with *H. pylori* (peptic ulceration and gastric cancer) decreases. Prospective studies following patients with functional dyspepsia show that the symptoms improve or remit in 30–70 per cent of cases. Patients who have had symptoms for more than two years, have lower educational attainment or higher psychological

vulnerability scores, or are infected with *H. pylori*, are less likely to experience remission of symptoms.

Costs associated with dyspepsia

Although only one in four patients with dyspepsia consults a physician, dyspepsia accounts for 3–4 per cent of general practitioner consultations and between 20 per cent and 40 per cent of all gastro-intestinal consultations. Symptom severity, fear of serious disease, and family history of gastro-intestinal malignancy influence the decision to consult a medical practitioner, but psychosocial factors such as anxiety, depression, and lack of family/social support are also important. The costs of prescribing for dyspepsia are high and account for over 15 per cent of all prescribing costs to general practice. Medication costs form only part of the National Health Service (NHS) costs of dyspepsia and, because so many patients manage dyspepsia without medical intervention, the true cost of dyspepsia to the community is much greater. The non-NHS costs of dyspepsia (over-the-counter treatments and time off work) have been estimated at £21 per person per year in the UK, totalling in excess of £1 billion, with the total NHS costs (consultations, investigations, and medication) estimated at £500 million.

9.2 *Helicobacter Pylori*

H. pylori is a Gram-negative spiral bacterium that infects human gastric mucosa. Approximately 50 per cent of the world's population are infected by *H. pylori*, making it the commonest chronic infection worldwide. However, infection rates vary substantially according to geographic region, age, and birth cohort. In developing countries, *H. pylori* is largely acquired in childhood and is almost universally present in adults. By contrast, the rate of childhood acquisition is much lower in developed countries and increases gradually by approximately 1 per cent per year into adulthood (Figure 9.2) (Pounder and Ng 1995). 🖳 The prevalence of infection declines with subsequent birth cohorts; in a study of sera collected in the UK in 1969, 1979, and 1989, the odds of being *H. pylori* seropositive decreased by 26 per cent per decade. This marked decline in the acquisition of *H. pylori* in recent decades in developed countries can probably be attributed to improved sanitation and living conditions (for example less overcrowding), which reduces the risk of infection during childhood.

Aetiology/risk factors

H. pylori infection is believed to be spread from human to human by the faeco-oral route, and in developing

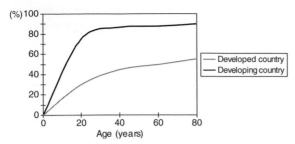

Fig. 9.2 Prevalence of *Helicobacter pylori* infection according to age of population in developed and developing countries. Source: Data from Pounder, R. E. and Ng, D. (1995). 'The Prevalence of *Helicobacter Pylori* Infection in Different Countries'. *Alimentary Pharmacology and Therapeutics,* **9**: 33–9.

countries spread may also be by contaminated water. The prevalence of infection increases with age but this mainly reflects a declining prevalence with successive birth cohorts (the birth cohort effect). There is no clear sex difference in the prevalence of infection. In the USA, Hispanics and African-Americans are three to four times more likely to be infected than Whites. Low socioeconomic status and poor living conditions during childhood are the most important risk factors for infection (Go 2002). 💻

Clinical significance

Although it had been known for more than 100 years that spiral organisms existed in the human stomach, their importance only became apparent in the early 1980s through the pioneering work of Warren and Marshall. (Marshall and Warren 1984). 💻 Not only were they able to identify and culture the organism, Marshall also ingested the organism, giving himself acute gastroenteritis. At gastroscopy, gastritis was seen and the organism was re-isolated from biopsies of his stomach. This experiment fulfilled Koch's postulates (see Chapter 1) indicating that *H. pylori* causes acute gastritis, and also recaptured the pioneer spirit of John Hunter, who had infected himself clinically with pus from a patient with gonorrhoea in the eighteenth century (Chapter 1). It has since been shown that infection with the organism causes chronic gastritis that may progress to gastric atrophy.

Duodenal and gastric ulceration

There is strong evidence that infection with *H. pylori* is an important causative agent in peptic ulceration that is unrelated to the use of aspirin or NSAIDs. *H. pylori* infection can be diagnosed in 90–100 per cent of

patients with duodenal ulcers and in 60–100 per cent of patients with gastric ulcers; infected individuals have an estimated lifetime risk of 10–20 per cent for the development of peptic ulcer disease, which is at least three- to fourfold higher than in uninfected subjects. Nested case–control studies have confirmed that infection precedes ulceration. In an Hawaiian study, individuals who were seropositive in blood samples collected during the 1960s were four times more likely to develop a duodenal ulcer over the next 20 years than subjects who were seronegative. Experimental studies have also shown that *H. pylori* eradication cures peptic ulceration (not caused by NSAIDs) and prevents its recurrence. Clearly, many people with *H. pylori* infection do not develop peptic ulceration, and, although it may be a '**necessary**' cause, it is not a '**sufficient**' cause (see Chapter 1) for ulceration, in common with most environmental risk factors for chronic diseases. Other factors such as genetic susceptibility or environmental/lifestyle factors, such as smoking, interact with *H. pylori* infection to cause peptic ulceration.

H. pylori is also an important risk factor for gastric adenocarcinoma (Helicobacter and Cancer Collaborative Group 2001) 💻 and gastric lymphoma. Paradoxically, it has been associated with a reduced risk of oesophageal adenocarcinoma.

> **Q1** Suggest possible study methods that could be used to investigate the relationship between *H. pylori* infection and gastric cancer. Discuss the strengths and weaknesses of the various options.

H. pylori and dyspepsia

For several reasons, it has proven difficult to determine whether there is a causal link between dyspepsia and infection with *H. pylori*. In addition to the definition and measurement problems associated with dyspepsia discussed previously, dyspepsia and *H. pylori* infection are both common and, therefore, frequently co-exist in the same person. Also, some patients with dyspepsia have peptic ulceration that is caused by *H. pylori* and is responsive to eradication of the organism. Studies designed to compare the benefit of *H. pylori* eradication against therapy with acid suppression alone for dyspepsia are the most robust studies examining this issue. Results from these studies are conflicting, but a recent meta-analysis concluded that there may be some benefit in testing for, and treating, *H. pylori* in dyspeptic patients (see Moayyedi *et al.* 2003). 💻 The authors of the meta-analysis calculated that the **number needed to treat** to cure one patient of dyspepsia was 15. This has to be balanced against the costs of the treatment and the disadvantages of widespread use of antibiotics in *H. pylori* eradication regimes, given that both dyspepsia and *H. pylori* are common.

9.3 Colorectal Cancer

Incidence/prevalence

Excluding non-melanoma skin cancer (see Chapter 15), colorectal cancer is the third most common cancer in men and the second most common cancer in women in the UK. In the year 2000, 18 700 UK men and 15 900 UK women developed this cancer, giving an incidence of 65.2 and 52.7 per 100 000, respectively. Colorectal cancer has a high fatality rate with 1-year and 5-year survival rates of approximately 70 per cent and 50 per cent, respectively. In the year 2000, 8500 men and 7700 women died from colorectal cancer in the UK, making it the second most common cause of death from cancer. Colorectal cancer has the highest incidence among pathological conditions of the large intestine other than diverticular disease (Table 9.1), and despite moderately high mortality rates, the prevalence of treated disease is high in the population. The incidence of colorectal cancer is almost 50 per cent higher in men than women. Incidence in both sexes increases with age, most markedly after 50 years (Figure 9.3).

Time trends and geographic distribution

The incidence of colorectal cancer in the UK has risen steadily in the past 30 years, more so in men than women. Between 1971 and 1997 the incidence in England and Wales increased by 20 per cent in men and by 5 per cent in women, while mortality fell by 24 per cent and 37 per cent, respectively, over the same period (Hayne *et al.* 2001). 🖥 Similar patterns have been seen in many developed populations, although the extent and timing of the increases in incidence vary between countries. The reasons for this are not fully understood although they may, in part, result from better detection of the cancer, for example after the introduction of colonoscopy. The difference in trends between the sexes is also ill-understood, although smoking may contribute to the sex difference.

There is a 10- to 20-fold variation in the incidence of colorectal cancer across the world. The highest rates are seen in North America, Western Europe, Oceania, and Japan (age standardized (world) incidence rates of 30–60 in men and 15–40 in women per 100 000), whereas

TABLE 9.1 Annual UK incidence, mortality, and prevalence (age-standardized per million population) of diseases of the large intestine

Disease	Incidence (per year)	Mortality (per year)	Prevalence
Colorectal cancer	588	276	1900[1]
Crohn's disease	83[2]	3.1	1448[2]
Ulcerative colitis	139[1]	3.5	2434[2]
Diverticular disease	282[3]	26	—

Mortality data are from the ONS (2001).

[1] from Hayne *et al.* (2001), estimate for 1993.

[2] from Rubin *et al.* (2000), estimates are for 1993.

[3] from Kang *et al.* (2003), based on hospital admission rates.

Office for National Statistics (2001). 'Mortality Statistics – Cause. Review of the Registrar General on Deaths by Cause, Sex and Age, in England and Wales, 2000'. Mortality Data Series DH2 No. 27. London: ONS.

Hayne, D., Brown, R. S., McCormack, M., Quinn, M. J., Payne, H. A. and Babb, P. (2001). 'Current Trends in Colorectal Cancer: Site, Incidence, Mortality and Survival in England and Wales'. *Clinical Oncology*, **13**: 448–52.

Rubin, G. P., Hungin, A. P., Kelly, P. J. and Ling, J. (2000). 'Inflammatory Bowel Disease: Epidemiology and Management in an English General Practice Population'. *Alimentary Pharmacology and Therapeutics*, **14**: 1553–9.

Kang, J. Y., Hoare, J., Tinto, A. *et al.* (2003). 'Diverticular Disease of the Colon on the Rise: A Study of Hospital Admissions in England between 1989/1990 and 1999/2000'. *Alimentary Pharmacology and Therapeutics*, **17**: 1189–95.

the lowest rates occur in India (age-standardized (world) incidence rates of 2.5–6 per 100 000 in both sexes). Substantial variation is seen between different ethnic groups: in the USA the highest rates are seen in the Japanese and in Blacks, and the lowest in American Indians; Jews have much higher rates of colorectal

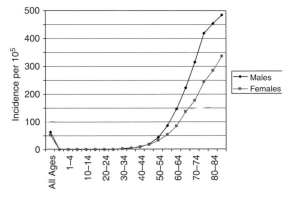

Fig. 9.3 Age-specific incidence of colorectal cancer, England 2000. Source: Office for National Statistics (2001). Mortality Statistics – Cause. Review of the Registrar General on Deaths by Cause, Sex and Age, in England and Wales, 2000. Mortality Data Series DH2 No. 27. London: ONS.

cancer than Arabs living within the same region in Israel. Studies of Japanese migrants to the USA show that colorectal cancer rates in US-born Japanese are up to twice those of native Japanese; these rates also exceed those of Whites born in the USA. The widespread variation in the geographic distribution of colorectal cancer, the recent secular trends, ethnic differences, and changes in the risk in migrants indicate the importance of environmental and lifestyle influences on risk of this cancer and suggest that the risk is modifiable, at least in part. However, genetic factors also predispose individuals to this cancer (see Chapter 15).

Aetiology

Genetics

Seventy-five per cent of colorectal cancers occur sporadically. Eighteen per cent of patients have a family history of colorectal cancer, but have no identified genetic predisposition, and 5 per cent of colorectal cancer patients have hereditary non-polyposis colorectal cancer (HNPCC, also called Lynch syndrome). In families with HNPCC, cancer usually occurs on the right side of the colon and at a younger age than sporadic colorectal cancer. Other cancers occur in these families, including cancers of the uterus, ovaries, stomach, urinary tract, small bowel, and bile ducts. HNPCC is caused by germ-line mutation of one of the mismatch repair genes (Calvert and Frucht 2002). One per cent of colorectal cancers occur in patients with familial adenomatosis polypi (FAP), who carry germ-line mutations of the *APC* gene (a tumour suppressor gene). In approximately one-third of these patients the mutations are spontaneous. Affected individuals have multiple colonic adenomas which, if untreated, inevitably undergo malignant change. Patients may also develop thyroid and other cancers, adenomas in other parts of the gastro-intestinal tract, and benign lesions of many organs. Prophylactic colectomy and routine endoscopic surveillance of the rectum are usually performed in patients with FAP to prevent the development of colorectal cancer. Patients with ulcerative colitis are at high lifetime risk of this cancer and contribute about 1 per cent of cases to its total.

Environmental/lifestyle risk factors

Most colorectal cancers occur in individuals without any known genetic predisposition, and several environmental/lifestyle risk factors have been identified. Intake of animal fat and meat has been consistently, positively related to the risk of colorectal cancer; for example data from the US Nurses' Health Study showed that women in the highest quintile of intake of animal fat had approximately twice the risk of colorectal cancer compared with those whose intake was in the lowest quintile. Also, women who ate meat every day were 2.5 times more likely to develop this cancer than women who ate meat less than once a month. The relation between fibre intake and risk of colorectal cancer is somewhat controversial. Data from the same study did not show any protective effect of dietary fibre on colorectal cancer; but recent data from the larger European Prospective Investigation into Cancer and Nutrition (the EPIC Study) showed a 40 per cent reduction in the risk of colorectal cancer for the highest compared with the lowest quintile of fibre intake (Bingham *et al.* 2003). Data relating to the association between intake of fruit and vegetables and risk of colorectal cancer are also inconsistent, although a generally low intake of fruit and vegetables appears to increase the risk of colorectal cancer. Collectively, epidemiological studies suggest an approximate 40 per cent reduction in the risk of colorectal cancer in individuals with the highest dietary folate intake compared with those with the lowest intake. High intake of calcium is also associated with reduced risk of colorectal cancer, and intervention studies have shown that calcium supplementation can reduce the occurrence of colorectal adenomas (Weingarten *et al.* 2004). Obesity is also a risk factor for colorectal cancer, obese individuals having about twice the risk of their lean counterparts. This seems to be particularly the case in men with central adiposity, and this may be mediated through insulin insensitivity. There is strong evidence from epidemiological studies that physically active men and women (taking 30–60 minutes per day of moderate- to vigorous-intensity activity) have a 30–40 per cent reduced risk of developing colon cancer, compared with inactive persons (Lee 2003). Physical activity is not associated with the risk of rectal cancer. Evidence is also accumulating that smoking is a risk factor for colorectal cancer. Epidemiological studies conducted before the 1970s in males, and before the 1990s in females, did not show this association, probably because an induction period of three to four decades is required between genotoxic exposure (from smoking) and the development of colorectal cancer.

Epidemiological studies have also shown that individuals reporting a regular intake of aspirin and other NSAIDs have a 40–50 per cent reduced risk of developing colorectal polyps and cancer. Intervention studies in high-risk patients (patients with colorectal adenomas and patients with colorectal cancer treated by curative resection) have shown a lower incidence of new colorectal adenomas in those treated with aspirin; however, this has not been demonstrated in subjects with normal or low risk (Herendeen and Lindley 2003). 🖥

Prevention

There is sufficient evidence to recommend that people should reduce their intake of meat and animal fat, increase their intake of fibre, fruit, and vegetables, maintain normal weight, and take regular physical activity of at least moderate intensity, to reduce their risk of colorectal cancer. Data at present are insufficient to recommend calcium or folate supplementation to prevent colorectal cancer, but these approaches show promise for the future. Too much controversy exists about the safety, efficacy, and optimal treatment regimen of NSAIDs to promote them as long-term chemopreventive agents in the general population, but their use may be appropriate in high-risk groups. Randomized controlled trials have confirmed that population screening of middle-aged men and women over the age of 50 years for non-visible (occult) blood in the faeces can reduce the mortality rate for colorectal cancer (Towler *et al.* 1998), 🖥 and plans are underway to introduce a national colorectal cancer screening programme in the UK (see Chapter 5).

9.4 Inflammatory Bowel Disease

Inflammatory bowel disease (IBD) includes ulcerative colitis (UC) and Crohn's disease (CD). Unlike the distinctive pathological features of UC and CD (see Box 9.3), the clinical features of the diseases are not sufficiently distinct to allow them to be separated with reliability. The main symptoms of both conditions include diarrhoea

---

> **BOX 9.3 PATHOLOGICAL DEFINITIONS OF MAJOR VARIETIES OF INFLAMMATORY BOWEL DISEASE**
>
> Ulcerative colitis is a chronic inflammatory disease of unknown cause which primarily affects the colonic mucosa. Inflammation is limited to the superficial layers and lack of extension to the muscularis and serosal structures is typical.
>
> Crohn's disease is a chronic, granulatomatous, inflammatory disorder of unknown cause which may involve any segment of the gastrointestinal tract from mouth to anus. Transmural inflammation is characteristic.

(which may be bloody and/or contain mucus), abdominal pain, weight loss, malaise, anorexia, fever, and lethargy. Both conditions tend to follow a relapsing and remittent course.

Prevalence/incidence

Measuring the prevalence or incidence of UC and CD presents some problems. Accurate diagnosis requires access to endoscopic and laboratory facilities to enable differentiation of these conditions from each other and from other disorders causing similar symptoms, for example infective gastro-intestinal diseases. This has implications for comparing the incidence of these diseases between countries, particularly between developed and developing countries. Also, mild UC may go undetected. Mortality is a poor measure of the incidence of these conditions, and outpatient management (especially in patients with mild UC) and repeated admissions to hospital (in CD patients) complicate the use of hospital admissions as measures of frequency of IBD. Population-based registers of IBD are uncommon (Rubin *et al.* 2000). 🖥 Estimates of the UK incidence and prevalence of UC and CD are shown in Table 9.1.

Time trends and geographic distribution

There is substantial geographic variation in the incidence of IBD. These diseases appear to be uncommon in developing countries but this may be due to under-ascertainment. In the developed world there is a north–south gradient in the incidence of IBD, both in Europe and the USA; the highest rates are seen in Scandinavia and in Scotland. A higher incidence of UC compared with CD is a fairly consistent finding in different populations. IBD most commonly presents in people in their late teens and twenties, with the peak age of presentation of CD being earlier than UC. The incidence of CD is higher in females, especially when presentation is at an early age (Figure 9.4). IBD, and in particular CD, is more common in urban than rural populations but there are no clear relations with socioeconomic status. The time trends in IBD are difficult to interpret because of changing diagnostic practices and the possibility of diagnostic transfer between the UC and CD categories. In Europe and the USA there appears to have been a sharp rise in the incidence of UC and CD after World War II, with the increase in the incidence of UC preceding that in CD by about 15–20 years. In most Western countries, the incidence of IBD appears to have levelled off towards the end of the twentieth century.

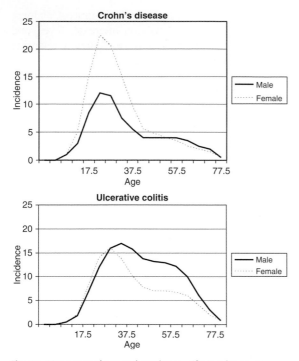

Fig. 9.4 Mean annual age and gender-specific incidence rates (per 100 000 inhabitants per year) of Crohn's disease and ulcerative colitis in South Limburg, The Netherlands (1991–1995). Source: Russel, M. G. (2000). 'Changes in the Incidence of Inflammatory Bowel Disease: What Does it Mean?' *European Journal of Internal Medicine*, **11**: 191–6.

Aetiology and risk factors

The aetiology of IBD is unknown but there is evidence that genetic susceptibility, environmental exposures, and host immune responses all contribute to development of these conditions. There is a high IBD concordance rate among monozygotic twins, especially for CD. IBD exhibits familial aggregation: the relative risk to a sibling is estimated to be between 15 and 35 for CD and between 7 and 17 for UC. Familial aggregation may reflect not only shared genes but shared environment, including exposure to infectious or other noxious agents. Other evidence of a genetic predisposition to IBD is provided by association with several well-defined genetic syndromes, such as Turner's syndrome. A susceptibility gene for CD has recently been identified; the CARD 15 gene. However, IBDs are genetically complex disorders and many other susceptibility genes are likely to exist, and remain to be identified (Tamboli *et al.* 2003). 🖳

Infection, or response to infection, may play a role in the aetiology of IBD. CD has been shown to be more common in people who, during infancy, live in houses with running hot water and separate bathrooms (Gent *et al.* 1994). 🖳 Improved living conditions in childhood and altered immune modulation resulting from later exposure to infections has been proposed to explain the rise in CD in industrialized countries, as has been suggested also in the case of asthma (Chapter 7). Some data suggest that breast-feeding may protect against IBD and that sensitivity to cow's milk is involved in the pathogenic process of IBD, but the evidence is far from conclusive. The high intake of refined sugar and starch may increase the risk of IBD, with stronger evidence available for CD risk than for UC risk. A lower intake of fruit, vegetables, and fibre has been shown in people with IBD, but it is uncertain whether this is a response to disease or whether these dietary components protect against IBD. Smokers have more than twice the risk of CD compared with non-smokers, and patients with CD who continue to smoke follow a more aggressive clinical course than non-smokers. In contrast, smokers have half the risk of UC compared with non-smokers, and UC patients who smoke have a better clinical prognosis than non-smokers. Nicotine has been proposed as a treatment for UC (Logan *et al.* 2002). 🖳 A meta-analysis of studies examining the relation between the use of oral contraceptives and IBD found only weak associations (relative risks below 1.3 for both CD and UC in users), and non-causal explanations could not be excluded.

IBD, particularly UC, is a risk factor for colon cancer; the risk is very high in patients in whom UC has been established for 10–20 years.

Prevention

Opportunities for the prevention of IBD are limited as the aetiology of these conditions is poorly understood. However, avoiding smoking may protect against CD, and patients with CD who smoke should benefit from stopping smoking. Conversely, patients with UC who smoke report that this reduces the likelihood of relapse. There is also some evidence that 'probiotics' (specific bacterial extracts) prevent relapse of UC.

9.5 Cirrhosis of the Liver

Cirrhosis is the end result of long-term liver damage. It results from the necrosis of liver cells and is characterized by formation of fibrous tissue, nodules, and scarring, which interfere with liver blood flow and liver

TABLE 9.2	Some causes of cirrhosis
Common causes	**Other causes**
Alcohol toxicity	Biliary cirrhosis (primary or secondary)
Chronic active hepatitis due to:	Autoimmune chronic active hepatitis
hepatitis C	Drugs, for example methotrexate
hepatitis B	Nonalcoholic steatohepatitis (NASH)
	Chronic heart failure
	Haemachromatosis
	Wilson's disease
	Alpha-1-antitrypsin deficiency
	Glycogen storage disease
	Idiopathic (cryptogenic)

cell function. Cirrhosis may lead to chronic liver failure and death. Some causes of cirrhosis are listed in Table 9.2. Alcohol and hepatitis C infection are the most common causes of cirrhosis in the UK but hepatitis B is the most common cause worldwide. In England, over 4000 people died from cirrhosis in 1999, two-thirds before the age of 65 years (Chief Medical Officer 2001). In the UK, deaths from cirrhosis have increased in the past three decades, especially among middle-aged males (Figure 9.5), with the most marked increases occurring in the 1990s. Binge drinking and drug use, with a risk of hepatitis, have been proposed to account for this.

Similar increases are seen in hospital admission rates for cirrhosis. In 1980, the mortality from chronic liver

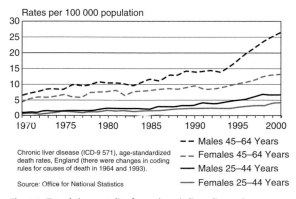

Chronic liver disease (ICD-9 571), age-standardized death rates, England (there were changes in coding rules for causes of death in 1964 and 1993).

Source: Office for National Statistics

-- Males 45–64 Years
-- Females 45–64 Years
— Males 25–44 Years
— Females 25–44 Years

Fig. 9.5 Trends in mortality from chronic liver disease in England, 1970–2000. Source: Chief Medical Officer (2001). *The Annual Report of the Chief Medical Office of the Department of Health.* London: Department of Health.

disease and cirrhosis in the UK was around 20 per cent that of the European Union (EU) but EU rates have fallen while UK rates have risen; in 2002 the UK rate was 70 per cent of the EU average and looks set to exceed that of the EU within the next decade (WHO 2002). Mortality data from the West Midlands for the 1990s suggested that the upward trend in cirrhosis mortality during this period resulted almost entirely from a threefold increase in alcoholic liver disease (Fisher *et al.* 2002). ⌨ Rates of increase in deaths from alcoholic liver disease were similar for men and women. A well-conducted case–control study in France found that women who drank heavily were more at risk of cirrhosis than men, and that they also developed cirrhosis at an earlier age (Tuyns and Pequingnot 1984). ⌨ There is also a genetic difference between the sexes in the levels of the enzyme alcohol dehydrogenase. This has implications for current and future trends in cirrhosis among women, as heavy drinking is increasing at a faster rate among women than men. In the UK the proportion of women drinking more than 14 units of alcohol a week increased by 50 per cent (from 10 per cent to 15 per cent) between the late 1980s and late 1990s whereas the proportion of men drinking more than 21 units remained stable at 27 per cent (Chief Medical Officer 2001). ⌨ Among middle-aged men, the pattern of alcohol consumption is very different in men from Northern Ireland and from France (Marques-Vidal *et al.* 2000) ⌨ although in younger adults trends may be tending to converge in Europe.

Hepatitis C is the second most common cause of cirrhosis in the UK. Around 250 000 people in England are thought to be infected by hepatitis C (Chief Medical Officer 2001). ⌨ Many of these people are unaware that they have the infection and will have a normal lifespan. However, in about 20 per cent, persistent chronic hepatitis will lead to the development of cirrhosis over a 20- to 30-year period. Consumption of alcohol is an important determinant of progression of hepatitis C infection to cirrhosis; high consumption of alcohol appears to confer more than a 10-fold increased risk of cirrhosis among infected persons.

Prevention of cirrhosis in the UK hinges on several separate strategies: tackling excessive alcohol consumption, especially among young people; reducing intravenous drug abuse; ensuring the safety of blood products; and instigating treatment to reduce the progression to cirrhosis among people infected with viral hepatitis. This disorder represents a considerable challenge to current and future clinical and public-health practitioners if trends are to be reversed.

9.6 Other Gastro-Intestinal Diseases

In this textbook lack of space prevents discussion of the epidemiology of other important diseases of the digestive tract. The epidemiological methods used to investigate gallstone disease, appendicitis, diverticular disease, coeliac disease, and pancreatitis are described elsewhere (Logan *et al*. 2002). 💻

Further Reading

Logan, R. F. A., Farthing, M. J. G. and Langman, M. J. S. (2002). 'Gastrointestinal Disease: Public Health Aspects', in R. Detels, J. McEwen, R. Beaglehole and H. Tanaka (eds.). *Oxford Textbook of Public Health*. Oxford: Oxford University Press.

References

References for this chapter can be found at www.oxfordtextbooks.co.uk/orc/yarnell. Where possible, these are presented as *active links* which direct you to an electronic version of the work. If you are a subscriber to that work (either individually or through an institution), and depending on your level of access, you may be able to peruse an abstract or the full article if available. 💻

Model answer

Study type	Advantages	Disadvantages
Case–control	Rapid, inexpensive	Cannot determine whether *H. pylori* infection preceded, or is the consequence of, gastric cancer
Cohort study	Can determine temporal sequence of infection and gastric cancer	Expensive, very time consuming. Long latent period between infection (normally in childhood) and development of gastric cancer (disease predominantly of the elderly)
Case–control study within a cohort (nested case–control)	Rapid, inexpensive, can determine temporal sequence of infection and gastric cancer	
Experimental study, for example RCT of eradication therapy	Could provide a definite answer?	Time consuming, expensive, very long follow-up period required, possibly decades. Preventing contamination of the control arm would be difficult. The disease process may be initiated at a very early stage with the result that prevention of infection rather than eradication is required to effect a reduction in gastric cancer occurrence

Renal system

In this chapter the epidemiology of acute and chronic renal failure are reviewed, and the high personal and economic costs necessary to cope with end-stage renal failure. A case study designed to estimate the population need for renal replacement therapy using a proxy indicator is reported. Other significant diseases of the urinary system are briefly reviewed.

Introduction

Adequate renal function is a prerequisite for a healthy life, but the kidneys are vulnerable to damage from many toxins, bacterial infections, circulatory stressors, and back pressure from post-renal obstruction. In a healthy adult, some 1.3 l of blood per minute (a quarter of cardiac output) pass through approximately two million glomeruli. About 180 l of glomerular filtrate containing water and soluble unbound simple chemicals is produced per day. The kidney has excretory, regulatory, endocrine, and metabolic functions; these all need to be addressed in patients with acute or chronic renal failure.

In the UK patients requiring renal replacement therapy (RRT) use about 1 per cent of the NHS budget (Beech *et al.* 2004) ⬛ but this is set to increase up to 4 per cent owing to an increasing proportion of elderly and vulnerable ethnic groups such as Afro-Caribbeans (prone to develop the renal complications of hypertension) and Indo-Asians (prone to develop the renal complications of diabetes). Opportunities clearly exist for improvements in primary prevention (control of hypertension and diabetes) but demand for RRT cannot be realistically reduced with an ageing population. Already in the UK the incidence of end-stage renal disease (ESRD) has doubled in the past 10 years but is lower than that registered in most European countries and in the USA (El Nahus and Bello 2005). 🖳

10.1 Acute and Chronic Renal Failure

The distinction between acute and chronic renal failure is important clinically for the investigations required, the management plan, and prognosis. In both forms of renal failure there is a reduced glomerular filtration rate (GFR). The fall in GFR may be asymptomatic and recognized only after a raised serum creatinine has been reported on a routine blood test. Serum creatinine is a common measure of renal function. Creatinine is derived from creatine released by skeletal muscle. Although serum creatinine is an imperfect measure of kidney function, and usually indicates extensive renal pathology, it has found widespread use in clinical practice due to its convenience and low cost compared with more accurate but cumbersome and expensive radioisotope methods. The absolute value of creatinine is influenced by muscle mass, which, in turn, is related to age, sex, and weight. Formula-based estimated GFR (eGRF) using a serum creatinine value is increasingly used in research and clinical practice. The formulae require simple input data such as the age, sex, ethnicity, and weight in addition to serum creatinine. Several websites provide easy access to these GFR calculators; for example, go to www.renal.org and click on 'GFR calculator'; alternatively, try www.bnf.org and click on 'BNF Extra' and go to 'Resources'.

Recently a similar marker of renal function, cystatin C, produced by all nucleated cells at a relatively constant rate, has been proposed as a more sensitive marker of renal function than plasma creatinine; but currently its primary role is in research, rather than in clinical practice.

Acute renal failure

Acute renal failure (ARF) is defined by a decline in GFR that occurs rapidly within a period of hours to a few weeks. ARF is generally reversible if promptly recognized, investigated, and managed appropriately. ARF is reported to complicate up to 5 per cent of all hospital admissions (Hou *et al.* 1983). 🖳 No single definition of ARF has been used in epidemiological studies.

Acute renal failure is traditionally explained in terms of pre-renal, renal, or post-renal factors. In pre-renal failure there is a decreased perfusion of histologically normal kidneys, for examle pre-renal failure occurs in hypotensive states such as hypovolaemic, cardiogenic, or septic shock. The kidneys respond to the reduced perfusion by activating the renin–angiotensin–aldosterone system, which results in enhanced renal sodium and water reabsorption, in an effort to restore perfusion to the kidneys. If the blood pressure improves and renal perfusion increases the GFR will rise and the ARF resolve. Prevention of pre-renal ARF requires careful management of the underlying cause; for example, fluid resuscitation if hypovolaemic, improving cardiac performance in cardiac shock, and appropriate treatment of sepsis in septic shock.

Post-renal failure or obstructive ARF occur when there is impaired drainage from the renal tracts or obstruction of the bladder outlet. The aetiology of obstructive ARF is age and gender related, and is commonly caused by obstruction to the bladder outlet owing to prostatic enlargement in older men. Ureteric obstruction may be insidious unless there are warning symptoms such as frank haematuria or pain. Clinical history and examination may yield important clues with symptoms such as hesitancy and poor urinary flow, suggesting bladder outlet obstruction and signs of a distended bladder on abdominal examination, or an enlarged prostate gland on rectal examination. The most useful investigation in determining obstructive ARF is an ultrasound scan, which can demonstrate dilated ureters, bladder distension, prostatic enlargement, and incomplete bladder emptying after micturition. Treatment directed at relieving obstruction could alleviate the renal impairment, but if urinary-tract obstruction was present for some time before being recognized, irreversible injury to renal structures may have occurred.

ARF can occur secondary to prolonged pre-renal insults, often as a complication of trauma or surgery in a hospital setting; commonly persisting hypotension results in hypoxic injury to renal cells and subsequent tubular necrosis. Acute tubular necrosis and pre-renal ARF account for 75 per cent of all ARF in the hospital setting. ARF may also occur owing to primary renal diseases such as proliferative glomerulonephritis or secondary to a systemic disorder such as small vessel vasculitis or multiple myeloma. On some occasions the injury is predominantly to the tubules and interstitial structures following an allergic reaction to drugs, for example proton-pump inhibitors or antibiotics. Prompt investigation of the cause of ARF, supportive management, withdrawal of all non-essential drugs, and treatment of the primary cause can stabilize and reverse the acute decline in GFR.

It is increasingly appreciated that ARF occurs in patients with pre-existing chronic kidney disease so called acute-on-chronic renal failure. This is best thought of as an acute deterioration in renal function occurring in an individual with limited renal reserve.

Chronic renal failure

Chronic renal failure is usually associated with chronic kidney disease (CKD) and typically causes a decline in GFR over months or years. This decline is usually irreversible and related to gradual reduction in functional nephron numbers (glomeruli and associated tubules). Many community-based surveys in the USA and the UK have highlighted that the prevalence of CKD is much higher than previously appreciated (Table 10.1).

10.2 End-Stage Renal Disease

End-stage renal disease (ESRD) is an irreversible loss of renal function and is fatal unless treated by RRT, either dialysis or transplantation. Usually ESRD is associated with an absolute reduction in GFR below 10 ml/min and an elevated serum creatinine above 500 µmol/l. Registries that collate information on incidence and prevalence of ESRD define a new patient as one who is accepted for treatment and dialysed or transplanted for more than 90 days (3 months). This definition would exclude an individual with newly diagnosed ESRD who died within three months and, therefore, leads to an underestimate of the true incidence of ESRD, which is compounded by exclusion of patients who have not been accepted for RRT.

Aetiology of end-stage renal disease

The commonest causes of ESRD in the UK and USA are shown in Table 10.2. In North America and most European countries, diabetic nephropathy has emerged as the most common cause (Feest *et al.* 2005). 🖳 Most patients with diabetic nephropathy have type 2 diabetes. Hypertension is present in most patients with ESRD, and the elevated blood pressure is secondary to chronic kidney disease.

A significant proportion of patients with ESRD present late with advanced renal failure, hypertension, and small kidneys on ultrasound scan. The precise aetiology of their renal disease is often undetermined although individual clinicians may attribute this to hypertensive nephrosclerosis or glomerulonephritis (unless confirmed by biopsy). Variation in clinical diagnostic practice and certainty will account for some of the apparent differences in clinical diagnoses when national ESRD registries are compared (see Table 10.2).

TABLE 10.1   Incidence of chronic renal failure (CRF) in UK population surveys of adults

Annual rate per million population	Definition of CRD (creatinine µmol/l)	Location	Study
11 444	>150 (single test)	Northern Ireland	Reaney *et al.* 2005
2435	>180 in men and >135 in women (single test)	Kent and Canterbury	John *et al.* 2004
1700	>150 (two tests)	Southampton	Drey *et al.* 2003
450	>300	Grampian	Khan *et al.* 1994
148	>500	Devon and northwest England	Feest *et al.* 1990
77	>500	Northern Ireland	McGeown 1990

Sources: Reaney *et al.* (unpublished data).

John, R., Webb, M., Young, A. and Stevens, P. E. (2004). 'Unreferred Chronic Kidney Disease: A Longitudinal Study'. *American Journal of Kidney Disease,* **43**: 825–35.

Drey, N., Roderick, P., Mullee, M. and Rogerson, M. (2003). 'A Population-Based Study of the Incidence and Outcomes of Diagnosed Chronic Kidney Disease'. *American Journal of Kidney Disease,* **42**: 677–84.

Khan, I. H., Catto, G. R., Edward, N. and MacLeod, A. M. (1994). 'Chronic Renal Failure: Factors Influencing Nephrology Referral'. *Quarterly Journal of Medicine,* **87**: 559–64.

Lamping, D. L., Constantinovici, N., Roderick, P. *et al.* (2000). 'Clinical Outcomes, Quality of Life, and Costs in the North Thames Dialysis Study of Elderly People on Dialysis: A Prospective Cohort Study'. *The Lancet,* **356**: 1543–50.

Feest, T. G., Mistry, C. D., Grimes, D. S. and Mallick, N. P. (1990). 'Incidence of Advanced Chronic Renal Failure and the Need for End Stage Renal Replacement Treatment'. *British Medical Journal,* **301**: 897–900.

McGeown, M. G. (1990). 'Prevalence of Advanced Renal Failure in Northern Ireland'. *British Medical Journal,* **301**: 900–3.

TABLE 10.2 Primary renal diagnosis for patients
starting renal replacement therapy in 2001

Diagnosis	UK[1] (%)	USA[2] (%)
Diabetes	17.6	44.6
Hypertension	6.1	24.0
Glomerulonephritis	9.8	11.1
Polycystic kidneys	6.3	3.2
Pyelonephritis	6.5	3.8
Renal vascular disease	7.0	2.9
Aetiology uncertain	21.9	10.4

Sources: [1]Ansell and Feest (2002); [2]United States Renal Data System (2003).

Ansell, D. and Feest, T. (eds.) (2002). *The Fifth Annual Report, The UK Renal Registry*. Bristol: UK Renal Registry.

United States Renal Data System (2003). 'Annual Data Report: Incidence and Prevalence of ESRD (2003)'. *American Journal of Kidney Disease*, **42** (Suppl. 5): S37–173.

Note: differences in relative percentage of diagnoses between UK and USA ESRD populations reflect multiple factors including diagnostic coding practices in each country, age structure of the ESRD population, ethnic mix, and acceptance rates for RRT.

Incidence of ESRD

The incidence of ESRD is rising worldwide. This reflects both a true increase in incidence of CKD and an increased acceptance of patients with ESRD for RRT. A true increase in incidence reflects demographic factors such as an ageing population and an increased prevalence of type 2 diabetes. Increased acceptance of ESRD patients for treatment has occurred owing to expansion in dialysis facilities and staff to provide appropriate care.

Acceptance rates in the UK have risen from 20 persons per million population (pmp) in the 1980s to 101 pmp in the year 2002 (Ansell and Feest 2002). 🖳 In the USA acceptance rates are higher, rising from 100 pmp in 1982 to 333 pmp in 2002 (US Renal Data System 2005). 🖳 There is also considerable worldwide variation in the incidence of ESRD. For instance, in 2002, incidence rates ranged from the lowest reported of 6 pmp in Bangladesh through intermediate rates (53 ppm Philippines; 129 pmp Korea; 170 pmp Belgium) to the highest rates of 251 pmp in Japan and 336 pmp in the USA (US Renal Data System 2005). 🖳

Trends in ESRD

The marked geographic variation in acceptance rates for ESRD between countries and within regions cannot be entirely explained by differences in population, age structure, ethnicity, or co-morbidity. Variation in the propensity to offer RRT reflects clinical, societal, and economic factors. Previously in the UK, older patients with ESRD were not accepted for RRT, but chronological age is not a bar to treatment and it is ethically unacceptable to deny life-sustaining treatment to elderly people. Indeed, the perceived quality of life of elderly dialysis patients is reported to be comparable to that in an age-matched population (Lamping *et al.* 2000). 🖳 Variations also exist within regions of the UK, with England in 2002 having lower acceptance rates than Wales, Northern Ireland, or Scotland, despite having a higher proportion of ethnic minorities (UK Renal Registry 2005). 🖳 People of Asian and Afro-Caribbean descent have higher rates of CKD. African-Americans have four times higher RRT acceptance rates compared with Whites related to a much greater prevalence of hypertension in the former (US Renal Data System 2005). 🖳

The total cost of RRT is, largely, dependent on the prevalence of ESRD. Prevalent cases of ESRD are sometimes referred to as the 'stock' of patients receiving RRT. Prevalence rates have risen from under 400 pmp in 1993 to 626 pmp in 2002 and are predicted to increase further. Furthermore, the relative proportions of ESRD patients treated by dialysis versus transplantation are changing. While renal transplantation provides the most cost-effective form of RRT, it is proving extremely difficult to significantly increase the overall rate of transplantation. Demand has continued to outstrip supply, and will continue to do so. Although living kidney donors (related, for example parent or sibling, or unrelated, for example partners) are increasingly being used, the number of cadaveric donor kidney procedures has fallen over the past 15 years (UK Transplant 2005). 🖳 In addition, many ESRD patients accepted for RRT are not suitable for transplantation because of their multiple medical problems and advanced age. It is currently unusual for renal transplantation to be performed in persons over 70 years of age as the supply of donor organs is limited.

Most ESRD patients will be treated by maintenance dialysis that is often provided by hospital-based haemodialysis; lower cost options such as continuous ambulatory peritoneal dialysis are also used (Beech *et al.* 2004) 🖳 but are unsuitable for more elderly patients with very poor renal function.

The annual mortality for a dialysis population approaches 15–20 per cent, which is worse than many neoplastic conditions. The high mortality reflects the excess cardiovascular risk in patients with CKD. Clustering of 'traditional' cardiovascular risk factors such as older age, male gender, hypertension, diabetes, and smoking account for some but not all of the increased risk. Novel 'renal' cardiovascular risk factors may include the adverse metabolic consequences of protein-uria, elevated homocysteine levels, dyslipidaemia, left ventricular hypertrophy associated with renal anaemia, and abnormal calcium-phosphate balance leading to widespread arterial calcification. Survival on dialysis is decreased also by advanced age, late referral for RRT, the type of renal disease, and the quality of the dialysis delivered. One measurement of dialysis quality is *ade-quacy*, which is mathematically determined by urea clearance during dialysis.

Primary renal diseases such as glomerulonephritis or polycystic kidney disease have a better prognosis than renal failure secondary to diabetic nephropathy or atheromatous renal vascular disease. A comparative **audit** between individual renal units or between countries is difficult to interpret without adjusting for **case-mix**, for example age and co-morbid medical problems. Attempts have been made to develop co-morbidity scores to determine the appropriate level of service provision (Chandna *et al.* 1999). ▢ Although this may have some validity at a population level, there is considerable individual variation, and occasionally prolonged survival of a person with an apparently dismal prognosis is seen.

Recent research has suggested that cardiovascular risk factors behave paradoxically in CKD. Serum choles terol levels fall as CKD progresses and those persons with ESRD and lowest cholesterol levels have the highest mortality. This inverse relation between cho-lesterol and mortality may reflect malnutrition and inflammation secondary to the uraemic state. Several randomized controlled trials are now addressing whether lipid-lowering with statin drugs improves outcome in CKD and ESRD patients. Similarly, ESRD patients with the highest homocysteine levels have the best survival, a finding that contrasts with the associa-tion between high homocysteine levels and increased risk of cardiovascular events in the population in general.

Future trends in CKD will be driven by the demo-graphic changes of an ageing population and increased incidence of type 2 diabetes (Chapter 8). Under-referral of patients with CKD has been uncovered in numerous community surveys (see Table 10.1). Appropriate investigation of persons with progressive CKD would allow at least some conditions, hypertension or urinary tract obstruction for example, to be effectively managed to slow progression of the renal disease.

It is unlikely that a steady state, where acceptance rates (reflecting referral) match the annual death rate of patients on RRT, will be reached within the next 10–20 years. Improvement in the quality of care delivered to patients with CKD and ESRD should improve individual survival. This in turn can lead to a further expansion in the stock of prevalent ESRD patients requiring RRT.

10.3 Estimating Unmet Need for Renal Replacement Therapy

Targeting Social Need (TSN) is a government initiative to direct resources to disadvantaged people, groups, and areas to reduce inequalities between rich and poor. Poverty and social exclusion result in poorer health, which is often compounded by reduced access to health services (see Chapter 17). Ensuring equitable access to services is therefore one of the key themes. As yet, little is known about whether unequal access to renal serv-ices is largely driven by variations in patient character-istics or in practice management styles at the primary care or secondary care level. However, in Scotland there was evidence of unequal access to the national transplant list (Oniscu *et al.* 2003). ▢ Access to services can be explored by using routine data sources that can yield patient data linked to geographic area. Strategies for the prevention of, or delay in the decline of, renal function will be better informed and more likely to succeed if service provision is appropriately applied and distributed.

As with many other diseases, chronic kidney disease shows a social class gradient, with patients in lower social classes experiencing worse outcomes, often as a result of late referral for specialist care. The conse-quences of late referral include a lower likelihood of transplantation and a greater risk of death. An analysis of patients receiving dialysis in Northern Ireland found that those from more deprived areas were younger at first dialysis than those from affluent parts of the Province, and that their subsequent survival was worse. This may have been because the rate of progression of disease is faster in less affluent patients or that their compliance with treatment for underlying morbidity is worse.

The research project reported below aims to iden-tify the determinants of referral to renal services in Northern Ireland by examining:

(i) the extent of under-referral to the renal service in Northern Ireland;

(ii) how referral varies according to patient age, sex, diagnosis, area of residence, and level of material deprivation;

(iii) how referral varies according to the practice and test-ordering characteristics of the patients' doctors.

To determine the level of under-referral to renal services, it is essential to know the incidence and prevalence of CKD in the population. Although the incidence and prevalence of ESRD have been reported in many countries (Berthoux *et al.* 1999; Lee 2003), ⌨ little is known about the incidence and prevalence of CKD, the usual pre-cursor of ESRD. A few studies of prevalence have been conducted in other countries (Coresh *et al.* 2003; Nissenson *et al.* 2001), ⌨ though these may not be generalizable to UK populations as the incidence and prevalence of CKD is known to vary with ethnicity (Roderick *et al.* 1994). ⌨ There is no commonly agreed definition of CKD; however, the current referral guidelines set by the Renal Association recommend that all patients with a serum creatinine level of 150–200 µmol/l should be assessed by a nephrologist. Even at this level, patients have already lost more than half of their renal reserve.

The project uses routine data on serum creatinine to identify those patients who meet the criteria for referral to renal services. Serum creatinine is part of the routine U and E (urea and electrolytes) test, which is performed pre-operatively or for medical patients in their general assessment. These and additional laboratory data listed below provide a readily accessible information source of patients with and without recognized renal disease, without having to undertake a special cross-sectional survey of the population.

Applying a single threshold for serum creatinine to define CKD is inequitable, because females and older people with lower muscle mass will have to reach a more advanced stage of renal failure before attaining the threshold. Estimated glomerular filtration rate (eGFR) takes these factors into account and may be a more accurate and equitable method of defining CKD. However, until routine reporting of eGFR is introduced (see section 10.1), general practitioners must rely on serum creatinine measurements when making decisions about referring a patient to a nephrologist.

Data were retrieved from all test results for serum creatinine, urea, albumin, urinary protein excretion, and haemoglobin AIc (HbAIc: a marker of adequacy of diabetic control (see Chapter 8)) performed in Northern Ireland laboratories between 1 January 2001 and 31 December 2002. This yielded the results of 2 892 340 blood and urine samples. Each patient may have had one or many samples taken during 2001 and 2002, so

individual blood or urine sample records were matched to produce a patient-level database. There were 656 002 unique patients who had tests of renal function or HbA1c performed in 2001 or 2002. All patients aged 20 years and over who had a creatinine test recorded in 2001 were selected from this database, yielding a total of 344 937 patients, which represents 29 per cent of the population of Northern Ireland in this age group. From these, we identified our study population of patients with CKD (aged 20 years or more with one or more blood samples tested for serum creatinine in 2001, where the test result was 150 µmol/l or above). (There were 19 286 patients who met this criterion.)

Although most patients with a serum creatinine level of 150 µmol/l or above will have CKD, some will have acute renal failure (ARF) after a severe illness, accident, or surgical operation. The project used the following arbitrary definition of acute renal failure: any patient with a serum creatinine greater than 300 µmol/l (twice the chosen threshold of 150 µmol/l) which returned to less than 120 µmol/l (the upper limit of normal laboratory range) within six months of the first elevated test. A further 824 patients who met this criterion were excluded from the database. The resulting cohort of 18 462 patients represents the CKD study population, giving a crude prevalence rate of 1.56 per cent of the population of Northern Ireland of adults aged 20 years and over. Figure 10.1 shows the age- and sex-specific rate for CKD.

Q1 Why may the data shown in Figure 10.1 underestimate the true prevalence of CKD in the population of Northern Ireland?

Q2 How would you estimate the theoretical maximum prevalence in the population?

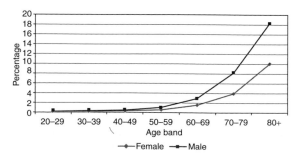

Fig. 10.1 Prevalence of laboratory-detected CKD by age and sex in a Northern Ireland population.
Source: Reaney *et al.* (unpublished data).

According to this study, between 18462 and 38532 adults in Northern Ireland merit referral to a nephrologist for assessment of CKD. There are currently 12 whole-time equivalent (WTE) nephrologists in Northern Ireland, who have a caseload of 1000 new patients per year and a stock of 1200 existing patients. Even if the number of nephrologists is increased to a total of 20 WTEs by 2010, it will be impossible to absorb these additional patients into the system.

This needs assessment of CKD in the population shows that the prevalence of CKD is greater than originally thought and that guidelines cannot be implemented as recommended. The project raises the further research question about which CKD patients progress to ESRD. If the factors that influence progression can be identified, then high-risk patients can be referred to nephrologists for specialist assessment and treatment, whereas GPs can manage the remaining patients in primary care.

The data were then analysed in more detail to ascertain which patients were more likely to be referred after a first raised serum creatinine test in 2001. Those subjects who had had any HbA1c test undertaken during the two year period were defined as diabetic. After exclusion of those who were already known to a nephrologist and those who had ARF, it was found that younger patients and diabetics were more likely to be referred, and that there was no difference in referral rates between males and females. There is, however, considerable under-referral of patients according to the guidelines, as only 7 per cent of all non-diabetic subjects and 19 per cent of diabetic patients were referred within 12 months of the first abnormal testing (see Table 10.3).

Cox's proportional hazards regression was used to test variation in the referred proportion according to age, sex, and whether diabetic or not (Table 10.4). Data on socioeconomic inequalities that examine general practitioner characteristics such as prescribing rates, practice size, and practice deprivation score (see Chapter 17), and their effect on referral, will be examined in future analyses.

10.4 Other Urinary Tract Diseases

Prostate cancer is the third commonest cancer in men and is reviewed in Chapter 15. **Bladder** (4.5 per cent of all cancers) and **kidney** (1.8 per cent of all cancers) are common sites in the urinary tract for neoplastic change, and the relative risk for these cancers is increased up to threefold by cigarette smoking. Bladder cancer risk is increased by occupational exposure to

TABLE 10.3 Cumulative risk of referral to a nephrologist within 12 months of initial abnormal creatinine result*			
	Age Group	Number	Cumulative proportion referred % (95% CI)
Non-diabetics	20–39	307	17 (12, 21)
	40–49	327	16 (12, 21)
	50–59	806	14 (11, 17)
	60–69	1746	10 (8, 11)
	70–79	4094	7 (6, 7)
	80+	5689	3 (3, 4)
	Total	12969	7 (6, 7)
Diabetics	20–39	74	42 (32, 52)
	40–49	95	25 (20, 30)
	50–59	279	26 (21, 32)
	60–69	801	26 (23, 29)
	70–79	1392	18 (16, 21)
	80+	1075	9 (7, 11)
	Total	3716	19 (18, 21)

*Patients previously known to the nephrology service have been excluded from the denominator.

Source: Kee, F., Reaney, E. A., Maxwell, A. P., Fogarty, D. G., Savage, G. and Patterson, C. C. (2005). 'Late Referral for Assessment of Renal Failure'. *Journal of Epidemiology and Community Health,* **59**: 386–8, reproduced with permission from the BMJ Publishing Group.

aromatic amines and other industrial chemicals used in the dyeing and rubber industries (a strong association was initially found with the use of aniline dyes but several highly carcinogenic amines were probably present in these dyestuffs as impurities). Occupational epidemiology has helped identify these carcinogens and removed them from the industrial environment in countries with strong regulatory controls.

Benign prostatic hyperplasia can be detected histologically in more than 50 per cent of men over 60 years of age, but only between 25 and 40 per cent of men present with significant symptoms of voiding or storage of urine (Neal *et al.* 2004). ⌨ About 25 per cent of men who have a prostatectomy present initially with acute retention of urine, a potentially life-threatening condition. Treatment rates are likely to rise in all countries with ageing populations and improved, cost-effective pharmacological and surgical treatments will be required to cope with predicted demand.

TABLE 10.4 Cox's proportional hazards regression of effects of age, sex, and diabetes on proportion referred within 12 months

Comparison		Relative hazard (95% CI)
Sex	Female versus male	1.08 (0.98, 1.20)
Diabetes	Yes versus no	3.11 (2.81, 3.43)
Age group (years)	20–39 versus 80+	5.81 (4.54, 7.44)
	40–49 versus 80+	5.31 (4.17, 6.77)
	50–59 versus 80+	3.79 (3.13, 4.58)
	60–69 versus 80+	3.19 (2.72, 3.74)
	70–79 versus 80+	2.21 (1.90, 2.56)

Source: Kee, F., Reaney, E. A., Maxwell, A. P., Fogarty, D. G., Savage, G. and Patterson, C. C. (2005). 'Late Referral for Assessment of Renal Failure'. *Journal of Epidemiology and Community Health*, **59**: 386–8, reproduced with permission from the BMJ Publishing Group.

Web Addresses

United Kingdom Renal Registry (2005), Annual Report, http://www.renalreg.com.

United Kingdom Transplantation (2005). Annual report. http://www.transplant.org.uk.

United States Renal Data System (2005). Database, http://www.usrds.org/atlas.htm.

References

References for this chapter can be found at www.oxfordtextbooks.co.uk/orc/yarnell. 🖳

Model answers

Q1 The prevalence of CKD in NI shown in Figure 10.1 is dependent on the underlying assumption that all cases of CKD in NI have had a serum creatinine measurement. This is unlikely, as many CKD patients will have no symptoms; they may not have attended their GP; or the GP may not have tested serum creatinine levels. The prevalence of CKD in NI therefore represents a minimum level of CKD in NI.

Q2 We then estimated a maximum prevalence of CKD in NI by making the assumption that the 344 937 patients who had creatinine tests performed are representative of the total population. Using those tested for creatinine as a denominator takes into account the differential rates of testing between age bands (14 per cent of 20- to 29-year-olds rising to 68 per cent of patients older than 80). Table 10A shows the age specific rates of CKD in this group of 344 937 patients and uses **direct standardization** to apply these rates to the population of Northern Ireland to calculate the expected number of CKD cases. This gives an expected number of 38 532 adults with CKD and an age standardized rate of 3.25 per cent in Northern Ireland.

Appendix

TABLE 10A Estimated rates of chronic kidney disease (CKD) in those with creatinine tests in 2001, applied to the Northern Ireland population

Age band (years)	Number of patients with criteria for CKD	Number with creatinine tests in 2001	Rate of CKD in those with creatinine tests (%)	Total males and females in Northern Ireland	Maximum number of CKD cases (applying rate to Northern Ireland population)
20–29	234	30 785	0.76	224 089	1703
30–39	422	43 757	0.96	257 156	2480
40–49	676	50 625	1.34	219 799	2935
50–59	1389	61 839	2.25	187 158	4204
60–69	3015	62 340	4.84	138 928	6719
70–79	5952	59 394	10.02	104 394	10 462
80+	6774	36 197	18.71	53 590	10 029
Total	18 462	344 937	5.35	1 185 114	38 532

Age standardized rate = 3.25 per cent (38 532/1 185 114).

Source: Reaney *et al.* (unpublished data).

Neurological disease

Chapter contents

This chapter deals with the major diseases considered to have a neurological basis in ICD-10 including Parkinson's disease, multiple sclerosis, epilepsy, and cerebral palsy. Dementia and Alzheimer's disease (Chapter 12) and vascular causes of neurological deficit (Chapter 6) are reviewed elsewhere.

Introduction

Neurological diseases are associated with damage to a particular region of the brain or nervous system. This group of diseases can be particularly difficult to diagnose. This poses problems, not only for the clinician, but also for epidemiologists. Difficulty in accurately diagnosing neurological disease hampers **case ascertainment**, thus reducing the robustness of incidence and prevalence data, precluding reliable assessment of secular trends, and reducing confidence in aetiological findings. Estimates of disease occurrence have been made for the wealthier countries, where patients and their families have full access to neurological services, the best estimates coming from large prospective studies. Available data are summarized in Table 11.1. In developing countries the problem is even more acute, because even death certification of neurological diseases is unreliable, and these diseases are very under-researched outside industrial nations.

At least 6 per cent of the population have a neurological disorder in their lifetime, and the prevalence of the disorders discussed in this chapter together exceed the lifetime prevalence rate for completed stroke (Table 11.1). Both cerebral palsy and multiple sclerosis contribute more strongly towards **disability-adjusted life-years (DALYs)**

TABLE 11.1	Epidemiological indicators for neurological diseases	
Disease	**Incidence rate (Age and sex-adjusted per 100 000 per year)**	**Lifetime prevalence per 1000**
Parkinson's disease	19	2
Multiple sclerosis	7	2
Epilepsy	46	4
Cerebral palsy	3	3
Stroke	205	9

Source: MacDonald, B. K., Cockerell, O. C., Sander, J. W. and Shorvon, S. D. (2000). 'The Incidence and Lifetime Prevalence of Neurological Disorders in a Prospective Community-Based Study in the UK'. *Brain*, **123 (4)**: 665–76.

because of their earlier ages of onset. Epilepsy is the commonest neurological disorder but, unlike other significant neurological disease, may remit completely in some patients. We look first at Parkinson's disease, the commonest of the movement disorders.

11.1 **Parkinson's Disease**

In his 1817 monograph '*The Shaking Palsy*' James Parkinson described the major features of the illness that now bears his name from his observation of patients in London. The pathology of Parkinson's disease begins on one side of the brain, principally in the basal ganglia, producing clinical manifestations in the contralateral limbs. The pathological hallmark of the condition is the loss of pigmented dopaminergic neurons in the substantia nigra with associated eosinophilic, cytoplasmic inclusions called Lewy bodies in the surviving neurons. The deficiency of dopamine in the brain, first described by Hornykiewicz in 1959, led to the therapeutic use of levodopa (l-dopa) and dopamine agonists that act directly on dopamine receptors within the brain, which today are the mainstays of the treatment of Parkinson's disease. Indeed, it is considered that if a patient has a response to l-dopa he or she is more likely to have classical (idiopathic) Parkinson's disease, the commonest form of the disease.

Diagnosis and clinical course

Parkinson's disease is the clinical syndrome of involuntary asymmetrical tremor (a rhythmic oscillation of one or more body parts) associated with poverty and slowness of movement (bradykinesia), cogwheel rigidity, and postural gait changes. Despite almost two centuries of research into this disease, the diagnosis is still based on clinical examination. Parkinsonism or 'secondary Parkinsonism' relates to a syndrome of many conditions similar to Parkinson's disease except that these conditions have an identifiable cause, such as neuroleptic drugs or carbon monoxide exposure; usually they have a more severe disease course, which may be manifested as early gait disorder. Falls tend to occur within the first year; urinary incontinence, orthostatic hypotension, dysarthia, or dementia are likely to follow within the first four years (Samii *et al.* 2004). 🖳 In a community-based series, idiopathic Parkinson's disease accounted for 75–80 per cent of all Parkinsonian syndromes with a prevalence of about 360 per 100 000 (Tanner and Ben-Shlomo 1999). 🖳 Several other degenerative brain diseases can produce manifestations of atypical Parkinsonism, including multiple system atrophy, progressive supranuclear palsy, corticobasal degeneration, and dementia with Lewy bodies.

As there is no diagnostic test, with autopsy remaining the best reference for diagnosis, it is important to determine the accuracy of clinical diagnosis. It has been shown that even practising neurologists cannot always distinguish between different forms of Parkinsonism. One hundred cases accumulated in the Parkinson's Brain Bank in London showed that only 75 per cent of Parkinsonian syndromes conformed pathologically to a diagnosis of idiopathic Parkinson's disease. The remaining cases had alternative pathologies, so cases confidently diagnosed by competent consultant neurologists were found to have atypical pathology. However, using more modern methods, the accuracy was recently reported to be 90 per cent (Hughes *et al.* 2002). 🖳

Inevitably, there is thus strong motivation to find biomarkers that reflect pathological change and response to treatment. Clinical, imaging, and biochemical and genetic factors are being actively sought; probably a combination of several biomarkers will be needed, the likelihood being that none will fulfil all the criteria listed in Box 11.1 (Michell *et al.* 2004). 🖳

Descriptive epidemiology

Parkinson's disease is a disease of ageing. Incidence is very low before age 50 years (less than 10 per 100 000 population), and is usually associated with a hereditary form of Parkinsonism after which there is a gradual increase in incidence rising steeply after the age of 60 years, and increasing to at least 200 per 100 000 at age 80 years (Tanner and Ben Shlomo 1999). 🖳

Prevalence is somewhat higher. In the USA, crude prevalence of Parkinson's disease for all ages is approximately 150 per 100 000, ranging from 30 per 100 000 in those younger than 50 years to 800 per 100 000 in 75- to 80-year-olds. It has generally been reported that mortality is higher in Parkinsonian patients than in the general population, although more recent analyses suggest that although the condition produces disability, it is largely in those with severe disease who do not respond to treatment, that life expectancy is shortened. Twentyfold worldwide variation in risk of Parkinson's disease has been reported, but whether this indicates genetic or environmental factors is not clear. Men have approximately twice the incidence and prevalence of Parkinson's disease as women. In a Finnish study, there was no difference in relative risk in men compared with women in 1971 but 20 years later men had an almost twofold greater risk, suggesting a possible environmental causative factor to which men may be more exposed or are more susceptible than women.

Aetiology

The 1917–18 influenza pandemic probably caused *encephalitis lethargica* – characterized by high fever, headache, double vision, delayed physical and mental response, and lethargy – which led to a severe form of Parkinsonism; more recent studies have failed to link infectious agents with Parkinsonism. In the 1980s a proportion of narcotics abusers on the west coast of the USA developed a severe l-dopa responsive form of Parkinson's disease after contaminated injections with a mitochondrial protoxin. Subsequent studies then

---

BOX 11.1 CHARACTERISTICS OF THE IDEAL BIOMARKER THAT IS DESIGNED TO REFLECT A CHANGE IN PATHOLOGICAL OR CLINICAL TRAIT X

Close (first-degree) association with X without relying on intermediate variables, thereby minimizing the risk of dissociation.

It must sensitively reflect even small changes in X.

Treatment has no direct effect on the biomarker; it only changes with a true change in X.

The biomarker changes linearly (either negatively or positively) in response to a change in X.

Measurements are reproducible at a different time or in a different centre.

The biomarker should ideally capture all changes in X so that no information is lost.

The optimal clinical biomarker should be cheap, non-invasive and quick to measure by untrained staff.

Appropriately thorough validation of the above (depends on the use of the biomarker and implications of error).

Source: Mitchell, A. W., Lewis, S. J. G., Foltynie, T. and Barker, R. A. (2004). 'Biomarkers and Parkinson's Disease'. *Brain*, **127**:1693–1705.

indicated that certain pesticides like paraquat and rotenone, which had similar activity, can reproduce the pathology of Parkinson's disease in animals, and a recent meta-analysis in human studies suggested an odds ratio of 1.94 (95% CI 1.49–2.53) for pesticide exposure in Parkinsonian disease.

People who have had a high dietary intake of foods rich in antioxidants, high exposure to caffeine and those who have smoked cigarettes are less likely to develop Parkinson's disease. The inverse dose–response association with smoking – heavier smokers having lower risk that lighter smokers – has been a consistent aetiological finding in both retrospective and prospective studies (Fratiglioni and Wang 2000). 💻

> **Q1** What explanations could there be for the negative association between smoking and risk of Parkinson's disease?

Genetic factors

Recently pedigrees of dominantly inherited 'Parkinson's disease' were reported, which were identified to be idiopathic Parkinson's. The genes associated with these pedigrees are called 'Park' genes and at least ten have been described (Feaney 2004). 💻 The product of these genes, α-synuclein, is a major protein component of Lewy bodies. It is hypothesized that the pathogenesis of Parkinson's disease involves the abnormal folding, aggregation, and deposition of α-synuclein as key steps in mediating neuronal dysfunction and degeneration, and that certain mutations may predispose to this.

As the population ages, Parkinson's disease is set to become more common. The challenge of making a valid diagnosis is probably largely responsible for the paucity of population-based studies providing accurate data about incidence, prevalence, and mortality. If adequate biomarkers can be uncovered, diagnostic reliability will improve leading to better studies which, with developing genetic insights, will allow wider scope for treatment and prevention of this important disorder.

11.2 **Multiple Sclerosis**

Multiple sclerosis is the commonest disabling neurological disease in young Caucasian adults, and is second only to trauma as the leading cause of acquired neurological disability. Worldwide there are around 2.5 million affected individuals. Annual health expenditure on this disease in the UK is approximately £1.2 billion including indirect costs such as loss of earnings, child care, and similar expenditure.

This is a chronic inflammatory disease of the central nervous system, characterized by large multiple focal areas of **demyelination**, and is so called because multiple areas of sclerosis (hardening) are observed at autopsy. The first evidence of pathology is a breakdown of the blood–brain barrier, which allows activated lymphocytes to leak into the brain, leading to inflammation and loss of myelin surrounding the axons of neurons. These lesions, or plaques, vary in age and are distributed throughout the central nervous system from the cerebrum through the length of the spinal cord, corresponding to the scattering of clinical symptoms in time and space. They were first noted in 1865 by the French neurologist Charcot. There is limited capacity for remyelination and, as the disease progresses over time, repeated episodes of inflammation and demyelination lead to loss of nerve cells and fibres, frequently culminating in severe disability. Although the pathological basis for these changes is unknown, the pattern is similar to that in autoimmune disorders.

Disease description and clinical course

The clinical course is characterized by episodes of variable activity called relapses, separated by remissions or periods of quiescence. Symptoms vary both between and within individuals, reflecting the functional anatomy of impaired axonal conduction at affected sites, and include limb weakness, disturbed vision, sensory loss or imbalance, bladder and bowel incontinence, pain, and fatigue. Moreover, cognitive disturbance is observed in up to 65 per cent of patients. The course is heterogeneous but two major subtypes are generally recognized: **relapsing-remitting**, seen in around 85 per cent of cases and **primary progressive** in the remainder. In the former there are usually phases of relapse with recovery, with gradually poorer recovery and accumulating residual deficit, culminating in **secondary progressive** disease in which, after about 15–20 years, there is increasing disability without any clear clinical relapses. For a proportion of relapsing–remitting patients the disease runs a **benign** course with full recovery between episodes and no significant disability up to 15 years after disease onset, although, even here, sufficient follow-up usually reveals disabling disease. About 5 per cent of patients have very rapid progression of disability, and this is labelled **acute** or the **Marburg variant**.

Diagnosis

Because no single clinical feature or test is sufficient for the diagnosis of multiple sclerosis, diagnostic criteria have included a combination of clinical and paraclinical studies. Revised diagnostic criteria incorporating evidence from magnetic resonance imaging (MRI) classify individuals into three categories: (i) multiple sclerosis, for which a minimum of two attacks affecting more than one anatomical site are required; (ii) possible multiple sclerosis; and (iii) not multiple sclerosis (McDonald *et al.* 2001; Polman *et al.* 2005). 🖳

Descriptive epidemiology

Accurately estimating the prevalence and incidence is not straightforward. Incidence and prevalence figures have largely been derived from cross-sectional surveys, yielding incidence rates of around one to ten per 100 000 person-years and prevalences of 120–200 per 100 000. It appears that the prevalence is increasing, probably in part due to increasing incidence (although the evidence for this is conflicting), and improved survival due to better management. Several studies have shown that multiple sclerosis is associated with an elevated risk of death. In a large study of patients from the Danish multiple sclerosis registry, the median survival time from onset was 10 years shorter for multiple sclerosis patients than for the age-matched general population, representing a threefold increase in the risk of death. More than half died from the disease itself, but excess mortality was also observed for several other diseases, and from accidents and suicide (Bronnum-Hansen *et al.* 2004). 🖳

> **Q2** Why is the prevalence of multiple sclerosis up to 500 times higher than disease incidence?

Greater precision in measuring disease burden can be gained from prospective studies. In the Danish registry, operating since 1948, nearly all Danish residents in whom the disease was diagnosed by a neurologist have been registered, and the diagnosis has been reviewed and classified, according to standardized diagnostic criteria, with overall diagnostic accuracy and completeness estimated at 94 per cent and 90 per cent, respectively. A UK study using capture–recapture techniques (see Chapter 2) demonstrated that the north–south gradient in the prevalence of multiple sclerosis was not an artefactual finding (Forbes and Swingler 1999). 🖳

Aetiology and risk factors

The cause of multiple sclerosis is unknown but it is clear that both environmental and genetic factors are involved. Significant geographical and ethnic differences in occurrence are observed. Among Eskimos, the Aboriginals of Australia, and the Bantu people of Southern Africa the disease is virtually unknown; and in Indians, Chinese,

and Japanese the distribution of lesions is different to that in people of European ancestry. These findings cannot be explained on the basis of population genetics alone. Outside Europe, prevalence rates among White people are half those documented for many parts of northern Europe. It has been suggested that adult immigrants retain the risk factor of their country of origin, whereas their children tend towards the risk factor of their host country. The hypothesis that an environmental factor acquired in childhood conveys a risk of developing multiple sclerosis in later life is supported by two **migrant** studies: firstly there is a low, second-generation risk in emigrants from high-risk countries such as the UK to South Africa; and secondly, that immigrants to the UK from areas of low risk (for example West Indies) have a low prevalence, but their British-born children have the same high prevalence as British Caucasians. Migrant studies and their methodological limitations have been reviewed in detail elsewhere (Gayle and Martyn 1995). 🖳

The **clusters** of the disease observed in several isolated populations, most notably the Faroe Islands, are considered by some to point to evidence for a transmissible agent, as the epidemic occurred after the occupation by British troops between 1941 and 1944.

It has been hypothesized that exposure to ubiquitous infectious agents may trigger the immune system to react against the brain; possible candidates include *Chlamydia pneumoniae*, human herpes virus 6, measles, herpes simplex, HSV-6, and Epstein–Barr virus (EBV). A meta-analysis by Ascherio and Munch (2000) 🖳 showed that the risk of multiple sclerosis was more than 10 times greater in EBV-positive individuals than in those who were EBV-negative. Non-infectious agents may also be implicated in disease risk or modulation, but evidence for a role for smoking or low antioxidant and vitamin D concentrations is weak or conflicting.

Increased disease risk is seen within families; risk is highest in identical monozygotic (MZ) twins (20–35 per cent), then dizygotic (DZ) twins and other siblings (2–5 per cent), then parents, and finally first cousins, whereas the frequency in adoptees is similar to that in the general population. If multiple sclerosis showed simple Mendelian inheritance, the risk in MZ twins would be close to unity, but as this is not so it indicates that multiple sclerosis is a complex trait in which susceptibility is determined by several genes acting independently (**epistatically**). In common with most other complex traits, no major susceptibility gene has been identified, but regions of interest have been provisionally identified. Multiple sclerosis affects twice as many women as it does men, mimicking the ratio seen in other putative autoimmune diseases. The lifetime risk for a young woman in Northern Ireland or Scotland of developing the disease is about 1 in 200 (McDonnell and Hawkins 1998). ⌨ Susceptibility seems to be conferred by genes within the major histocompatibility complex, although recent studies indicate that other loci are also involved. The relative rarity of multiple sclerosis, and the complexities and heterogeneity of the disorder, suggest that large studies and pooled data from several investigations will be required to properly elucidate its genetic nature. Along with these, advances in technology are likely to make genetic studies more fruitful. Nevertheless, multiple sclerosis presents major obstacles for both patient and researcher, and there is much to understand before preventive and therapeutic modalities can be designed.

Therapy

There have been considerable recent advances in the treatment of multiple sclerosis. In particular, interferon-beta has been demonstrated in several independent, multicentre clinical trials to lower unequivocally the biological activity of relapsing–remitting and secondary progressive disease, and of clinically isolated syndromes. The results of these trials have been consistent, demonstrating a reduction in both disease activity and cumulative disability, using a combination of clinical MRI outcome measures and, more recently, measures of brain atrophy (Miller 2004). ⌨ On balance, convincing evidence is provided to support the notion that there is a clinically relevant dose–response in the use of interferon-beta to treat patients with relapsing/remitting disease, although this remains an active area of current research.

> **Q3** You have resources to set up a register for multiple sclerosis. What factors are important to maximize the potential of the register?

11.3 **Epilepsy**

The term **epilepsy** encompasses several syndromes whose cardinal feature is a predisposition to recurrent unprovoked seizures. Although epilepsy is the most common serious neurological condition, affecting 40 million people worldwide, its epidemiology remains poorly understood. Various factors contribute to this deficiency; differences in inclusion criteria can elevate (for example inclusion of febrile seizures) or deflate (exclusion of non-active epilepsies) prevalence figures,

cases ascertained using hospital records may underestimate true community levels, while coding errors also lead to inaccuracies.

Definition and classification of epilepsy

An epileptic **seizure** is an intermittent, stereotyped disturbance of behaviour, emotion, motor function, or sensation accompanied by an abnormal cortical neuronal discharge, which may lead to altered consciousness. Anyone can have a seizure if the circumstances are appropriate, and triggers such as hormonal changes, stress, or fever may provoke onset. Those with a low seizure threshold are more at risk of developing epilepsy. An isolated seizure does not necessarily warrant the diagnosis of epilepsy, which is specifically defined as a disorder in which the individual has a tendency to experience spontaneous and *recurrent* seizures. For most epidemiological studies, two unprovoked seizures on separate occasions are necessary to define the disease (Hauser *et al.* 1998). ⌨ For many patients, epilepsy is relatively short-lived, over two-thirds entering early remission, after which relapse is uncommon.

Essential for epidemiological investigation, accurate **classification** of seizures is also required to ensure appropriate management. Unfortunately, this is not straightforward. The most widely used classification, developed by the International League Against Epilepsy, and recently revised, takes account of the clinical manifestations of a seizure, which depend on where in the brain the discharge originates and spreads. The two main types are: (primary) **generalized** in which both cerebral hemispheres are affected simultaneously, usually resulting in loss of consciousness and motor or sensory symptoms, and **partial** (or focal) affecting only part of the brain, sometimes without impaired consciousness. **Secondary generalized** seizures are partial seizures that spread to become generalized. Electroencephalograph (EEG) recordings may assist the clinical classification as different seizure types are usually accompanied by characteristic EEG changes. However, **inter-ictal** EEGs (between attacks) tend to be of limited value.

> **Q4(a)** Accurate case definition is an essential part of epidemiology, but diagnosing seizure may not be straightforward. What other conditions may be confused with seizure?
>
> **Q4(b)** Apart from drug toxicity what other *personal* issues would arise from being (mis)diagnosed with epilepsy?

Descriptive epidemiology

A meta-analysis of incidence studies of epilepsy reported an overall incidence rate (omitting febrile and single convulsions) of around five per 10 000 per year (Kotsopoulos *et al.* 2002). 🖳 In the 1958 UK national child development study cohort, based on over 17 000 children born in March 1958, the cumulative incidence of confirmed epilepsy was 8.4 per 1000 by the age of 23 years, with an active prevalence of 6.3 per 1000. Lifetime prevalence has been estimated at 2–5 per cent, far in excess of the active prevalence of 6–10 cases per 1000, confirming the self-limiting nature of most seizures. Of the approximately 160 000 people in the UK with active epilepsy, around 25 000 have more than one major seizure per month, and over double this number have a similar rate of minor attacks. Up to 20 000 have advanced disease with attendant handicaps that may necessitate institutional care. Risk at birth is about 1 per cent until the age of 20 years, rising to 3 per cent by the age of 75 years (cumulative incidence). Summary descriptive data by age are shown in Figure 11.1.

Individuals with epilepsy are known to have greater risk of death than the general population, particularly among the young and in the first five to ten years after diagnosis. The UK National General Practice Study of Epilepsy, a prospective, population-based study of people with newly diagnosed epilepsy, estimated that life expectancy can be reduced by up to two years for people with a diagnosis of idiopathic/cryptogenic epilepsy, and the reduction can be up to ten years in people with symptomatic epilepsy. Reductions in life expectancy are highest at the time of diagnosis and diminish with time (Gaitatzis and Sander 2004). 🖳 After 1950, epilepsy mortality declined steeply in people younger than age 20 years. For young and middle-aged adults, the rate of decline was lower, whereas in people aged 65 years and over, mortality initially declined but rose again from 1974 onwards. There was general evidence of a fall in epilepsy mortality with each successive birth cohort after 1905, in parallel with improvements in antenatal care and perinatal mortality (O'Callaghan *et al.* 2000). 🖳

Aetiology and risk factors

Onset of epilepsy is age-related, with many seizures occurring in infancy and childhood, but the incidence is also high in later life (see Figure 11.1); there is also an upward secular trend in epilepsy among individuals aged 60 years and above, probably because of an ageing population with longer life expectancy and increased risk of diseases such as stroke. A 34 per cent increase in the proportion of incidence cases in those aged 65 years or more between 1985 and 1994 has been described in the Rochester, Minnesota, population.

Environmental factors

In most cases of epilepsy no specific cause can be found (60–70 per cent) (idiopathic epilepsy), but a national UK study found the following aetiologies: cerebrovascular disease 15 per cent, cerebral tumours 6 per cent, alcohol 6 per cent, trauma 2 per cent, developmental 8.0 per cent; any other causes, including specific epilepsy syndromes, were rare. However, age of diagnosis was very important in determining cause, with epilepsy in children largely due to developmental conditions, infections, and, to a lesser extent, trauma. In young adults, trauma was the major risk, whereas in middle age, trauma and tumour accounted for the bulk of disease, with cerebrovascular aetiology becoming steadily more important with advancing age. In this latter group, degenerative conditions also led to epilepsy.

Febrile convulsions in infancy, particularly complex febrile convulsions, are associated with subsequent risk of epilepsy in cohort studies, and a recent community-based study reported a twofold increase in risk of epilepsy in the most socioeconomically deprived fifth of the population in a UK region (Heaney *et al.* 2002). 🖳 These latter findings suggest associations with birth defects, trauma, infection, and poor nutrition, which are known to be more common in non-affluent populations.

Brain injury accounts for approximately 13 per cent of epilepsy of presumed cause; the severity of the injury is directly related to the subsequent incidence of

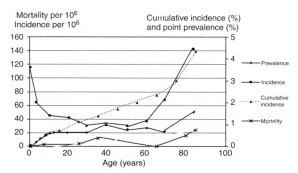

Fig. 11.1 Epidemiological indicator for epilepsy by age in population-based studies in Rochester, Minnesota.
Source: Redrawn from Annegers, J. F. (2004). 'Epilepsy', in L. M. Nelson. C. M. Tanner, S. K. Van Den Eeden, and V. M. McGuire, (eds.), *Neuroepidemiology. From Principles to Practice.* Oxford: Oxford University Press.

epilepsy, but the period of risk appears to be limited to five years after the insult. A similar period of risk follows bacterial meningitis, with a fivefold increase in risk. Viral encephalitis carries a tenfold increase in risk and the period of risk is 15 or more years. Taken together, all brain infections are believed to account for up to 5 per cent of epilepsy cases. Cerebrovascular disease is the major cause of seizures in the elderly, but there are few valid data on the magnitude of the effect or its duration. Seizures occurring for the first time in late life, without a predisposing cause, may indicate increased risk of stroke (Cleary *et al.* 2004). ⬚ Brain tumours account for around 12 per cent of acquired epilepsy, with risk being greatest in 25–64 year-olds. Almost one-third of individuals with newly diagnosed brain tumours develop seizures, although these are rarely persistent. Developmental and degenerative diseases also increase the risk of epilepsy.

Genetic factors

Although seizure disorders aggregate in families, there are very few Mendelian seizure disorders. On the other hand, mutations in over 70 genes now define biological pathways leading to epilepsy, and the list of genes will certainly expand (Noebels 2003). ⬚ Better understanding of the molecular and cellular circumstances that predispose to seizure could have implications for prevention and development of more effective anticonvulsive treatments, possibly including gene therapies. An unresolved puzzle is why risk is higher in children whose mother has epilepsy rather than the father. At least 12 forms of epilepsy have been demonstrated to possess some genetic basis. For example, LaFora disease (progressive myoclonic, type 2), an autosomal recessive disorder and a particularly aggressive epilepsy, is characterized by the presence of glycogen-like Lafor bodies in the brain.

Treatment and prevention

Although a novel (medical or surgical) treatment option for epilepsy was marketed almost every year during the past decade, many patients still experience uncontrolled seizures or have adverse effects (Nguyen and Spencer 2003). ⬚ Treatment effectiveness can be monitored by seizure diaries, and quality of life scales have also been designed for people with epilepsy.

Epilepsy raises additional problems in women of child-bearing years; female hormones can influence seizure control and drug treatments can affect hormonal contraception, fertility, and the developing embryo. Previous studies have shown an increased risk of major congenital malformations (neural tube defects in particular) from prenatal exposure to phenytoin and sodium valproate, as these inhibit folate metabolism. Folate supplementation is now given routinely to all female patients of child-bearing age who are taking these drugs. Teratogenic effects of current and newer drugs and possible effects on cognitive and behavioural development of the offspring are increasingly being explored. A UK register of women who take epilepsy drugs during pregnancy has been set up to allow better monitoring of the effects on mothers and their offspring and to ultimately enable more informed recommendation of seizure medication (Craig and Morrow 1997). ⬚ Similar initiatives have been established in the USA (NEAD Study 2003). ⬚

As noted previously, both in the UK and in the USA there has been a decline in mortality from epilepsy, possibly linked to improvements in antenatal care (O'Callaghan *et al.* 2000), ⬚ but improvements may also have occurred in secondary care. Epilepsy can perhaps be best viewed as a heterogeneous disorder with different aetiologies in the young and in the elderly and consequently requiring differing strategies towards prevention.

> **Q5** Table 11.2 shows mortality data from community-based studies of epilepsy. Why do you think there is such disparity in the risks of death?

11.4 **Cerebral Palsy**

Introduction

Cerebral palsy is a disorder of voluntary movement and posture caused by damage to the developing brain and is relatively rare, affecting 2–2.5 per 1000 of the population in the developed world (SCPE 2004). ⬚ However, it is the commonest cause of severe physical disability in childhood and is often associated with other impairments affecting intellect, vision, hearing, and communication, and can include seizure disorders. As might be expected, those with the more severe and complex forms of cerebral palsy are at higher risk of early mortality, although developments in medical care, for example artificial feeding, antibiotics and respiratory management, have increased life expectancy. Consequently, an estimated 85 per cent or more of people with cerebral palsy survive to age 20 years, and this has implications for health and social services provision as well as medico-legal settlements (Hemming *et al.* 2005). ⬚

TABLE 11.2 Community-based studies of all-cause mortality in epilepsy

Study setting	Methods	Follow-up	Age	SMR (95% CI)
Rochester Minnesota, USA	Retrospective incidence cohort	34 years	All	2.1 (1.9–2.5)
UK	Prospective incidence cohort	14 years	All	2.1 (1.8–2.4)
Iceland	Retrospective incidence cohort	30 years	All	1.6 (1.2–2.2)
Sweden	Prospective incidence cohort	11 years	All?	2.5 (1.6–3.8)
France	Prospective incidence cohort	1 year	All	9.4 (8–11)
Switzerland	Retrospective incidence cohort	10 years	All	7.0 (6.2–8.4)
Wales	Retrospective incidence cohort	6 years	All	2.1 (1.7–2.6)
Canada	Retrospective incidence cohort	15 years	Children 1 month–6 years	8.8 (4.1–13.4)

SMR – Standard Mortality Ratio.

Source: Adapted from Gaitatzis, A. and Sander, J. W. (2004). 'The Mortality of Epilepsy Revisited'. *Epileptic Disorders*, **6**, 3–13.

Definition

The term 'cerebral palsy' refers to a collection of disorders affecting voluntary movement and posture resulting in loss of motor function. Cerebral palsy is generally caused by damage to the developing brain some time during pregnancy, delivery, or in the neonatal period, and is sometimes referred to as 'congenital' cerebral palsy. With developments in neuroimaging it is becoming apparent that cerebral palsy is often associated with observable neuropathology; that is, static lesions or brain malformation evident with MRI (Krageloh-Mann et al. 1995). ▭ Although the damage to the brain is non-progressive, the clinical presentation of cerebral palsy can change over time as a result of growth and maturation, sometimes leading to improved function, but at other times giving rise to complications such as muscle contractures, bony deformities, and deteriorating abilities. Cerebral palsy can also occur after the neonatal period in 'early childhood'; this is called 'acquired' or postneonatal cerebral palsy. This subgroup accounts for 7–14 per cent of all cases and, from an aetiological perspective, is a distinct group with childhood infections, trauma, surgical complications, and non-accidental injury as the main causes.

Clinical presentation

There are three main cerebral palsy subtypes. Spastic cerebral palsy is the commonest (85–90 per cent of cases), and presents with velocity-related increased muscle tone in one or more limbs. Spastic cerebral palsy is associated with damage to the motor cortex and internal capsule of the brain. Dyskinetic cerebral palsy (fewer than 10 per cent of cases) presents with slow, writhing and involuntary movements, with fluctuating tone and total body involvement due to damage in the basal ganglia. Ataxic cerebral palsy (fewer than 5 per cent of cases) presents as short and jerky movements with low tone, and is associated with damage to the cerebellum. It is also possible to have 'mixed' subtypes (for example spastic–dyskinetic or spastic–ataxic), where there is increased tone, usually in the legs, accompanied by slow and writhing, or short and jerky, movements as a result of damage to the pyramidal and extrapyramidal structures of the brain.

Aetiology

The following discussion is confined to congenital rather than to postneonatal cerebral palsy, because, as noted above, the latter forms a distinct aetiological group. In contrast, the precise causes of congenital forms of cerebral palsy are unknown and the opportunities for primary prevention remain limited (Nelson 2003). ▭ This is because the timing of adverse events during foetal and infant development is difficult to assign, and is also associated with many possible biological factors. However, it is important to distinguish between those born at term (37+ weeks), those born preterm (less than 37 weeks), and very prematurely (less than 32 weeks). These scenarios represent different causal pathways in cerebral palsy (Stanley et al. 2000). ▭ For example, most cerebral palsy in term infants (more than 75 per cent) is believed to be of prenatal origin related more to cerebral malformations, intra-uterine infection, or placental insufficiency, whereas fewer than 10 per cent are related to possible intrapartum events, of which suboptimal care is only one possibility (Blair and Stanley 1993). 💻 Evidence to support prenatal aetiology includes an excess of congenital malformations and growth restriction among infants with cerebral palsy born at term when compared with the unaffected population. Most cerebral palsy in preterm babies (75–90 per cent) is believed to be of perinatal origin. Evidence to support perinatal aetiology includes abnormal brain scans taken in the first week of life in infants who subsequently develop cerebral palsy.

The preterm brain is prone to damage of the white matter caused by bleeding and ischaemia due to inadequate regulation of cerebral blood flow. These complications can span the antenatal, intrapartum, and postnatal periods, but in preterm babies most complications are thought to occur postnatally (Stanley *et al.* 2000). 💻 The periventricular region of the brain is particularly vulnerable to fluctuations in perfusion during weeks 26–36 of development (Hagberg and Hagberg 1993). 💻 This contrasts with the brain of babies born at term, where regulation of the cardiovascular system is well established, but the brain's oxygen requirements are greater. At term, several areas of the brain are particularly sensitive to the effects of asphyxia and oxygen deprivation; these include the cortical and subcortical areas, the basal ganglia, and thalamus.

Risk factors

It is well established that birthweight and gestational age are strongly inversely associated with cerebral palsy. Although gestational age is the single, strongest determinant of cerebral palsy (Stanley *et al.* 2000), 💻 birthweight-specific rates are most often cited in epidemiological studies. Birthweight is used as a proxy for gestational age (or maturity) as it is easier to measure and more readily available. Figure 11.2 shows the relation between birthweight and cerebral palsy. These data are from the geographically defined case register, the Northern Ireland Cerebral Palsy Register, and comprise 893 congenital cases born during 1981–97 when there was a total of 412 256 livebirths, giving an overall prevalence of 2.2 (95% CI 2.0–2.3) per 1000 livebirths (Parkes *et al.* 2005). 💻

> **Q6** The risk of cerebral palsy increases with decreasing birthweight. Why then in Figure 11.2 is the rate of cerebral palsy among the 1000–1499 g group greater than the <1000 g group?

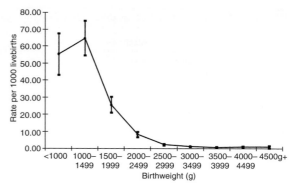

Fig. 11.2 Birthweight-specific prevalence of cerebral palsy per 1000 livebirths for the birth period 1983–97 in Northern Ireland (excludes 1988).

Birthweight and gestation have independent effects on the risk of cerebral palsy and represent the scenarios of being born too small and/or too soon. The relative risk of cerebral palsy among babies born very prematurely (less than 32 weeks) is up to 100 times greater than risk in those born at term (37+ weeks). The risk of cerebral palsy among babies born very small (less than 1500 g) is about 70 times greater than that in those of normal birthweight (2500 g+). These higher risks are particularly evident if the rate of cerebral palsy is expressed per neonatal survivors and not livebirths. This is because mortality is highest among the smallest and most premature infants (up to 50 per cent for the most extreme groups). Rates based on neonatal survivors tend to be higher than rates based on livebirths as the population 'at risk' has been depleted. However, the attributable risk of very premature and small babies developing cerebral palsy is small, as these births constitute only about 1 per cent of all livebirths in developed countries.

The risk of cerebral palsy also increases when the weight for gestational age is well above the norm (large for gestational age) or below the norm (small for gestational age) (Jarvis *et al.* 2003). 💻 The risk increases tenfold in the case of babies who are small for gestational age, although this increase mainly affects those born at term (37+ weeks) or moderately preterm (32–37 weeks) but not the premature (less than 32 weeks).

Another important risk factor for cerebral palsy is multiple birth, mainly related to the higher rate of premature birth among this group. Twins (who represent around 2 per cent of all births) constitute about 10 per cent of all cerebral palsy cases, and the rate of cerebral palsy among this group is sevenfold that for singletons (Williams *et al.* 1996). 💻 The origin of cerebral palsy in multiple births stems from poor uterine growth, complications of preterm delivery, congenital malformations, placental complications and, in monozygotic multiple pregnancies, from problems related to shared blood supply and, if monochorionic, to cord entanglement. It has been postulated that the death of a monozygotic co-foetus may be a significant cause of spastic cerebral palsy (Pharoah and Cooke 1997). ▯ This is associated with the increased risk of sharing a vascular supply and developing twin-to-twin transfusion syndrome, which has a poor outcome. The early detection and recording of multiple pregnancies and their outcome (including early losses) is important, and could provide important clues about the causal mechanisms.

Trends in prevalence

It is difficult to be definitive about trends in cerebral palsy between 1950 and 1970 because reports conflict. The Surveillance of Cerebral Palsy in Europe project (SCPE 2002) reported an increase in the overall rate of cerebral palsy during the 1970s, which stabilized during the late 1980s. The apparent, but relatively small, increase during this time has been attributed to an increase in the survival of low and very low birthweight babies. Secular trends in the prevalence of cerebral palsy can only really be understood when rates are stratified by birthweight or gestational age. Most case registers of cerebral palsy have reported statistically significant increases in the rates of cerebral palsy among the very low birthweight group (less than 1500 g) in the 1980s, but before 1985 in particular. It is unclear

to what extent these increases represent improved survival of already compromised babies or the improved survival of babies at higher risk of developing cerebral palsy because of their prematurity, or elements of both.

Establishing reliable prevalence rates of cerebral palsy

Surveillance of cerebral palsy cannot be based on a simple case count as the condition varies by type, severity, aetiology, and pathology and is difficult to define and classify in a standardized way. The ability to group together similarly defined cases of cerebral palsy and clinical subtypes is essential to reliably monitor geographic and temporal trends, undertake aetiological research and plan services. Several important methodological issues are worthy of note in the interpretation or compilation of statistics on cerebral palsy (see Box 11.2).

Routine child-health information systems have been found to be incomplete and are an unreliable source of information on children with cerebral palsy, partly because they tend to adopt a simple case-count approach. In contrast, successful case registers of cerebral palsy tend to use predetermined inclusion criteria, multiple and overlapping sources of ascertainment, a standardized approach to classification, and active surveillance of a geographic population over time (Cans et al. 2004). ▯ In particular, follow-up of infants up to five years of age at least is important to establish eligibility for inclusion, and monitoring the population for emigration, migration, and death also assists accuracy.

BOX 11.2 METHODOLOGICAL ISSUES WHEN COMPARING CEREBRAL PALSY PREVALENCE RATES BETWEEN POPULATIONS

Case definition	• Conforms with international definition (SCPE2000)
	• Inclusion/exclusion criteria stated
	• Differentiation of congenital and postnatal cases
Case ascertainment	• Geographically defined register with multiple sources of ascertainment
	• Professional and voluntary sectors should be checked for cases
Denominator data	• Match to case-register geographic area
	• Basic data required are livebirths, infant and child mortality, and population at risk
Incidence and prevalence	• Prevalence is preferred measure as cases may only be detected at five years of age or more
	• Based on neonatal survivors
Age at ascertainment	• Incomplete registration may result if cases ascertained before five years of age
Deaths, immigration, and emigration	• Flagging of cases using NHS central register may be useful to follow removals within the UK

Conclusions

Cerebral palsy is likely to affect 2–2.5 per 1000 of the population for the foreseeable future. Continued surveillance of cerebral palsy over time is required to monitor the effect of improved survival of very small and premature infants, the severity of the condition, and the effect of new technologies such as assisted reproduction. International collaborative work in the epidemiology of relatively rare conditions such as cerebral palsy offers an important way forward.

Further Reading

Nelson, L. M., Tanner, C. M., Van Den Eeeden, S. K. and McGuire, V. M. (eds.) (2004). *Neuroepidemiology*. New York, NY: Oxford University Press.

Stanley, F., Blair, E. and Alberman, E. (2000). *Cerebral Palsies: Epidemiology and Causal Pathways. Clinics in Developmental Medicine*. London: Mac Keith Press, 151.

Web Addresses

Cerebral Palsy Registers, http://www.liv.ac.uk/Public Health/ukcp/UKCP.htm.

European Collaboration on Cerebral Palsy, http://www-rheop.ujf-grenoble.fr/scpe2/site_scpe/index.php.

Parkes *et al.* Report on Cerebral Palsy for Northern Ireland, http://www.qub.ac.uk/nur/cpconf.htm.

References

References for this chapter can be found at www.oxfordtextbooks.co.uk/orc/yarnell. Where possible, these are presented as *active links* which direct you to an electronic version of the work. If you are a subscriber to that work (either individually or through an institution), and depending on your level of access, you may be able to peruse an abstract or the full article if available. 🖥

Model answers

Q1

(a) The association may be due to chance: but over 40 studies, some prospective, have reported the same finding.

(b) Reverse causality is also ruled out because in prospective studies individuals without disease would have been non-smokers long before disease onset; prospective studies also overcome the problem of recall bias which can occur in case–control studies.

(c) The association may be real, and animal studies suggest that nicotine protects against experimental Parkinsonism.

(d) Alternatively, it has been suggested that decreased smoking in Parkinson's disease is a sign of the conservative personality that has been noted in patients before their diagnosis.

Q2 Incidence is rare, but as multiple sclerosis often occurs in young people and has no cure and a relatively low excess mortality, patients generally survive for a long time after diagnosis, thus making the number of people with the disease much higher than the number of new cases.

Q3

● Accurate demographic data to determine denominator: for example, census.

● Sources of data: inpatient and outpatient clinics, individual physicians, especially neurologists, health insurance organizations, multiple sclerosis societies, and support organizations.

● Diagnostic criteria to validate diagnosis.

● Success depends on the probability that an individual with multiple sclerosis is diagnosed and that this individual is identified by the search, which is determined in part by the completeness of the provider lists.

Q4

(a) Syncope, pseudo-seizures, transient ischaemic attack, breath-holding episodes, and narcolepsy, etc.

(b) A diagnosis of epilepsy may preclude certain types of employment and, unless treatment renders the patient seizure-free continuously for a minimum period of 12 months, a driving licence cannot be issued.

Q5 Because the population at risk appears to be similar for all cohorts it is likely that differences in the case-definition of epilepsy in the various studies account for the discrepancies in the mortality rates.

Q6 It is likely that the pre-natal mortality rate is higher in foetuses under 1000 g in weight. Additionally these deaths are likely to occur as miscarriages (before 24 weeks) rather than as stillbirths (after 24 weeks).

Mental disorders

Chapter contents

Four major disorders of mental health are discussed in this chapter, focusing on the problems of disease definition and their descriptive epidemiology: schizophrenia, depression and anxiety, dementia, and learning disability. In addition the epidemiology of suicide is described as it is frequently associated with mental disorder (although the International Classification of Disease (ICD) includes it under 'accidents, poisonings and violence', based on the external cause of death).

Introduction

'Mental disorder' or mental illness is an umbrella term that is used to describe many different psychiatric conditions with various causes and effects. The word 'mental' tends to elicit negative connotations, and stigma is a serious problem encountered by people with a mental illness, not least because it may pose a major obstacle to seeking help. To an individual, mental health is just as important as physical health, and a recent systematic review of one type of mental disorder – depression – concluded that depressive disorders account for the fourth most common disease burden in women and the seventh most common in men; thus mental disorders represent a major public-health challenge (Ustun *et al.* 2004). 🖳 The systems of classifying mental or psychiatric illnesses are based on a description of symptoms and natural history rather than on causes, mainly because the causes appear to be multifactorial: genetic, physical, psychological, and social factors have all been reported to contribute to these disorders.

There are significant problems involved in defining and measuring mental disorders and, therefore, in determining incidence and prevalence rates in the population. For example in the USA, the Epidemiological Catchment Area Study found a lifetime prevalence rate for mental disorder of around 38 per cent compared with 48 per cent reported in the National Co-morbidity Survey (Kessler *et al.* 1994). 🖳 Clearly, psychiatrists, psychologists, and epidemiologists need to improve the methods of measuring mental disorders by standardizing operational definitions, to produce reliable and consistent epidemiological estimates of mental disorders in the population. Prevalence estimates, based on 'treated' populations, often underestimate the 'true' population prevalence. Furthermore, population surveys using questionnaires or rating scales, in common with all continuously distributed variables, are based on a cut-point or threshold value denoting 'disease'. This chapter should be read with these methodological problems in mind.

Mental illness is often conceptualized in terms of psychoses or neuroses. People who experience a psychotic mental illness such as **schizophrenia** tend to lose their grasp or understanding of reality. Neuroses such as **anxiety** and depression tend to be less severe, though more common than psychoses. The category of 'mental disorders' used in the ICD system includes various types of psychotic and neurotic illness, as well as conditions relating to developmental or behavioural irregularities (collectively termed **learning disabilities**) in addition to drug misuse, eating problems, sexual difficulties, and personality disorder. Mental illness may be conceptualized also in terms of **organic** versus **functional** disorders. An organic disorder, such as **dementia** (experienced by 1 in 20 or more people aged over 65 years), is a condition that appears due to physical changes in the brain. However, most mental disorders are labelled 'functional' in that they are not due to structural abnormalities of the brain, nor do they have any known biological cause. This chapter focuses on the epidemiology of the major disorders including: schizophrenia; depression, which commonly coexists with anxiety; dementia; and learning disability. The estimated point prevalence of each is shown in Box 12.1. Suicide and parasuicide are more appropriately described using mortality and incidence; they are discussed in the concluding section of the chapter.

12.1 Schizophrenia

Definition

Schizophrenia is a complex brain disorder first recognized by the European psychiatrists Kraepelin and Bleuler in the late nineteenth century. It was Bleuler who

---

BOX 12.1 PREVALENCE ESTIMATES FOR MAJOR MENTAL DISORDERS IN THE GENERAL POPULATION

Type of disorder	Prevalence (%)
Any mental disorder	28–29
Schizophrenia	0.7–1.0
Unipolar depression	1.9–3.2
All forms of depression	9.6–20.4
Anxiety (generalized)	3–5
Dementia	5–8 (>65 years); 20–34.5 (>85 years)
Learning disability	0.3–0.4 (severe); 2.5–3.0 (mild)

Data from: Kessler *et al.* (1994); WHO (2001); Launer *et al.* (1999); Fryers (2002). 🖳

originated the term schizophrenia from the Greek words 'schizein', meaning, 'to split' and 'phren', meaning 'mind'. This captures the fundamental nature of the condition, which is characterized by marked and sometimes bizarre disturbances in cognitive, emotional, and social functioning, all of which may profoundly affect the quality of life of patients and their families (see Wilkinson et al. 2000). Broadly, the symptoms include: disordered thinking, attention, and perception; flat or inappropriate affect (the formal psychiatric term for mood); and social withdrawal.

Schizophrenia is the most heterogeneous and debilitating of all the mental disorders, with a clinical picture and aetiology that may vary widely from one individual to the next; the ICD-10 classification of mental disorders describes nine different sub-types, including paranoid schizophrenia and simple schizophrenia. The course of the illness, which may be continuous or episodic in nature, also shows high inter-individual variability. Despite continuing controversy and difficulties surrounding its diagnosis, the key clinical features are typically categorized into *positive* and *negative* symptoms, both of which may co-exist. The former are most closely identified with the disorder and usually accompany an acute episode. They include incoherent speech, delusions (that is, false unrealistic beliefs) and hallucinations (that is, sensory experiences not shared by others, such as hearing voices). The more chronic negative symptoms reflect an absence, or a reduction in normal behaviour and refer mainly to flat affect (impaired or absent emotional expression and responsiveness), apathy and severe social impairment.

The disorder may affect many aspects of patients' lives, placing them at increased risk of developing problems related to homelessness, depression, substance abuse, and suicide. Substance abuse, in particular, has been estimated to occur in more than one-third of people with schizophrenia in the UK, whereas estimates from the USA suggest a figure closer to 50 per cent. The treatment of such co-morbidity presents considerable difficulties for addiction and mental health services, not least because they tend to operate within different ideological frameworks. Furthermore, there is, as yet, little evidence to inform appropriate service development in this area (Weaver et al. 1999).

Descriptive and aetiological epidemiology

The lifetime prevalence of schizophrenia is approximately 1 per cent, with an incidence rate of approximately two cases per 10 000 population per annum. Its prevalence and incidence are broadly similar across different cultures, although developing countries report better outcomes. Onset typically occurs in late adolescence or early adulthood; men and women appear to be equally at risk, although men tend to have poorer long-term outcomes. It has been estimated that approximately 13 per cent of those with mental disorders who present to their general practitioner have schizophrenia; but many of these patients, owing to the nature of the illness and the continuing perceived stigma, may avoid contact with both primary and secondary services for many years.

Multiple factors appear to be involved in the aetiology of schizophrenia. Convincing evidence has accumulated from family, twin and adoption studies to illustrate the significant contribution of genetic factors, while biological influences (for example obstetric complications) have also been implicated (Thomas et al. 2001). The risk of developing schizophrenia increases dramatically if a sibling or parent has the diagnosis (around nine and twelve times higher, respectively, than in the general population); recent research suggests that at least seven genes may be involved (Harrison and Owen 2003). However, epidemiological studies have identified several other socioeconomic and cultural factors that may interact with genetic influences including social class, membership of (non-White) ethnic minorities, nutritional deficiencies, and a history of taking drugs such as lysergic acid diethylamide (LSD) and heavy use of cannabis (see Chapter 17). Importantly, social class has been identified repeatedly as a significant risk marker for schizophrenia. Research has shown that those in lower socioeconomic groups are around five times more likely than others to be diagnosed with schizophrenia and have less favourable outcomes. This is widely thought to be due to downward social *drifting* caused by the cumulative impairments in functioning that result from developing the illness (the **socio-genic hypothesis**). However, the role of social class *at birth* on relative risk, or on the course of the disorder remains unclear.

Mulvaney et al. (2001) used a case–control design to investigate the effect of social class of origin on the risk of schizophrenia and age at first presentation. Almost 400 patients with first presentation of schizophrenia were matched with the next registered same-sex birth from the same birth registration district and compared on several outcome measures. The authors reported no statistically significant differences between cases and controls in terms of social class distribution. However, people in the lower social classes tended to present later (mean age 33.1 years) than those in higher social classes (mean age 24.8 years), suggesting that social class influences the age at which treatment is first received.

Prevention

The strong genetic predisposition to schizophrenia makes attempts at primary prevention difficult. However, the **stress-vulnerability model** provides a useful framework within which psychosocial and environmental factors may mediate this genetic vulnerability and ultimately prevent the full-blown expression of the illness. According to this model, the development and natural history of schizophrenia depend on a delicate balance between vulnerability and stress on the one hand (to which people with schizophrenia are particularly sensitive), and the individual's strengths and environmental supports on the other. Within this framework, it is desirable to reduce, as far as possible, any environmental stressors in the lives of those who are most at-risk, or in the early stages of the illness to prevent the development of, or reduce, symptoms. It is also important that patients effectively manage any stress that they do encounter in their lives through the development of appropriate coping skills and/or participation in meaningful daytime activities.

A large body of research has found an association between 'expressed emotion' among family members and relapses (but not onset) in their relatives who have been diagnosed with schizophrenia. Thus, the type and amount of social and emotional stress (for example, hostility or emotional over-involvement) to which people with schizophrenia are exposed within the family milieu may often influence their path of recovery. However, research focusing on attempts to detect at-risk individuals so as to implement early interventions is in its infancy. Consequently, pharmacological treatment and maintenance regimens remain the mainstay of secondary prevention with psychosocial interventions (designed to improve social and daily living skills) and/or rehabilitation such as specialist day care or training and supported (sheltered) employment schemes (McGilloway and Donnelly 2000). 🖳

The above interventions are important, not only in promoting recovery, but also in helping to prevent the typically high rates of suicide among people with schizophrenia. Approximately 5 per cent die prematurely in this way (Mueser and McGurk 2004), 🖳 while the lifetime occurrence of attempted suicide (parasuicide) in this group has been estimated to range from 18 per cent to 55 per cent. The risk of both is significantly increased by the presence of depressive symptoms and/or substance abuse. The fatality rate of suicide attempts has also been reported to be greater in people with schizophrenia when compared with those with other psychotic illnesses. Furthermore, the risk of suicide is compounded by the tendency for people with schizophrenia failing to present to their general practitioner, or to avoid contact with them after discharge from psychiatric hospitals. However, the development in recent years of more accessible and less stigmatized community-based psychiatric clinics has gone some way towards remedying this.

12.2 Depression and Anxiety

Definition and heterogeneity

Depression is one of the most prevalent and costly of all the mental disorders and a leading (and growing) cause of disability worldwide, affecting as many as one in four people over their lifetime. Commonly described as **unipolar depressive disorder**, it is broadly categorized within ICD-10 into **depressive episode** and **recurrent depressive disorder**. Each has several sub-types rated according to severity (for example mild, moderate, and severe) and the presence of other psychiatric symptoms. Depressive symptoms may also be seen in **bipolar affective disorder**. This describes a condition characterized by episodes of mania (that is, euphoria, irritability, and distractibility) or both mania and depression. However, all types of depression are characterized by a prevailing feeling of sadness and varying degrees of emotional and social withdrawal, often involving a loss of (or impaired) self-esteem, sleep, concentration, appetite, and/or libido. Symptoms may vary from mild to severe and are usually of an episodic and recurrent nature, although approximately 20 per cent of sufferers have chronic depression without remission (Thornicroft and Sartorius 1993). 🖳

A depressive episode may also be caused, or exacerbated, by co-morbid chronic physical conditions such as stroke or heart disease, diabetes mellitus or Alzheimer's disease. Elderly people with depression are also more at risk of developing Alzheimer's disease and of being admitted to nursing-home care than their non-depressed counterparts. Unfortunately, many depressive disorders in the elderly population go undetected and untreated because they tend to be viewed as part of the ageing process and/or are not reported by older people. Additionally, the presence of depression in all age groups can lead to a myriad of attendant physical symptoms such as chronic pain, headaches, and digestive disorders. It is also the mental disorder that is most frequently linked to suicide (see section 12.5). It has been estimated that one in six of all patients with clinical depression take their own life (Gunnell and Frankel 1994) 🖳 but this figure excludes the potentially large 'at-risk' group of people who do not seek or receive treatment.

Paradoxically, the risk of suicide increases when treatment is started as most relevant medications cause motor symptoms which can increase anxiety levels.

Depression co-exists commonly with **anxiety**, an overwhelming, uncontrollable and irrational apprehension and/or fear experienced during normal day-to-day activities. Clinical anxiety may cluster with other mental disorders and is much more intensive, debilitating, and longer-lasting than periods of anxiety that may be experienced as part and parcel of everyday life. According to ICD-10, **anxiety** refers to a family of disorders, some of which may also co-occur and which may share common diagnostic criteria and aetiologies. Major categories include **phobic anxiety disorders** and **other anxiety disorders** as well as reactions to severe stress such as **post-traumatic stress disorder (PTSD)**. The second grouping includes generalized anxiety disorder, which is one of the most common (and often untreated) forms of anxiety. The sufferer may be described as a 'chronic worrier' who is persistently and uncontrollably anxious about everyday matters and events irrespective of their perceived importance. Together, anxiety and depression make a significant contribution to the global burden of disease (GBD) (see Chapter 17) and are estimated to become the second most common cause of disability by the year 2020.

Descriptive and aetiological epidemiology

Both depression and anxiety (or at least certain forms of anxiety such as generalized anxiety disorder) are almost twice as common in women as in men and may occur at any point in the lifespan. However, there is increasing evidence to suggest that these disorders are becoming more prevalent among teenagers and adolescents, many of whom rarely seek help. The most recent estimates from the GBD show a lifetime prevalence for unipolar depressive episodes of 3.2 per cent for women

compared with 1.9 per cent for men (WHO 2001). However, when all forms of depression (stand-alone or co-morbid) are taken into account, these figures rise dramatically to 20.4 per cent for women and 9.6 per cent for men (WHO 2001). The corresponding prevalence rates in any 12 month period are 9.5 per cent and 5.8 per cent, respectively. Similarly, the lifetime prevalence for generalized anxiety disorder in the general population has been reported to be as high as 5 per cent (Wittchen *et al.* 1994).

A UK-based survey of 10 000 adults in private households (OPCS 1995) found that one in seven had a psychiatric disorder, the most common of which included anxiety-depressive disorder (7 per cent) and generalized anxiety disorder (3 per cent). The higher prevalence of both depression and anxiety among women appears to be due to a complex interplay of biological, sociocultural, and psychological/behavioural factors.

Many people may develop neurotic illnesses such as depression and anxiety without ever being treated or receiving a formal diagnosis. However, the prevalence rates for (diagnosed) depression and anxiety, as well as age at onset and the course of the illness, vary widely across populations. Several social and economic factors have been identified as important in explaining this variation, the most important of which would appear to be poverty and deprivation. It is now well known that the risk of developing depression (and indeed mental illness in general) is higher in poorer, developing countries than in the richer, developed world where levels of physical health and nutrition are generally better and health services are more richly resourced. However, Figure 12.1 indicates that the prevalence of depression is higher in low-income groups in both developing and developed countries.

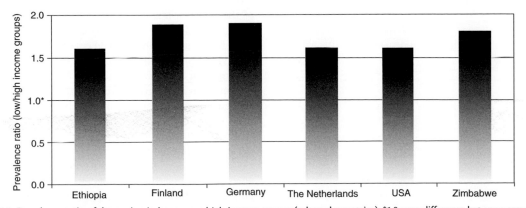

Fig. 12.1 Prevalence ratio of depression in low-versus high-income groups (selected countries). *1.0 = no difference between groups.

However, the relation between poverty and mental health is not straightforward and involves many potentially mediating factors. A recent Swedish follow-up study of first psychiatric admissions during 1997–1999 showed that the incidence of depression (and psychoses) increased significantly with rising levels of urbanization, after controlling for age and gender (Sundquist *et al.* 2004). 🖵 Level of urbanization was assessed by dividing the study population (4.4 million) into five equal groups according to the population density of area of residence. The authors found that those living in more densely populated areas had a 12–20 per cent greater risk of developing depression than those in more sparsely populated regions (Table 12.1). Depression was defined using several diagnostic codes within the ICD-9 and ICD-10 classification systems as well as additional specialized classification systems for mental disorder.

The relation between poverty and mental disorders such as depression and anxiety is multi-dimensional and may encompass other socioenvironmental risk factors such as political instability and conflict. Natural disasters and major epidemics may also play an important role. For example, a diagnosis of human immunodeficiency virus/acquired immunodeficiency syndrome (HIV/AIDS) often gives rise to extreme stigma and discrimination and, in turn, to high levels of depression and/or anxiety among sufferers and their families. Major life events such as bereavement or marital breakdown, and the extent of social support, are additional risk factors for developing depression and anxiety.

> **Q1** Previous studies of possible urban–rural differences in mental health are inconsistent. Why do you think this might be?

Prevention

Most depressive and anxiety disorders tend to be self-limiting but can, nonetheless, be extremely debilitating and distressing. There is little evidence for the effectiveness of approaches to primary prevention per se (WHO 2001), 🖵 but a range of interventions has been shown to be effective, not only for reducing symptoms of depression and anxiety, but also in screening, educating, and supporting at-risk groups such as mothers with post-natal depression (Cooper and Murray 1998). 🖵 However, these kinds of initiatives are relatively uncommon, especially within primary care where most of these disorders are first recognized and treated.

Thus, antidepressant and anxiolytic (anti-anxiety) medication remain the most commonly used forms of treatment designed to reduce or alleviate symptoms in the short term, to prevent a relapse and ultimately (and more challengingly) to promote a full recovery. However, these do not work for everyone and there is evidence to suggest that they are more effective for the treatment of moderate and severe depression than for milder forms of the illness (National Institute for Clinical Excellence (NICE) 2004). 🖵 Some people may also experience adverse side effects such as physical addiction, especially if medicated for a prolonged period. Furthermore, evidence on the apparent links between newer anti-depressant medication, such as selective serotonin re-uptake inhibitors and an increased risk of suicide, has led to a ban on their use in children (under 18 years of age) (Gunnell and Ashby 2004). 🖵 However, increased prescribing of these drugs has coincided with an overall drop in the suicide rate in many countries, but the evidence is weak owing to the difficulty in disentangling the effects of medication from the many other factors that may influence suicide rates. Clearly, further research in

---

TABLE 12.1 Population and age-adjusted incidence rates for depression in a general population aged 25–64 years in Sweden[1]

Variable	Female rate (95% CI)	Male rate (95% CI)
Urbanization		
Q1 (lowest)	84 (82–86)	67 (65–69)
Q2	87 (85–89)	66 (64–68)
Q3	90 (88–92)	66 (64–68)
Q4	107 (104–109)	71 (69–73)
Q5 (highest)	122 (120–125)	87 (85–90)
Marital status		
Living alone	135 (133–138)	103 (100–105)
Married/co-habiting	79 (76–81)	53 (51–54)
Education		
Low	129 (126–132)	88 (86–90)
Middle	93 (91–95)	68 (66–70)
High	82 (80–84)	58 (56–59)

[1]Incidence rate per 100 000 person-years.

Source: Sundquist, K., Frank, G. and Sundquist, J. (2004). 'Urbanisation and Incidence of Psychosis and Depression'. *British Journal of Psychiatry*, **184**: 293–8.

this area is required to determine the long-term safety of antidepressant prescribing.

General practitioners and other health professionals are also increasingly recognizing the value of psychological therapies in the treatment and management of both depression and anxiety; cognitive behavioural therapy (CBT), interpersonal psychotherapy (IPT), and various forms of counselling are all used as forms of treatment, often with medication. Beck's cognitive therapy (CT) (a form of CBT) is primarily aimed at changing negative and maladaptive thought patterns. IPT, on the other hand, helps patients to improve their interpersonal and social skills and to derive greater benefit from their social interactions. Both of these forms of therapy have been found to be effective, to a greater or lesser degree, in alleviating the symptoms of depression. The evidence for their effectiveness is derived mainly from several controlled studies, one of the largest and most widely cited of which was conducted by the National Institute for Mental Health in the USA (Elkin *et al.* 1985). 💻 The findings indicated that, although pharmacological therapy led to a more rapid improvement during the 16-week treatment period, all three forms of treatment including CT and IPT achieved significant and equivalent degrees of success when compared with the placebo group. Many other studies have since been conducted (for example Ward *et al.* 2000) 💻 which suggest that some time-limited therapies such as CBT and non-directive counselling can be as effective as medication, but only for mild to moderate depression. However, the efficacy and effectiveness of other therapies relative to medication remain controversial.

12.3 Dementia

Definition and heterogeneity

Dementia is a syndrome characterized by a progressive decline in cognitive and functional abilities. Onset is usually gradual and the main symptoms include: a loss of recent memory; a decreased ability to perform activities of daily living; impaired judgement; disorientation; changes in personality; a deterioration in language skills; and behavioural disturbance. Affective changes such as depression are also common. It is important to evaluate the nature and degree of co-morbidity among older people when assessing their mental health status. In particular, it is necessary that epidemiological and clinical assessments take account of the possibility of misclassifying depression as dementia (so-called pseudo-dementia).

Descriptive and aetiological epidemiology

Dementia refers to a range of different diseases, although there is considerable uncertainty about their aetiology. Kukall and Bowen (2002) 💻 provide a comprehensive list of the causes of dementia under several major categories including: idiopathic (for example Alzheimer's disease); focal central nervous system pathology (for example multi-infarct dementia); infections (for example HIV); toxins (for example side effects of medication); inherited disease (for example Huntingdon's disease); systemic disease (for example cardiac); movement disorders (for example Parkinson's disease); and deficiency (for example vitamin B12 deficiency). There is some variation between studies in estimates of different types of dementia. Alzheimer's disease appears to be the most common dementia, accounting for up to two-thirds of cases. Post-mortem examination of people who had the disease indicates significant brain damage in the form of 'plaques and tangles' around the brain cells. The second most common type of dementia is vascular dementia (accounting for an estimated 20 per cent) and it is characterized by the death of cells in certain areas of the brain because of cerebrovascular disease. Approximately 10 per cent of cases have other forms of dementia such as Lewy-body dementia (see Chapter 11).

A key task in psychiatric epidemiology is to identify and describe disorders such as dementia. Thus, several scales and interview schedules have been developed to assess the presence of dementia and other disorders. For example, the Composite International Diagnostic Interview (CIDI) is used by clinicians and non-professionals to assess prevalence; and the Mini-Mental State Exam (MMSE) is an interviewer-administered scale or questionnaire that is used to screen for cognitive impairment, particularly in community-based studies. Individuals who score above a certain cut-point on the MMSE obtained in validation studies are designated a 'case', indicating that they have significant cognitive impairment. There is some uncertainty about which cut-point should be used to define a 'case': a common methodological problem in epidemiology for most risk factors based on continuous distributions, whether measured by questionnaire or using a physiological measured variable. Different cut-points will lead to variations in estimates of prevalence and incidence. However, in general, research suggests that the widely used MMSE appears to be a valid test for detecting dementia. For example, a cut-point of 21/22 on the MMSE had a sensitivity of 96 per cent and a specificity of 80 per cent for a diagnosis of dementia in community epidemiological studies (see Chapter 5). Some studies suggest that higher cut-points may be required with graduates or other similar professional and literate populations.

Both the incidence and prevalence of dementia increase exponentially with age (Launer *et al.* 1999). 🖳 Overall, approximately one in twenty people over 65 years and one in three people over 85 years old have dementia, while around only 1 in 1000 people under 65 develops the illness. Clearly, dementia is a disease of old age. Current estimates indicate that the number of people diagnosed with dementia in the UK is in excess of 700 000 and will increase to 855 000 by the year 2020 (Department of Health 1997). 🖳 Reviews of the epidemiology of dementia tend to report variation in prevalence rates (probably owing to the different methods used to detect cases), and a consistent relation between age and dementia across studies, with prevalence doubling approximately every five years. As noted earlier, dementia may be mistaken for other conditions such as depression or for poor cognitive performance; particular attention needs to be paid to the specific difficulty associated with the diagnosis of mild dementia, which some research reports describe as a 'chameleon-like entity' (Mowry and Burvill 1998). 🖳 Prevalence and incidence rates for dementia overall appear to be comparable between countries, and rates for men and women seem to be similar, though there are more women with dementia because of the larger population of elderly women.

Epidemiological studies on risk factors for dementia have tended to use retrospective case–control designs and, as noted in Chapter 2, the findings from these kinds of studies may be unreliable if proper account is not taken of methodological problems such as survival bias, recall bias, and the difficulties associated with collecting reliable information about exposure. Studies that use a prospective design provide a more robust investigation of risk and protective factors. For example, the Canadian Study of Health and Aging (CSHA) is a population-based, multi-centre, prospective study into the epidemiology of dementia and associated risk factors (Lindsay *et al.* 2004). 🖳 It found that the main risk factors for Alzheimer's disease were increasing age, fewer years of education, and the presence of the *ApoE4* gene. Family history did not appear to be related to risk (though an association had been observed in an earlier case–control component of CSHA). There was no supporting evidence in CSHA for smoking or a history of depression as risk factors. For vascular dementia, the main risk factors included: age; the *ApoE4* gene; depression; diabetes; hypertension in women; heart problems

in men; taking aspirin; rural residence; and occupational exposure to pesticides. There was no relation between vascular dementia and sex, education, smoking, or alcohol use.

> **Q2** Why do you think there have been fewer incidence studies than studies of the prevalence of dementia?

Large population-based epidemiological surveys should provide the kind of information that is required to estimate the prevalence and incidence of dementia and to identify significant trends if appropriate case-finding methods are used. Prevalence estimates provide important information for service planning and provision; incidence data are used in the identification and appraisal of possible risk factors. The extent to which the results from any study may be generalized to the wider patient population with the particular illness or condition in question is an important indicator of the quality and utility of research in mental health. Therefore, both **internal and external validity** are particularly relevant in the design of epidemiological studies of mental health.

Notwithstanding, many factors that confound epidemiological studies may be reduced or eliminated in studies of special populations because of their relative homogeneity. For example, a longitudinal investigation of dementia in a population of 678 Catholic nuns was able to control for a range of potential confounding factors because the nuns were all unmarried, without children, and had similar social activities and support, occupations (teachers and educationalists), income, and socioeconomic status (Snowdon 2003). 🖳 In addition, the nuns drank only a moderate amount of alcohol and did not smoke. The fact that the study investigated the entire population of nuns (who were aged 75–102 years at the beginning of the study in 1991, with the oldest Sister surviving to 107 by 2002), meant that there was considerable variation in terms of cognitive ability, physical functioning, health and disease status, and survival time. Data were collected from a rich combination of different sources including: (1) early-, mid- and late-life events and conditions from convent archives; (2) annual medical (including psychiatric) examinations of each nun to chart changes in cognitive and physical functioning; and (3) post-mortem assessments of the structure and pathology of the nuns' brains. Low linguistic ability in early life was associated with increased risk; in later life stroke increased both the risk and severity of Alzheimer's disease.

Treatment and prevention

Currently, there are no fully effective treatments for dementia, though in recent years a variety of approaches have been developed. NICE has recommended the use of several cholinesterase-inhibiting drugs, particularly in early or mild dementia. Non-pharmacological or behavioural approaches, such as reality orientation, reminiscence therapy and validation therapy (Neal and Briggs 2003) 🖳 are also available, but further research is required about their overall effectiveness. Current treatment options do not offer a 'cure' for dementia, but instead delay or control symptoms. Consequently, an assessment of **quality of life** is a more meaningful outcome measure with which to assess the effectiveness of the interventions and available services, rather than traditional clinical outcomes such as mortality.

Significant protective factors for Alzheimer's dementia include the use of non-steroidal anti-inflammatory drugs, wine consumption, coffee consumption, and regular physical activity. For vascular dementia, possible protective factors are eating shellfish and regular physical activity, particularly for women (see Lindsay *et al.* 2004). 🖳 In addition, recent clinical trials found that anti-hypertensive treatment was associated with a lower incidence of dementia and vascular dementia (Hanon and Forette 2004). 🖳 Physical activity is a common protective factor for all dementias (and other conditions) and thus an important component of any preventive strategy. In a prospective cohort study, men who had walked less than a quarter of a mile per day had 1.8 times the risk of dementia than men who walked more than two miles per day. The Nurses' Health Study (Weuve *et al.* 2004) 🖳 repeated questionnaires and telephone interviews two years apart to test the cognition, verbal memory, and attention of 18 766 women aged 70–81 years. The results showed that women who walked for at least 1.5 hours per week had better levels of cognitive performance than women who walked less than 40 minutes per week, indicating that sustained, regular physical activity helped to prevent cognitive decline in older women. Also, several longitudinal studies of both the general and special populations, such as religious congregations, have found that frequent participation in activities that are cognitively stimulating is associated with a reduced risk of cognitive decline and dementia. A recent review of research concluded that '... social engagement, intellectual stimulation and physical activity play a key role in maintaining cognitive health and preventing cognitive decline' and it is likely that better cognitive health will be observed in individuals who make lifestyle changes earlier rather than later (Butler *et al.* 2004). 🖳

12.4 Learning Disability

Definition and heterogeneity

In the UK, the term 'learning disability' has replaced the term 'mental handicap' to refer to people with intellectual impairment and impaired functioning or adaptive behaviour. Learning disability is a permanent condition that tends to be present from birth and has a lasting effect on development. Intellectual impairment is usually defined as an IQ score lower than 50 for individuals with severe disability and between 50 and 70 for those with the milder form (see Fryers (2002) 🖳 for discussion of key issues including the problems associated with definition). In addition, up to 40 per cent of people with this disorder also have a mental illness, and there is a high level of physical ill health. For example, people with learning disability tend to have higher levels of epilepsy, sensory impairments, osteoporosis, musculoskeletal problems, dysphagia, and nutritional problems when compared with the general population.

There is a lack of consensus about the most appropriate way to define and describe people with this disorder. 'Developmental disabilities' is a term that is used commonly in the USA; other popular labels include 'intellectual disabilities' and 'learning difficulties'. The inadequacy of using any single definition is evident from epidemiological studies, which tend to report significant levels of variation and complexity in impairments and disabilities among people with the disorder. While these terms may be stigmatizing to varying degrees, it is important to try to arrive at an accurate definition for the purposes of planning, organizing, and delivering appropriate and necessary services. Epidemiology can provide a framework within which to conduct a needs assessment of the population with learning disabilities and to plan the provision of health and social services (Rees *et al.* 2004). 🖳

Descriptive and aetiological epidemiology

Fryers (2002), 🖳 in his overview of the difficulties surrounding the definition, categorization, and epidemiology of learning disability, noted that much of the literature is 'useless for comparison or application elsewhere' and that only the research literature relating to severe disability is reliable. The incidence and prevalence is variable and changes owing to its heterogeneous nature, the many different types, the wide array of aetiological factors, and the dynamic processes of inception, mortality, and migration. These points should be borne in mind when reading epidemiological studies of the disorder.

In general terms, reviews of prevalence studies of people with learning disability known to service providers have found three to four people with severe disability and between 25 and 30 people with less severe disability in every 1000 of the general population. Studies that have screened whole populations of people with severe disorder have found 6 per 1000 of the population. Prevalence rates vary according to gender, age, ethnic background, and socioeconomic circumstances. Lesser disability is more common among people from families with low incomes and adverse or unstable backgrounds. Evidence for the relation between severe disability and socioeconomic group is mixed (Fryers 2002). 💻

Learning disability comprises a very heterogeneous group of syndromes and conditions with different aetiologies. Down syndrome represents the largest single cause. A social model of disability tends to view the disorder in terms of developmental delay that is due to differences in learning opportunities and receipt of appropriate interventions rather than to biological causes per se (Chappell *et al.* 2001). 💻 Screening for Down syndrome is discussed in Chapter 5, and congenital anomalies are described in Chapter 14. The varied aetiology is summarized in Box 12.2.

Severe disability is associated with genetic or biological factors such as Down syndrome and fragile X syndrome. Causes may also be classified according to the time (ante-, peri-, or post-natal) of damage to the development of the central nervous system. Antenatal factors such as rubella or toxins (for example foetal alcohol syndrome) contribute 50–70 per cent of cases. Perinatal damage such as asphyxia during birth accounts for 10–20 per cent of cases whereas post-natal damage (5–10 per cent) may be due to factors such as meningitis, encephalitis, and accidental or deliberate injury. Severe learning disability in four out of five children is caused by genetic and biological factors compared with between one and two out of five with less severe disability. The aetiology of the latter is more likely to involve a combination of genetic and environmental factors.

There is considerable developmental variation among people with the same genetic condition; also, social factors have a bearing on development and on the severity of the impact of a biological impairment. For example, early intervention strategies may be successful in ameliorating the effects of Down syndrome

---

BOX 12.2 AETIOLOGY OF LEARNING DISABILITIES

Genetic exposures

Dominant genes causing gross disease of the brain
Tuberose sclerosis, Neurofibromatosis.

Recessive genes causing metabolic disorders affecting
Amino acids (for example phenylketonuria, homocystinuria), urea cycle (citrullinuria, aminosuccinic aciduria), lipids (Tay–Sachs, Gaucher's and Niemann–Pick diseases), carbohydrate (galactosaemia), mucopolysaccharidoses (Hurler's syndrome).

Chromosome abnormalities
Down syndrome, Klinefelter syndrome, Turner syndrome.

X-linked disorders
Fragile X syndrome, Lesch–Nyhan syndrome.

Cranial malformations
Hydrocephalus, microcephalus.

Polygenic factors influencing the normal distribution of intelligence
Non-specific learning disability.

Ante-natal exposures
Infections (rubella, cytomegalovirus, syphilis, toxoplasmosis), intoxications (lead, certain drugs, alcohol), physical damage (injury, radiation, hypoxia), endocrine disorders (hypothyroidism, hypoparathyroidism), foetal malnutrition (including iodine deficiency, a common cause in developing countries, see Chapter 8).

Peri-natal exposures
Birth asphyxia, kernicterus, intraventricular haemorrhage.

Post-natal exposures
Injury (accidental, child abuse), infections (encephalitis, meningitis), lead intoxication.

Adapted from: Gelder, M., Gath, D. and Mayou, R. (eds.) (1994). *Concise Oxford Textbook of Psychiatry*. Oxford: Oxford University Press.

(Cunningham 1996) 💻 although few controlled studies have been conducted. The personality, family background, and social environment of each individual with the disorder, as well as the nature and degree of their disability, will determine the kind of life that they will experience. The majority (around 80 per cent) are classified as 'mild' and most tend to be able to live in their respective communities without needing support or supervision, in contrast to people with 'severe' disability who require formal services and support from health and social services and other agencies (and the committed support of families). Children with mild disease may not be identified or detected formally until they attend school whereas people with severe disability tend to be known from birth. Indeed, Fryers (2002) 🖳 makes the important point that mild learning disability is socially determined to a large degree.

Treatment and prevention

Disability that is due to causes such as hypothyroidism, phenylketonuria, rubella infection, and kernicterus can be successfully prevented using public-health measures such as rubella immunization and neonatal screening; disability from other causes such as chromosome defects, rare single gene disorders, drug exposures, exposure to lead, and head injury can be reduced by methods such as the use of educational programmes, genetic counselling, prenatal and neonatal diagnosis, and other prevention strategies. (See Table 12.2 for a list of relevant services for prevention.) While the diagnosis or detection of the disorder and the identification of genetic conditions are very important tasks, the prognosis or the quality of life of individuals may be influenced significantly by the availability of opportunities in areas such as specific interventions, education, vocational training and employment, and support to live 'ordinary lives' (Gates 2002). 🖳

12.5 Suicide and parasuicide

Definition

Suicide refers to acute self-inflicted death which, in the UK, can only be labelled as such after a coroner's investigation, and frequently an open or accidental verdict is made which falls short of suicide. This practice varies considerably between different countries owing to legal, cultural, and religious factors, thereby making comparisons of suicide rates difficult. The same is true for attempted suicide (parasuicide), although comparisons over time can be made within countries. The term 'parasuicide' was coined to describe deliberate self-harm inflicted with no intent to die. In practice, 'intent' can be difficult to evaluate and the distinction between attempted suicide and parasuicide is frequently blurred in epidemiological studies. In most countries, attempted suicides are referred to the psychiatric services for assessment and possible intervention, and most studies suggest that attempted suicide/parasuicide is a highly heterogeneous disorder

TABLE 12.2 Services for the prevention of learning disabilities
(a) Pre-conceptual services
Immunization of adolescent girls against rubella
Genetic counselling
General advice on diet, avoidance of tobacco and alcohol consumption, and avoidance of drug abuse and HIV
(b) Pre-natal
Identification of 'at risk' pregnancies
Monitoring alpha-fetoprotein (AFP) levels, etc., provision of amniocentesis
Blood tests
Diagnostic ultrasound services
Advice and counselling on termination of pregnancy
(c) Perinatal/neonatal
High quality obstetric and neonatal care
Neonatal screening and treatment of specific conditions
Surgical intervention to prevent or reduce impairments
Injection of anti-D immunoglobulin to prevent antibody formation in mothers at risk of future rhesus incompatibility
Phenylketonuria (PKU) screening
(d) Post-natal
Immunization
Control of infection and complications in children already suffering a specific impairment
General support to families at risk

Adapted from: Felce, D., Taylor, D. and Wright, K. (1994). 'Learning Disabilities', in A. Stevens and J. Raffery (eds.). *Health Care Needs Assessment: The Epidemiologically Based Needs Assessment Reviews* (1st edn). Oxford: Radcliffe Medical Press.

with considerable variation in the level of intent and the possibility of repeated attempts.

Descriptive and aetiological epidemiology

Suicide is one of the three leading causes of death among 15- to 34-year-olds in the developed world. However, in many countries, even in Europe, the incidence is several-fold higher in the elderly, particularly in men (see Figure 12.2). 'Global' mortality rates from suicide have been

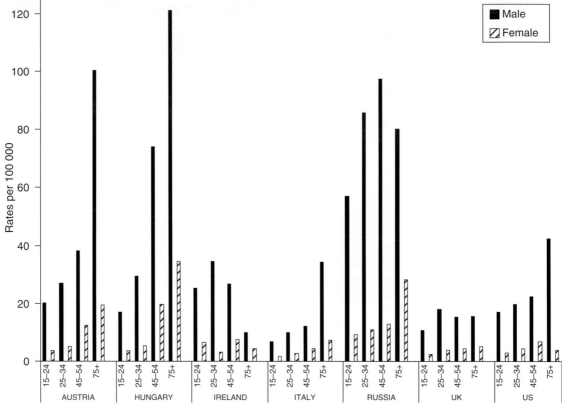

Fig. 12.2 Mortality from suicide in selected age groups by country in the year 2000. (Data obtained from the World Health Organization.)

estimated to be as high as 16 per 100 000 whereas the rate of attempted suicide may be up to 20 times more common again (WHO 2001). ▢ Suicide rates worldwide vary considerably and, as noted above, are notoriously difficult to estimate, compare, and interpret. Recent data from the World Health Organization (WHO) data are shown in Figure 12.2.

Parasuicide, in contrast, is much more common, particularly among females, and the highest rates are found in young adults. Repeated episodes are common, but parasuicide is also a major risk factor for completed suicide with 30–47 per cent of such cases having had an episode of parasuicide (Welch 2001). ▢ A recent national British survey indicated that suicidal thoughts are more common in women than men, possibly because of different patterns of help-seeking behaviour and/or the use of more lethal methods by men (Gunnell *et al.* 2004). ▢ However, Gunnell *et al.* indicate that fewer than 1 in 200 of those who develop such thoughts actually go on to

commit suicide. Nonetheless, these gender-related differences may be important for identifying at-risk individuals and developing appropriate measures for suicide prevention.

Potential for prevention

Several important risk factors for suicide – in addition to depression and schizophrenia – have been identified. These include: alcohol/substance abuse; previous and/or family history of suicide; childhood abuse; deliberate self-harm; and chronic physical illness (Torphy 2005). ▢ Arguably, the heterogeneous nature and methods of suicide coupled with its multifactorial aetiology hinder attempts to develop adequate and systematic preventive measures. However, the strong links between suicidal behaviour and mental ill health suggest that the effective, timely, and appropriate identification and treatment of mental disorders, including depression, represent an important element of any suicide prevention programme. Evidence from the UK suggests that more than a fifth of suicides among people with mental illness are preventable (Department of Health 2001). 🖳 As mentioned previously, there remains considerable debate as to whether or not the increased prescribing of anti-depressants, in particular, has led to a reduction in suicidal behaviour. The evidence, so far, remains circumstantial (Gunnell and Ashby 2004). 🖳

There is good evidence to suggest that suicide can be prevented by the early and appropriate treatment of some mental disorders such as depression (WHO 2001). 🖳 However, prevention of suicide, especially among young people, is controversial because, in large part, of the paucity of population-based studies and a failure to take account of the multiple risk factors involved. Dedicated strategies to prevent suicide aimed at developing and promoting effective clinical practice have also been implemented. These include, primarily, training and education programmes for general practitioners and other health professionals designed to improve the recognition, assessment, and treatment of individuals presenting a risk of suicide. For example, a Swedish study by Rutz *et al.* (1995) 🖳 reported a decline in suicide rates after the implementation of a training programme for general practitioners. Similarly, public awareness and education programmes have been designed to overcome the stigma commonly associated with suicide and mental illness in general, but few appear to have been evaluated. Other more specific preventive interventions aim to address the means by which people commit suicide, such as the removal of all ligatures to prevent hanging (traditionally the most common method of suicide) in institutional settings and the screening of at-risk groups. Only the former has had any measure of success, although the findings from a recent randomized trial indicate that post-crisis contact between mental health professionals and individuals at risk for suicide (and who refuse ongoing treatment) was effective in reducing suicide rates during the two-year period after discharge from hospital (Motto and Bostrom 2001). 🖳 On balance, however, it is still difficult to find convincing systematic evidence for the effectiveness of any single suicide prevention programme, and much more work in this area is needed.

Conclusion

Because of an increasing prevalence and public awareness, future epidemiological studies, based on biological and socio-psychological measures, will be required to improve our understanding of mental disorders and their possible prevention.

Further Reading

Gelder, M. G., Lopez-Ibor, J. J. and Andreasen, N. C. (eds.) (2000). *New Oxford Textbook of Psychiatry*. Oxford: Oxford University Press.

The Nun's Study, www.neuroanatomy.wisc.edu/selflearn/Nunsandalzheimers.htm.

Tsuang, M. T. and Tohen, M. (eds.) (2002). *Textbook in Psychiatric Epidemiology*. New York, NY: Wiley.

References

References for this chapter can be found at www.oxfordtextbooks.co.uk/orc/yarnell. Where possible, these are presented as *active links* which direct you to an electronic version of the work. If you are a subscriber to that work (either individually or through an institution), and depending on your level of access, you may be able to peruse an abstract or the full article if available. 🖳

Model answers

Q1 Firstly, the relation between the two is complex owing to the potential range of other influential factors (for example socioeconomic status, gender, and ethnicity) that most studies are unable to account for in their entirety. For example, social networks are generally better developed in rural than in urban areas and these may act as a 'buffer' against the more adverse living circumstances and daily life stress typically encountered in cities. This may, in turn, result in fewer psychiatric admissions from rural areas. Methodologically, however, it is difficult to obtain a measure of social support within large-scale studies other than perhaps marital status, which is too simplistic and differs by gender. Despite the potentially greater likelihood of supportive relationships, rural living may also be typified by factors that may, in the long term, precipitate mental ill health, such as limited access to appropriate support services. A second methodological difficulty relates to how urbanization is measured. In the study by Sundquist *et al.*, it was calculated (correctly) as population density, but other studies have used self-report estimates or the number of addresses per unit area, neither of which is a sufficiently precise or unbiased measure of the actual number of people in any area (Sundquist *et al.* 2004). 🖳 Thirdly, the number of psychiatric beds may differ across urban and rural areas and may, therefore, bias the results (although this was not found in the above study) as would perhaps the effects of selective urban–rural migration.

Q2 Incidence studies tend to be more difficult and costly because they involve identifying and selecting a large cohort of people who do not have dementia at the outset of a study and then following-up these study participants and assessing them over a significant period.

Musculoskeletal diseases

This chapter reviews the epidemiology of four of the most common musculoskeletal disorders: rheumatoid arthritis, osteoarthritis, osteoporosis, and backache.

Introduction

Musculoskeletal disorders are extremely common and include more than 150 different diseases and syndromes. The most common worldwide are rheumatoid arthritis, osteoarthritis, osteoporosis, spinal disorders (backache), and limb trauma. These disorders have a major impact on society owing to their frequency, chronicity, and resultant disability. Approximately 5 per cent of adults in Western populations have a musculoskeletal-related disability, with a higher prevalence in women and the elderly. Furthermore, the prevalence of these disabilities is set to increase markedly in coming decades as the world's population continues to age. Musculoskeletal conditions are the second most common reason for consulting a doctor in most countries, are the commonest cause of long-term sickness absence in developed countries, and are one of the most common reasons for claiming disability benefit. Patients suffering from these disorders experience greatly reduced quality of life (QoL), especially in physical functioning (Figure 13.1), and the associated pain and physical disability also affect the social functioning and mental health of patients.

In Figure 13.1 standardized QoL scales (see below) have been used in different patient groups in a total of 15 000 patients. Physical and mental functioning have been compared for various disorders. Healthy individuals (data not shown) tended to have higher scores on both scales. In general, the results suggest that many diseases have an impact of similar magnitude on the physical and mental QoL, although it should be

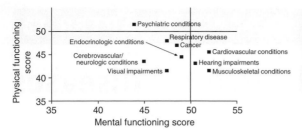

Fig. 13.1 The position of disease clusters with respect to physical and mental functioning.
Note: Mean scores have been set at 50 to facilitate comparison of the two aspects of functioning.
Source: Sprangers, M. A., de Regt, E. B., and Andries, F. (2000). 'Which Chronic Conditions are Associated with Better or Poorer Quality of Life?' *Journal of Clinical Epidemiology*, **53**: 895–907.

BOX 13.1 **ADAPTED FROM THE REVISED 1987 AMERICAN COLLEGE OF RHEUMATOLOGY CRITERIA FOR RHEUMATOID ARTHRITIS. FOUR OF THE FOLLOWING MUST BE PRESENT, WITH 1–4 PRESENT A MINIMUM OF 6 WEEKS**

1 Morning stiffness for at least 1 hour.
2 Arthritis of three or more joint groups simultaneously.
3 Arthritis of one or more of 14 joints in hands or wrist.
4 Simultaneous involvement of some joint areas on both sides of the body.
5 Rheumatoid nodules over bony prominences or extensor surfaces or in juxta-articular regions.
6 Positive serum rheumatoid factor (RF).
7 Radiographic changes including erosions or bony decalcification localized in, or adjacent to, the involved joint.

Source: Arnett, F. C., Edworthy, S. M., Bloch, D. A. *et al.* (1988). 'The American Rheumatism Association 1987 Revised Criteria for the Classification of Rheumatoid Arthritis'. *Arthritis and Rheumatism*, **31**: 315–24.

recognized that these assessments are based on the subjective assessments of patients and may also reflect, in part, coping behaviours.

13.1 **Rheumatoid Arthritis**

Definition

Rheumatoid arthritis (RA) is a chronic, multisystem, autoimmune disorder of unknown cause, the major characteristic of which is chronic symmetrical erosive synovitis, usually involving the peripheral joints. There are no unique clinical or laboratory features that define the disease, and RA is distinguished from other rheumatic disorders by application of the revised 1987 American College of Rheumatology criteria for rheumatoid arthritis (Box 13.1).

Non-articular manifestations of RA include subcutaneous nodules, vasculitis, pericarditis, pulmonary nodules, intestinal fibrosis, neuritis, and episcleritis or scleritis.

Incidence and prevalence

RA occurs throughout the world and affects all races. Most studies of the occurrence of RA have examined prevalence rather than incidence of the disease and estimates of point prevalence in developed countries vary between 0.5 and 1 per cent (500–1000 per 100 000 population). Throughout the world, RA is more common in women than men with a female:male ratio of disease prevalence of approximately 2.5:1, although there is variation between populations. In the UK, the annual incidence is 36 per 100 000 in women and 14 per 100 000 in men (Symmons 1994). 🖥 The age and sex

distribution of incidence of RA is shown in Figure 13.2. Incidence increases with increasing age but appears to fall in elderly women. The disease occurs at an earlier age in women than in men: peak age of incidence is around 55–64 years of age in women and 10 years later in men.

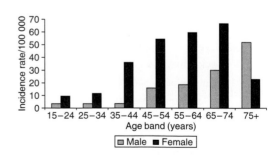

Fig. 13.2 Age- and sex-specific incidence of rheumatoid arthritis.
Source: Symmons, D. P., Barrett, E. M., Bankhead, C. R., Scott, D. G. and Silman, A. J. (1994). 'The Incidence of Rheumatoid Arthritis in the United Kingdom: Results from the Norfolk Arthritis Register'. *British Journal of Rheumatology*, **33** (8): 735–9.

Time trends and geographic distribution

Evidence from skeletal remains indicates that RA occurred in native North American populations for several thousand years but was unknown in Europe before the fifteenth century, when it may have been imported by early explorers of the 'New World' (Rothschild *et al.* 2004). 🖳 The incidence of RA in Europe appears to have increased rapidly during the nineteenth and early twentieth centuries, possibly related to industrialization, but has fallen in Westernized populations over the past 50 years. There is substantial geographic variation in the prevalence of RA. It is rare in rural Africa, and in urban and rural settings in China, Indonesia, and the Philippines (around 0.4 per cent), whereas the prevalence in India is similar to that in the West (approximately 0.75 per cent). The highest prevalence has traditionally been seen in Pima Indians in North America, although there have been declines in the prevalence in this group in the past few decades. The geographic distribution and time trends underline the contribution of environmental and lifestyle factors to the development of this disease.

Aetiology and risk factors

The aetiology of RA is unknown but probably results from an interaction between exposure to environmental agents and genetic susceptibility. Family studies indicate a genetic predisposition; 10 per cent of patients have a first-degree relative with the disease and monozygotic twins are four times more likely to be concordant for disease than dizygotic twins. Approximately 70 per cent of patients with RA express the class II major histocompatibility complex (MHC) gene product HLA-DR4, compared with 28 per cent of control subjects; this association has been seen in many populations but is strongest in Caucasians. Other genetic factors and autoimmunity are also under investigation.

Hormonal factors are thought to be important in the development of RA. Women have a higher incidence than men, onset during pregnancy is rare, and pregnancy is associated with remission of disease, while exacerbations may occur post delivery. However, a meta-analysis of studies examining the association between oral contraceptive use and development of RA has failed to demonstrate that oral contraceptives protect against RA (Pladevall-Vila *et al.* 1996). 🖳 Smokers of both sexes have an increased risk of developing rheumatoid factor (RF) positive, but not RF negative, RA. The increased risk occurs after a long duration, but moderate intensity, of smoking and may remain for several years after smoking cessation. There is evidence from population-based case–control studies that obesity is a risk factor for RA, and that consumption of alcohol is protective, but these findings have not been confirmed in a recent prospective study of middle-aged and elderly women. The role of diet in the epidemiology of RA has been infrequently investigated. Fish oils have a beneficial effect on the symptoms of established RA, but it is not known whether they reduce the risk of developing the disease. There is emerging evidence that high intake of fruit and vegetables and antioxidants may be protective against RA (Cerhan *et al.* 2003). 🖳

Many patients attribute their RA to either physical or psychological trauma but there is no robust evidence to support this notion, and, although recent infection has been implicated in triggering RA, no specific organism has been identified. Although environmental exposures are undoubtedly important in the development of RA, the evidence is insufficient to identify possible preventive measures.

Natural history

The course of RA varies considerably between patients; some experience only a brief mild oligo-articular arthritis with minimal joint damage whereas others develop a chronic destructive arthritis with marked functional impairment and disability. Within a decade of diagnosis between 50 per cent and 60 per cent of patients are too disabled to remain economically active. Several factors appear to be associated with the development of disabling disease. Patients who are RF-positive are more likely to develop erosive disease than those who are RF-negative. Later onset of the disease is associated with more rapid progression and women have a worse functional outcome than men, although sex does not appear to influence radiological progression. There is no evidence that use of oral contraceptives or hormone replacement therapy has any long-term effect on the outcome of RA among women. Socioeconomic disadvantage is also associated with a worse clinical course (and earlier mortality) in RA patients, which does not appear to result from systematic differences in treatment but probably from differences in individual susceptibility and lifestyle factors.

Patients with RA have been shown to have approximately twice the mortality rate of the general population and a life expectancy reduced by 5 to 10 years. Risk of death from a variety of causes is increased, including gastrointestinal, respiratory, cardiovascular, and infectious diseases, with cardiovascular disease contributing up to 40 per cent of the observed excess mortality.

Quality of life

Management of RA is aimed at relieving symptoms, modifying the disease process and minimizing disability associated with the disease; the overall goal is to maximize the patient's QoL. As the course of RA can extend over many years, with periods of remission and relapse, and because early and continuous treatment with toxic drugs has now become standard management, the measurement of health-related QoL in this patient group has assumed increasing importance. There is an increasing consensus that the evaluation of health and health care should comprise an assessment of (1) health status and (2) QoL as well as (3) the usual physiopathological measures relating to the presence, nature, and severity of a disease. According to Gill *et al.* (1995), ☐ these three dimensions provide doctors with a comprehensive outcome assessment, a better understanding of the complex relationship between physiological and psychosocial health, and a measure of the effect of illness and chronic disease on a patient's life. Because of the long-term nature of the disease, clinical outcomes such as mortality, survival, and relapse rates are less appropriate and less informative for RA and other chronic conditions in which the main goal of treatment and care is to improve, or at least maintain, QoL. In addition, clinical outcomes tend to be assessed by doctors, whereas health status and QoL tend to be self-assessed, thereby providing a patient perspective of the consequences of a disease. Health-status measures such as the Short-Form 36 health survey questionnaire (Ware and Sherbourne 1992)☐ provide important information (usually in a self-report format) about aspects of the quality of a patient's health, for example pain, functioning, and mood. Health status may be assessed by a health-care professional or a family carer as well as by a patient, whereas each individual patient assesses QoL. Thus, QoL measures provide an opportunity and means of eliciting and recording the unique perspective of each patient on their condition and how it affects their daily life. Measures tend to be questionnaire based. It is important that a relevant, condition-specific measure is applied to the appropriate patient group which is sufficiently sensitive to assess each patient's status and which can also detect any changes in QoL over time. For example, it would not be appropriate to use a generic measure or a measure that had been designed specifically for use with schizophrenia, to assess patients with RA. Fortunately, many compendiums of QoL scales and similar outcome measures are readily available (see, for example, Bowling 1995). ☐

> **Q1** What is the most important reason for the use of QoL scales for the clinician specializing in musculoskeletal disease?
>
> **Q2** For which other diseases may QoL scales be especially relevant?

13.2 Osteoarthritis

Definition and natural history

Osteoarthritis (OA), until relatively recently, was considered to be part of normal ageing, which is reflected in terms such as 'degenerative' or 'wear-and-tear'. Currently, despite some controversy, OA is defined as a disease characterized by focal areas of loss of articular cartilage within synovial joints, which are associated with hypertrophy of bone (osteophytes and subchondral bone sclerosis) and thickening of the capsule. Clinically, the condition is characterized by joint pain, tenderness, limitation of movement, crepitus, occasional effusion, and, as reflected in the name, inflammation. It can occur in any joint but is most common in the hip, knee, and the joints of the hand, foot, and spine. Inclusion in the disease definition of changes made visible by X-ray cannot distinguish between symptomatic and relatively asymptomatic OA. However, in an attempt to reduce overestimation of disease burden, epidemiological studies use definitions that combine X-ray findings and joint pain.

Most people with OA have relatively mild symptoms, but for an appreciable minority, the condition is more aggressive. In this group, fraying and fibrillation of cartilage results in development of synovitis, which is probably responsible for much of the more severe pain in the disorder. Unfortunately, it is not yet possible to accurately identify those individuals who will develop severely symptomatic disease, or indeed, benefit from any preventive treatment that might be found. However, more recent studies suggest that narrowing of joint spaces apparent on X-rays of knees is a strong predictor of future progression, and is also a significant predictor of total joint arthroplasty (Wolfe and Lane 2002). ☐

Incidence and prevalence

OA was estimated to be the eighth leading non-fatal burden of disease in the world in 1990, accounting for 2.8 per cent of total years of living with disability. In general, it is more prevalent in Europe and the USA than in other parts of the world.

Few data are available on the incidence of OA because of the difficulty of defining it and in determining its onset. A study from Australia which sought to calculate the incidence indicated that the disease is more common among women in all age groups (2.95 per 1000 population versus 1.71 per 1000 in men). For women, the highest incidence is among those in the 65–74 year age-group, reaching 13.5 per 1000 population per year, whereas for men, the highest incidence occurs among those aged over 75 years (9 per 1000 population per year). More recent radiological longitudinal surveys in the UK suggest that the incidence may be much higher, with 20–30 women per 1000 aged 50–60 years developing new radiological knee, hip, or spinal OA each year (Hassett et al. 2003). 🖳

Prevalence is also problematic to measure accurately. Worldwide estimates are that 9.6 per cent of men and 18.0 per cent of women aged 60 years and above have symptomatic disease. Most attempts to estimate the prevalence are based on radiographic surveys of populations and indicate that prevalence increases indefinitely with age; changes are uncommon in persons under the age of 40 years but are seen in more than 50 per cent of people over the age of 65 years and almost universally after 85 years. Men are affected more often than women among those aged less than 45 years, whereas in the over 55-year-old age group it is women who experience more disease. Radiographic studies of North American and European populations aged over 45 years show higher rates for OA of the knee: 14 per cent for men and 23 per cent for women. Symptomatic, radiographically proven OA of the knee has been found among 3 per cent of women aged 45–65 years. Hip OA is slightly less common, with a radiographic prevalence of 1.9 per cent among men and 2.3 per cent among women aged 45 years or more in one Swedish survey (Danielsson and Lindberg 1997). 🖳

Time trends

Not surprisingly, because of the difficulty of defining and measuring the disease, there are few data on trends in the incidence of OA, and whether incidence is changing is not clear. Two Nordic studies used proxy measures to assess trends. The first, from Norway, reported that the incidence of OA-specific disability pensions increased over the 30 years from 1968 to 1997 while the second, an Icelandic study, found an increase in the rate of new hip replacements from 1982 to 1996. However, it has been suggested that this reflects improved access to surgery rather than an upward trend in incidence.

In the USA, pharmacological treatment for OA decreased from 49 per cent of visits (1989–91) to 46 per cent (1992–94) to 40 per cent (1995–98), which supports this view. As the incidence and prevalence of the disease rise with increasing age, extended life expectancy will result in greater numbers of people with the condition. The burden will be the greatest in developing countries, where life expectancy is increasing and access to arthroplasty and joint replacement is poor.

Risk factors

The main risk factors are age, a positive family history, female sex, obesity, and joint trauma. Modifiable factors, including obesity, injury, quadriceps strength, malalignment of the joint, and occupational activities, contribute to the onset and progression of joint disability.

Obesity is a risk factor for the development of OA of the hand, knee, and hip and for progression in the knee and hip. It was generally believed that the obesity was secondary to inactivity brought about by the painful joints. However, well-designed epidemiological studies now show that the risk begins as early as the third decade of life. For every two units increase in body mass index (BMI) (equivalent to about 5 kg), the risk of OA of the knee is increased by 36 per cent. Conversely, for every 5 kg decrease in body weight during the preceding 10 years, the risk of OA of the knee declines by more than 50 per cent. People classified as obese (BMI > 30 kg/m^2) have a 20-fold risk of developing bilateral OA of the knee (Hart et al. 1999). 🖳

Trauma and certain physically demanding activities or occupations are also risk factors for the development of OA of the knee and hip. Farming presents the greatest relative risk: 4.5 for those who work in farming for 1–9 years and 9.3 for those who farm for more than 10 years. The strongest association with occupational activity has been shown with OA of the knee in men. It is estimated that up to 30 per cent of OA in this joint is attributable to occupational activity that involves repeated knee bending, kneeling, squatting, or climbing. These activities increase the risk two- to fourfold and, if combined with heavy lifting of more than 25 kg on a regular basis, increase risk fivefold. Strong interactions are shown between occupational knee bending and obesity (risk increased 10–15 times) and between age and injury to the knee.

Family history is a well-documented risk factor, with the occurrence of Heberden's nodes having almost autosomal dominant inheritance. Despite this strong association, no single gene defect has been identified.

Studies of twins now suggest that the heritability component of osteoarthritis may be as high as 60–65 per cent for hip and hand osteoarthritis, and around 40–50 per cent for knee osteoarthritis.

All **races** can be affected by OA, but some Asians have a much lower prevalence in the hip and hand, but a higher prevalence in the knee. More disease is seen in the knee in Chinese women when compared with North American women, and is independent of weight and anatomical alignment of the lower limbs. Why this might be so is suggested in a study that investigated the association between squatting and risk of OA, a common daily posture in China (Zhang *et al.* 2004). 💻

Treatment issues

Although pharmacotherapy has a major role in treatment of OA, hip and knee joint replacements are also of great importance as they are among the most cost-effective interventions available. Ninety per cent of total hip replacements and over 95 per cent of total knee replacements are performed for OA. The difficulties in measuring incidence and prevalence of OA complicate the assessment of **population need** for total joint replacement surgery. Many aspects need to be considered, not only incidence and prevalence, but also disease progression, and patients' preferences for surgery and doctors' propensity for recommending it. Such factors were considered in studies of the need for total hip and knee surgery in England. The authors estimated that, whereas hip replacement rates were closely in line with need, a doubling of the current rate of knee replacement surgery would be required just to meet existing need (Juni *et al.* 2003). 💻 This **unmet need** was not just the result of health-care services' inability to keep up with demand, but also of patients and doctors not considering, or offering, knee replacement as a treatment option.

13.3 Osteoporosis

Osteoporosis (OP) is a systemic skeletal disease characterized by progressive age-related loss of bone strength that leads to increased risk of fracture of both long bones and vertebrae. This is of particular importance in the elderly who are at risk of falling, often causing fracture of the neck of the femur at the hip joint, or Colles' fracture of head of the radius at the wrist joint. Hip fracture (neck of femur) carries a high case fatality rate of up to 24 per cent at one year (NIH Consensus Development Panel 2001). 💻 In young adults, bone strength far exceeds the loads that are normally applied to bone during activities of daily living. Thus there is a large

'safety factor' in this age-group. However, with increased age there is a marked reduction in bone mass and destruction of bone architecture, leading to sizeable decreases in strength.

Bone strength is thought to be influenced by bone quality, which encompasses characteristics such as trabecular micro-architecture, bone remodelling rate, micro-damage, and the degree of mineralization of the matrix (NIH Consensus 2001). 💻 Bone strength cannot be determined directly *in vivo*, and bone mineral density (BMD), which accounts for about 60–80 per cent of whole bone strength, is commonly used as a proxy indicator.

Evaluation of BMD measurements

Several technologies now exist which measure BMD, including single and dual energy absorptiometry, dual-energy X-ray absorptiometry and quantitative computed tomography. They vary in their accuracy, which can be compared to a 'gold standard' where BMD is measured in animals, and animal bone is then evaluated chemically (WHO 1994). 💻 Accuracy may also depend on the precise skeletal site being assessed and the amount of fat tissue interposed between the instrument and the bone. However, when evaluating the usefulness of different screening techniques it is also important to consider the population variance in BMD. The distribution of BMD in young adults is shown in Figure 13.3.

Osteoporosis is defined as a bone mineral density more than 2.5 standard deviations below the young

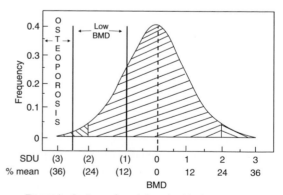

The curve describes the normal range for bone mineral density expressed as percentage positive or negative deviation from the mean, or in units of standard deviation (SDU).

Fig. 13.3 Distribution of bone mineral density (BMD) in a young, normal population and definition of osteoporosis.
Source: Adapted from World Health Organization (1994).
Assessment of Fracture Risk and Application to Screening for Postmenopausal Osteoporosis. WHO Technical Report Series No. 843. Geneva: World Health Organization.

adult reference mean. Standard deviation units are termed *z*-scores and allow comparisons of methods with different units of measurements and other populations such as the young and elderly. It has been estimated that 70 per cent of women aged 80 years or more in the USA have BMD greater than 2.5 standard deviations below the mean. A *z*-score between –1 and –2.5 is defined as low BMD in young adults, but clearly cannot guide treatment in the elderly. The evaluation of a patient with suspected OP must involve a thorough clinical history, physical examination, and BMD measurement. Table 13.1 illustrates some of the more important modifiable and non-modifiable risk factors for OP.

There has been much debate about the value of BMD measurement as a screening tool. The National Screening Committee (2002), 🖳 however, has not been able to recommend this based on current methods and evidence. It is true that combinations of risk factors multiply the risks of sustaining a fracture (Table 13.2), but most people with these risk factors will not experience an adverse outcome. Thus, among the key reasons for the decision of the National Screening Committee, is the relatively poor ability of the test to predict which *individuals* will sustain a fracture. It is crucial, when any diagnostic or screening test is being evaluated, to consider its place in a clinical pathway designed to improve patient outcomes. No test should be ordered unless the result will be likely to affect the outcome for the patient. Screening of all women is not recommended, but selected high-risk women are routinely screened in North America. Arguments for (Dequeker and Luyton 2001) 🖳 and against (Wilkin and Devendra 2001) 🖳 the use of bone densitometry as a screening tool have been recently proposed. An evaluation of four different selection criteria in a cohort of 2365 post-menopausal women from Canada showed that an alternative set of decision rules was superior to that recommended in national guidelines to predict risk of hip fracture (Cadarette *et al.* 2001). 🖳

Prevention of hip fractures

Sustaining a fracture, particularly a hip fracture in old age, is not a trivial affliction. Any strategy to prevent or treat OP therefore, must incorporate a programme to prevent falls as an element. Intensive multifactorial preventive strategies that include exercise, reduction in medications, and environmental modifications can reduce falls by 30 per cent (Carter *et al.* 2001). 🖳 At a minimum, the risk factors for falls to predict hip fracture should be recorded and acted upon for all frail elderly, whether in hospital or community. Some of these risks are illustrated in Table 13.3 and many are amenable to simple interventions.

However, the condition needs to be tackled on multiple fronts, with, for example, advice on diet (and calcium supplementation where necessary) and effective treatment (with modern bone strengthening agents such as bisphosphonates) for established disease. An important lesson to be drawn from the debates about the measurement of BMD must be that the outcome of any intervention (whether diagnostic or therapeutic) must be seen against a broad canvas: the benefit of a **systems approach** lies in seeing our actions and intervention to combat the consequences of OP in their place, as part of a system or environment that can either enhance or erode our health (See Box 13.2).

13.4 Backache

More than two-thirds of adults in Western countries will at some time suffer from low back pain (LBP) (Deyo and Weinstein 2001) 🖳 but, fortunately, although LBP consists of a variety of entities with somewhat different aetiologies, most episodes are of limited duration. Nevertheless, the condition is a leading cause of sickness absence and retirement due to ill health. The epidemiology and management of the condition were well reviewed in the 1990s by the Clinical Standards Advisory Group (1994) and by the Royal College of General Practitioners (1996), and the guidance emerging from

TABLE 13.1 Risk factors for osteoporosis

Not modifiable	Possibly modifiable
Personal history of adult fracture	Low bone mineral density
History of fracture in first-degree relative	Current cigarette use Low body weight (<127 pounds or 57 kg)
Caucasian and Asian race	Oestrogen deficiency including menopause onset at younger than 45 years
Advanced age	Alcoholism
Female sex	Lifelong low calcium intake
Glucocorticoid use	Recurrent falls
Dementia	Inadequate physical activity
Poor health/frailty	Discontinuation or non-compliance of anti-resorptive therapy

TABLE 13.2 Population relative risk of fracture by number of risk factors

Women aged 50–60 years			Annual absolute fracture risk for women aged:	
Risk factors	Prevalence of factor (%)	Relative risk if have factor versus average risk	50–54 years (%)	55–59 years (%)
No risk factors	58.3	0.5	0.7	0.8
One risk factor	32.8	1.2	1.5	1.9
Two risk factors	7.6	2.7	3.5	4.3
Three risk factors	1.4	5.9	7.6	9.4
After bone densitometry				
One risk factor, BMD > mean	14.3	0.6	0.8	1.0
One risk factor, BMD in second quarter	8.5	1.1	1.5	1.8
Two risk factors, BMD > mean	2.9	1.4	1.7	2.8
One risk factor, BMD in lowest 1/4	10.1	2.0	2.5	3.2
Two risk factors, BMD in second lowest quarter	2.0	2.4	3.0	3.8
Three risk factors, BMD above mean	0.4	2.8	3.6	4.5
Two risk factors, BMD in lowest quarter	2.6	4.0	5.2	6.5
Three risk factors, BMD in second lowest quarter	0.1	4.8	6.2	7.6
Three risk factors, BMD in lowest quarter	0.9	7.8	10.1	12.5

The non-spine fracture incidence for Caucasian British women aged 52 years is 1.3 per cent, and for women aged 57 years is 1.6 per cent.

Modified from: Torgerson, D. J., Igesisias, C. P., Reid, D. M. (2001). 'The Economics of Fracture Prevention', in D. H. Barlow, R. M. Francis and A. Miles (eds.), *The Effective Management of Osteoporosis*. London: Aesculapius Medical Press, 111–21.

these is still valid. Surveys have shown that the equivalent of nearly 2 per cent of all people in employment have lost at least one day in the past four weeks from LBP, whereas the estimate for total working days lost in Britain is around 52 million days. The cost of disability benefits and lost production exceeds £5 billion annually (Clinical Standards Advisory Group 1994). 💻

Epidemiology

Any strategy to reduce morbidity has to start with an appreciation of the epidemiology and risk factors. In a review of studies, the population annual prevalence was reported to lie between 15 per cent and 45 per cent and the point prevalence averaged 30 per cent. In surveys of the general population, LBP is found equally in men and women and is most common in the elderly (Andersson 1999). 💻 Up to 60 per cent of people with LBP will also have neck pain, and LPB is frequently associated with other complaints. There is conflicting evidence for a relation between LBP prevalence and social class, and this may be largely related to occupation. It seems clear that back pain is more common in people in heavy manual occupations who undertake heavy lifting, and it has been reported to be more common among smokers. On both counts, the health service itself needs to target its training programmes towards especially vulnerable staff such as nurses.

Psychological factors are often quoted as being important to the aetiology of LBP, but it is difficult to distinguish those that preceded acute symptoms from those that followed. Nevertheless, such factors have to be borne in mind when decisions about patient management are being made in primary care. In a longitudinal study in the UK, it was noted that 90 per cent of patients were no longer consulting their general practitioner three months after the initial consultation, but, on interview, most had continued symptoms and disability 12 months later.

TABLE 13.3 Host risk factors for falls among the elderly for which the evidence is strong or moderate

Demographic characteristics

Older age

Female sex

Functional level

Limitations in activities of daily living and instrumental activities of daily living

Cane/walker use

History of falls

Gait, balance, strength

Slow walking speed

Postural sway

Low lower-extremity strength

Low upper-extremity strength

Impaired reflexes

Sensory

Poor vision

Lower-extremity sensory perception

Chronic illnesses

Parkinson's disease

Other neuromuscular disease

Stroke

Urinary incontinence

Arthritis

Acute illness

Medications, alcohol

Several medications used

Hypnotics

Sedatives

Antidepressants

Antiparkinsonism drugs

Mental status

Cognitive impairment

Depression

Kelsey, J. L. and Sowes, M. F. (2004). 'Musculoskeletal Diseases', in R. Detels, J. McEwen, R. Beaglehole, and H. Tanaka (eds.), *Oxford Textbook of Public Health* (4th edn). Oxford: Oxford University Press. Modified from Grisso *et al.* (1991).

BOX 13.2 A SYSTEMS APPROACH TO THE EVALUATION OF BONE DENSITOMETRY

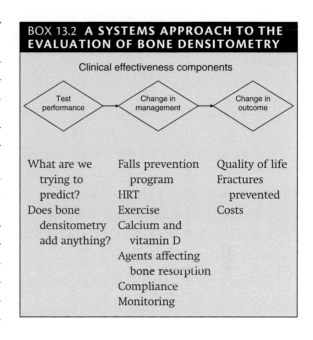

Clinical management

The most important underlying principle to guide management of LBP in primary care is early and effective triage (French: *trier*, to sort). Box 13.3 summarizes the main points for triage and initial management. Most cases can and should be managed without recourse to secondary care, which should be reserved for those who have failed to settle within six to eight weeks. Consensus evidence suggests that there should be a gradual increase in physical activity with no initial bed rest (Royal College of General Practitioners 1996). The types of hospital service most likely to prove effective are those that offer multi-disciplinary assessment from the outset, including psychosocial and vocational advice and input from rehabilitation and pain management specialists. In certain defined cases, manipulative treatment or surgery can be beneficial. A recent review suggested that evidence on prognosis is limited, which will also have implications for the evaluation of effective interventions. Small trials of early intervention suggest that early and manual (Wand *et al.* 2004) interventions are more successful at leading to improvement than passive or waiting models of care or exercise interventions respectively. In a randomized controlled trial, chiropractors were more successful than hospital outpatient departments in achieving pain relief and general satisfaction with the outcome of treatment (Meade *et al.* 1995).

BOX 13.3 **DIAGNOSTIC TRIAGE**

Diagnostic triage is the differential diagnosis between:

- Simple backache (non specific low back pain)
- Nerve root pain
- Possible serious spinal pathology

Simple backache: specialist referral not required

- Presentation 20–55 years
- Lumbrosacral, buttock, and thighs
- 'Mechanical' pain
- Patient well

Nerve root pain: specialist referral not generally required within first 4 weeks, provided resolving

- Unilateral leg pain worse than low back pain
- Radiates to foot or toes
- Numbness and parathesia in same distribution
- SLR reproduces leg pain
- Localized neurological signs

Red flags for possible serious spinal pathology: prompt referral (less than 4 weeks)

- Presentation under age 20 or onset over 55 years
- Non-mechanical pain
- Thoracic pain
- Past history: carcinoma, steroids, HIV
- Unwell, weight loss
- Widespread neurology
- Structural deformity

Cauda equina syndrome: immediate referral

- Sphincter disturbance
- Gait disturbance
- Saddle anaesthesia

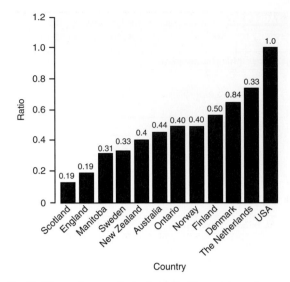

Fig. 13.4 Rates of surgery for back pain in 11 countries and Canadian provinces as a proportion of those in the USA. Source: Anderson, G. B. J. (1999). 'Epidemiological features of chronic low back pain'. *The Lancet* **354**: 581–5.

A recent review of trials of primary prevention in the workplace concluded that there was little evidence to support the use of education in lifting techniques or for lumbar supports but there was some evidence to recommend an exercise programme (van Poppel *et al.* 2004). 🖥

Q3 How would you interpret the data shown in Figure 13.4?

Q4 What additional data would be helpful?

Further epidemiological studies and RCTs will be required for all musculoskeletal disorders because of their uncertain aetiologies, the general lack of effective treatments (joint replacement surgery may provide an exception to this statement), and a likely increase in the prevalence of these disorders in an ageing population. In addition, QoL outcome measurements for these disorders will require further development.

Model answers

Q1 Musculoskeletal disease does not cause death in the short term; however, pain and disability can severely restrict movement and the ability to perform activities of daily living. This will have an effect on QoL, so QoL scales are an important means of assessing remission, progression of disease, and response to treatment.

Q2 Similarly, other diseases that may be long term and debilitating include mental disorders, certain cancers, chronic cardiovascular diseases such as angina and stroke, and chronic lung and kidney disease.

Q3 There is a more than 10-fold difference between rates for surgical intervention for back pain between the UK and USA. In part this may reflect a conservative attitude towards intervention on the part of the UK surgeons (and also those in Manitoba), but it may also reflect the availability of the service. It would be helpful to know where the optimal intervention rates lie in relation to the current evidence-base for surgical intervention.

Q4 From the perspective of audit it would be helpful to have an estimate of the complication rate of surgery.

References

References for this chapter can be found at www.oxfordtextbooks.co.uk/orc/yarnell. Where possible, these are presented as *active links* which direct you to an electronic version of the work. If you are a subscriber to that work (either individually or through an institution), and depending on your level of access, you may be able to peruse an abstract or the full article if available. 🖳

Maternal and child health

This chapter introduces the topics of fertility (its influence on population structure), infertility, and maternal mortality. Major causes of death in neonates, infants, and children are discussed for developed countries and for developing countries with inadequate levels of health care. Surveillance and screening for congenital anomalies conclude this chapter.

Introduction

The delivery of a healthy baby who survives to adulthood is not only a potentially desirable outcome for any mother, it is one of the most valuable assets a community can enjoy. Each year over 10 million children in the world die below the age of five years (Black *et al.* 2003) ⌨ and over half a million women die from complications of pregnancy, child-bearing, or unsafe abortion. Most of these deaths occur in developing countries, where poverty is widespread, effective public-health programmes and clinical care services are often poor or absent, and malnutrition, both overt and at subclinical and micronutrient level, affects many women of child-bearing age and their infants. The health of both is jeopardized by the resulting impaired immunity to infectious disease and the suboptimal physical and mental development that ensues.

While defining and measuring health may raise philosophical and practical questions, the reproductive performance of women and the survival of the infants they bear are widely accepted in all countries as summary markers of the general health status of a population. Measurement of these markers provides some insights into the range and quality of health-care services for women and their infants, and facilitates the monitoring of the impact of changing health-care practices (for example the introduction of antenatal screening programmes). They also improve our understanding of the health effects of changes in other sectors such as agriculture, education, and fiscal policy (see also Chapter 1, Figure 1.1 and Chapter 21).

The key indicators to be considered here relate to the patterns of fertility, maternal, perinatal, and infant mortality, and congenital malformation in the population.

14.1 Fertility and Infertility

The capacity to control or improve fertility is the outcome of a range of inter-related factors. Contraceptive practice and effectiveness, marriage and cohabitation trends, sexual mores and practice, female expectations and aspirations, availability of abortion, and social and economic circumstances, all influence the pattern of reproduction.

While some information about fertility in England and Wales has been collected since registration of live births was introduced in 1838, comprehensive data were not recorded throughout the UK until 1974. Figure 14.1 shows the trend in the general fertility rate in England and Wales since reliable records began. This reflects the net effect of many factors including political stability and economic growth (rising rate), war and economic depression (declining rate), and widespread availability of contraception (declining rate).

This fall has been the result of a marked reduction in childbearing among younger women. Reproductive rates have risen among older women, suggesting a postponement of childbearing to the thirties or forties

(Botting *et al.* 2001). 🖥 In the past 25 years the proportion of births in England and Wales in women age 30 years or above has doubled, and the proportion to mothers aged 35 years or more has trebled in the past 10 years; but the net effect of the changes has been that **total period fertility rate** (**TPFR**: a standard measure which gives the total number of children a woman would bear if she experienced the age-specific fertility rates for the year in question) has been declining. In Western countries a TPFR of 2.1 is required to maintain long-term population levels, assuming no migration. The rate in all parts of the UK is now below two. This fall in 'replacement' population coupled with the increasing longevity of the current population raises important social and economic questions.

Population structure

Declining fertility in many economically well-developed countries and improved survival of both the very young and the elderly has led to alteration in the **demographic** profile of such countries. Recent population structures for some Western countries are shown in Figure 14.2 with current fertility rates. The figure also includes two Middle Eastern countries, Egypt and Iraq, which portray the classical '**population pyramid**', and finally two African countries, one significantly affected by acquired immunodeficiency syndrome (AIDS), which has been responsible for many deaths in young adults.

Population structures are available electronically for most countries from the US Census Bureau (2005). 🖥

Mortality or morbidity rates, which compare different countries, clearly require adjustment for differing population age structures. The World Health Organization (WHO) uses two standard reference populations to which rates can be adjusted; the **World and the European standard populations** which reflect averages for the two regions, the World standard population conforming to the classic pyramidal structure (reflecting a high fertility rate and a greater proportion of infants and children than adults), and the European standard population reflecting similar proportions of young and old.

Apart from the social and cultural factors influencing fertility, two 'medical' interventions have had an important role. These are developments in **assisted reproduction techniques** and the **legalization and liberalization of abortion**.

Assisted reproduction

Human fertility is low compared with most other species, and the chance of pregnancy per menstrual

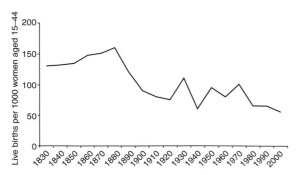

Fig. 14.1 General fertility rate, England and Wales, 1830–2000. Source: Office of National Statistics (1998). www.statistics.gov.uk.

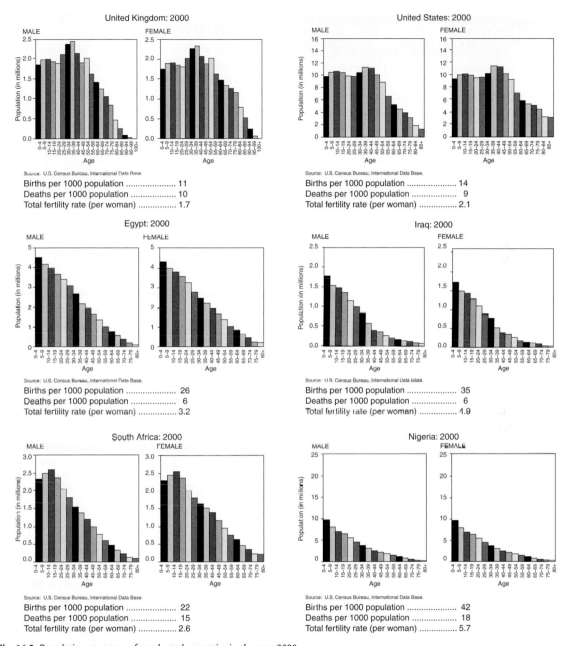

Fig. 14.2 Population structures for selected countries in the year 2000.
Source: US Census Bureau (2005). International database, summary statistics available at: www.census/gov/ipc/idbsum.html.

cycle in the most fertile couples is about 33 per cent. Within a year of regular intercourse, 90 per cent of fertile couples should become pregnant, but a delay of more than one year is usually the accepted criterion to define sub-fertility and initiate investigations. A woman's fertility declines with age, and one effect of

choosing to defer childbirth to later years has been to increase referrals for infertility investigations and treatment. Many technologies for assisted conception exist with a bewildering array of acronyms, but all with the aim of bringing sperm and egg together to promote fertilization, achieve pregnancy, and to see that result

BOX 14.1 **ABOUT THE HUMAN FERTILISATION AND EMBRYOLOGY AUTHORITY**

The Human Fertilisation and Embryology Authority (HFEA) was set up in August 1991 by the Human Fertilisation and Embryology Act 1990. The first statutory body of its type in the world, the HFEA's creation reflected public and professional interest in the potential future of human embryo research and infertility treatments, and a widespread desire for statutory regulation of all related procedures.

The HFEA's principal tasks are to license and monitor clinics that carry out *in vitro* fertilization, donor insemination, and human embryo research. The HFEA also regulates the storage of gametes (sperm and ova) and embryos.

in a healthy baby. The three main types of assisted conception are:

1 **Intrauterine insemination (IUI)**: prepared sperm are pipetted in the uterus at a time when ovulation is likely or assisted.

2 *In vitro* **fertilization (IVF)**: Fertilization is aided by mixing sperm and eggs in the laboratory.

3 **Intracytoplasmic sperm injection (ICSI)**: A single sperm is injected directly into the egg cytoplasm to achieve fertilization.

All patients considering an assisted pregnancy must be informed of the live birth rate per treatment cycle started, sometimes called the '**take home baby**' rate for the centre providing the service; all clinical pregnancies and their outcome from these various techniques must be reported to the Human Fertilisation and Embryology Authority (HFEA).

The live birth rates from the different techniques vary but are around 20 per cent per treatment cycle started. The cause of the infertility, ages of partners, sperm quality and duration of infertility all affect the outcome but maternal age is a major determinant of success, whatever the method. Only 1 per cent of live births in the UK are from assisted conceptions, but an increasing proportion of multiple births stem from these procedures. For women under 40 years of age, HFEA has proposed that a maximum of two eggs are used per treatment cycle (three or more can be used in women over 40 years of age).

14.2 **Abortion**

Spontaneous abortion or miscarriage is a common outcome of pregnancy with an international average of approximately 15 per cent (Vogel and Motulsky 2002); if occurring very early in pregnancy it may be unrecognized but, for epidemiological and legal purposes in the UK, it is defined as the expulsion of a foetus or dead-born infant occurring before 24 weeks of pregnancy. Spontaneous abortion is associated with a higher than average prevalence of congenital anomaly, often due to chromosomal abnormalities. In England, Wales, and Scotland the Abortion Act of 1967, which came into effect on 27 April 1968, allows termination of pregnancy by a registered medical practitioner, subject to certain conditions. These include: risk to the life of the woman, risk of injury to her physical or mental health or that of her existing children, and substantial risk that the infant would be born with such physical or mental abnormalities as to be seriously handicapped. Later, in 1990, amendments to the 1967 legislation came into force through the Human Fertilisation and Embryology Act, making the time limit of abortion 24 weeks on certain statutory grounds, and without time limit on certain others. So far, there have been almost five million terminations under the Abortion Act. Legal termination accounted for the outcome of almost 20 per cent of pregnancies in the past decade (Table 14.1).

In England and Wales in 2001 some 17 women per 1000 in the age group 15–44 years had legal terminations and fewer than 1 per cent were on the basis of risk of serious handicap in the infant.

One of the major benefits of the Abortion Act has been the eradication of the toll of maternal death associated with the illegal abortions to which many desperate women had hitherto resorted. Legality and safety are highly correlated. In global terms, dealing with unwanted pregnancy is a major maternal health problem. The latest estimates suggest that some 19 million unsafe abortions are performed annually, and that they account for some 13 per cent of maternal deaths in developing countries (WHO 2003). It has been further estimated that if all women who say they want no more children were able to stop childbearing the number of births would be reduced by 35 per cent in Latin America, 33 per cent in Asia, and 17 per cent in Africa. If this happened, maternal mortality would be expected to fall proportionately.

The widespread availability of effective contraception and of safe termination of unwanted pregnancies have a strong influence on maternal reproductive behaviour

TABLE 14.1 Estimated triennial pregnancy outcomes (in thousands) in the UK, 1991–99

Triennium	Maternities	Legal abortions	Spontaneous abortions	Ectopic pregnancies	Total estimated pregnancies
1991–93	2317.3	525.6	266.4	30.2	3139.5
1994–96	2197.6	519.1	164.7	33.5	2914.9
1997–99	2123.6	564.1	153.6	31.9	2873.3
Percentage	73.9	19.6	5.3	1.1	100.0

Source: Botting, B., on behalf of the Editorial Board (2001). *Trends in Reproductive Epidemiology and Women's Health*. Confidential Enquiry into Maternal Deaths in the United Kingdom. 5th Report. London: Royal College of Obstetricians and Gynaecologists.

and outcome. The methods available in the developed world may prove difficult to introduce or practise in countries where religious, cultural, and economic factors limit the availability or acceptability of some services.

> **Q1** Summarize the methods of birth control, their relative effectiveness, advantages and disadvantages (suggest constructing a table).

14.3 Maternal Mortality

Before the second half of the twentieth century, it was recognized that pregnancy and childbirth were often hazardous times for both mother and baby. Effective treatment of common, serious complications of pregnancy was extremely limited, regular antenatal supervision was unusual, and the specialty of obstetrics was undeveloped. In the UK at the end of the nineteenth century, five women died in every 1000 pregnancies. Recent figures from developing countries range from 17–18 deaths per 1000 live births (Sierra Leone and Afghanistan) to 2–6 per 1000 live births (Philippines and India). In the UK and other industrialized countries this was largely the picture until the 1940s, when several key scientific and social developments occurred which have reduced the maternal mortality to 0.14 per 1000 'maternities' (total pregnancies; miscarriages, stillbirths, and livebirths). Here, we can use a more precise denominator because the data for miscarriages, stillbirths, and livebirths are available, although miscarriages may be estimated. In developing countries only data for live births are commonly available. Measures to prevent or treat the sepsis, haemorrhage, and toxaemia, which had hitherto threatened the lives of many women, were of major importance but, so too were the establishment of routine antenatal care, and a

wide range of schemes related to education and social welfare. Together these improved not just the nature, availability, and organization of maternity care but also the health of the women who required it. In the UK an important development was the introduction in 1952 of a Confidential Enquiry into Maternal Deaths, which focused attention on collecting comprehensive, valid information on all the deaths. It was recognition of the importance of monitoring, examining, and summarizing events, so that avoidable factors could be identified and the scope for improvement fully realized.

The Enquiry collects information on all maternal deaths, from whatever cause, occurring during pregnancy and for up to one year after delivery. The classification of deaths in the UK Confidential Enquiry into Maternal Deaths is shown in Box 14.2.

Maternal mortality has fallen by 80 per cent since the Confidential Enquiries began and now stands at 13.5 per 100 000 maternities (RCOG 2001). 🖥 Hypertensive diseases of pregnancy, pulmonary embolism, abortion, and sepsis were the main causes of death in early reports but deaths directly attributable to complications of pregnancy, labour, or the puerperium now account for less than 50 per cent of all maternal deaths. The most recent report cites thromboembolism, heart disease, and suicide as the most common reasons for maternal death (Figure 14.3). Although a great deal has been achieved, the Confidential Enquiries indicate that women continue to die from potentially treatable conditions, and that there are patterns of practice, service provision, and public-health issues that need to be addressed. Since 2003, in the UK maternal and infant deaths have been reviewed collectively as the Confidential Enquiry into Maternal and Child Health (CEMACH 2005). 🖥

Maternal death is one end of a spectrum of what is, for most women, a natural and uncomplicated process.

BOX 14.2 **CLASSIFICATION OF MATERNAL DEATHS (UK)**	
Direct	From obstetric complications of the pregnant state (pregnancy, labour and puerperium) from interventions, omissions, incorrect treatment, or from a chain of events resulting from any of the above.
Indirect	From previous existing disease or disease that developed during pregnancy and which was not due to direct obstetric causes, but which was aggravated by the physiologic effects of pregnancy.
Late	Between 42 days and one year after termination of pregnancy, miscarriage or delivery that are due to Direct or Indirect maternal causes.
Coincidental	Deaths from unrelated causes that happen to occur in pregnancy or the puerperium.

Source: Royal College of Obstetricians and Gynaecologists (2001). *Why Mothers Die 1997–99*. The 5th Report of the Confidential Enquiries into Maternal Deaths in the United Kingdom. London: RCOG Press.

The risk of death, complications, or other unsatisfactory outcome is related to a range of factors, both physical and social. For maternal age and parity the association is J-shaped, rates being lowest for women aged 20–24 years and then rising with age, particularly for mothers aged 35 years and over. The pattern with parity is that the lowest rate for women is in their second pregnancy. Analysis of the social class differences in mortality and morbidity have demonstrated that for many women their reproductive life and that of their infants would be much improved if they had a better education, adequate income, good housing, a balanced diet, a stable relationship, and sound general health and family medical history. Mortality rates among the socially disadvantaged, including women from lower socioeconomic groups, many single mothers, teenagers, and some ethnic groups, are higher than among the population as a whole. Those in the most deprived circumstances are at substantially greater risk of dying than women from professional or managerial groups (Figure 14.4).

Other newer factors that merit further exploration are: obesity, access to care, violence in the home, multiple pregnancy, and *in vitro* fertilization. The health service can have little direct role in changing these factors once pregnancy has occurred, but it has a duty to ensure that such disadvantages are recognized and that the clinical care is focused on ameliorating their effect, so far as is possible. Risk recognition, clinical

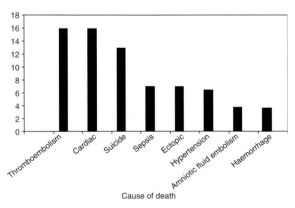

Fig. 14.3 Major causes of maternal deaths by rate per million maternities.
Source: Royal College of Cause of death Obstetricians and Gynaecologists (2001). *Why Mothers Die 1997–99*. The 5th Report of the Confidential Enquiries into Maternal Deaths in the United Kingdom. London: RCOG Press.

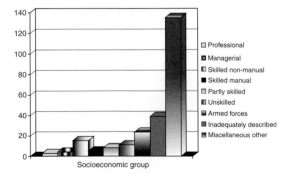

Fig. 14.4 Maternal mortality by social class in the UK 1997–99.
Source: Botting, B., on behalf of the Editorial Board (2001). *Trends in Reproductive Epidemiology and Women's Health.* Confidential Enquiry into Maternal Deaths in the United Kingdom. 5th Report. London Royal College of Obstetricians and Gynaecologists.

protocols, and guidelines for care can all help but it is the public-health challenge which these social inequalities pose that must be met if there is to be further reduction in maternal mortality.

14.4 Perinatal and Infant Mortality

At the beginning of the twentieth century **infant mortality (deaths in the first year of life)** in Britain was about 140 per 1000 live births, although it was more than double this rate in parts of Russia and Germany. Effective preventive or therapeutic measures to combat infection were not available, malnourishment was widespread, and the particular requirements of the premature infant were not understood. Just as with maternal mortality, the second half of the twentieth century saw the mortality rate in infants begin to fall steeply, and between 1950 and 2000 it fell from 30 to 6 per 1000 live births (ONS 2004). As noted in Chapter 1, most of the decline in infant mortality occurred long before the introduction of immunization against childhood infections.

As rates fell, an increasing proportion of the deaths occurred in the early postnatal period. Over 50 per cent of infants who die now do so in the first week of life, the majority on the first day. The longer a baby lives the greater its chances of continuing to survive. It was recognized that these very early postnatal deaths were often part of a continuum of threats to the foetus, and, whether a particular infant died shortly before or after birth, was often largely a matter of chance. Therefore a new measurement (**perinatal mortality**) was introduced, which encompassed stillbirths and deaths in the first week of life, and has become an important marker of foetal and neonatal health.

Stillbirth recording, introduced in England and Wales in 1927 (1939 in Scotland and 1961 in Northern Ireland), was but the belated application of an important observation made many centuries before (see Box 14.3).

The perinatal mortality rate in England and Wales has fallen from an initial rate of over 60 per 1000 total births when first recorded to eight in the year 2000, stillbirths accounting for five of these. The rates have been stable over the past decade (Figure 14.5).

In 1999 the most common identifiable causes of stillbirth were malformation and maternal complication of pregnancy, for example antepartum haemorrhage. Over 50 per cent were described as unexplained antepartum foetal deaths, that is, the death could not be attributed to any discernible foetal pathology or maternal condition (Table 14.2).

Whether 'unexplained' actually means inexplicable is questionable. Some may be unexplained because no post-mortem was performed or, if they occurred in women at apparently low risk of unfavourable outcome, there may have been little detailed examination for signs of foetal distress. Failure to detect these foetuses at risk raises several questions: whether they are truly undetectable, the utility of current risk assessment measures, and whether the routines of standard antenatal care are the most appropriate and reliable ways of detecting signs of foetal disorder.

In the normally formed infant, birthweight is the major determinant of survival. The immature infant, born too small, accounts for almost 50 per cent of **neonatal mortality** (deaths within 28 days of birth) (Figure 14.6), and over 10 per cent of **post neonatal mortality** (deaths between 28 days and one year).

Low birthweight may be the result of failure to grow appropriately *in utero* or of delivery at an early **gestational age**. For infants who thrive appropriately, but are born early, a clinical reason for the premature onset of labour is not clear in about 50 per cent of cases; but characteristics associated with pre-term birth include multiple pregnancy, smoking, history of previous pre-term birth, and non-White ethnic origin

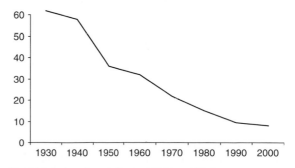

Fig. 14.5 Perinatal mortality per 1000 total births.
Source: Office of National Statistics (2004). www.statistics.gov.uk.

TABLE 14.2 Causes of stillbirth in UK (2001)	
Cause of stillbirth	**Percentage**
Congenital malformation	12.6
Intrapartum asphyxia	7.3
Other specific cause	5.7
Infection	2.4
Unclassifiable	0.6
Accident	0.1
Maternal obstetric complication	21.2
Unexplained antepartum death	50.1

Source: Maternal and Child Health Research Consortium (2001).
8th Annual Report. Confidential Enquiry into Stillbirths and Deaths in Infancy. London: Maternal and Child Health Research Consortium, www.cemach.org.uk.

(RCOG 2003). 🖳 The reasons for failure of an infant to grow appropriately *in utero* may be congenital or environmental, foetal or maternal in origin. The sex of the infant, maternal parity and size, smoking, ethnicity, maternal disease, and nutrition are contributory factors.

The social class (see Chapter 17) of a mother is a summary indicator reflecting a range of circumstances

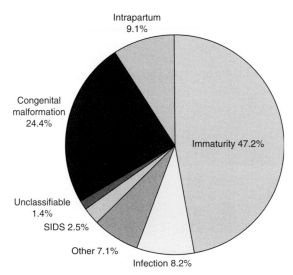

Fig. 14.6 Neonatal deaths in England, Wales, and Northern Ireland in 1999.
Source: Maternal and Child Health Research Consortium (2001). 8th Annual Report. Confidential Enquiry into Stillbirths and Deaths in Infancy. London: Maternal and Child Health Research Consortium. Available at: www.cemach.org.uk.

and behaviours that affect the foetus and neonate. Social class differences in low birthweight and in perinatal and infant mortality have long been described, and these differences have not narrowed in the past decade.

Developments in neonatal intensive care in particular and, more recently, the growing specialty of foetal medicine have contributed enormously to improved survival of the premature newborn. Infants born at 27/28 weeks of gestation now have survival rates of almost 90 per cent (RCOG 2003). 🖳 To what extent this increased survival seen in recent years equates with subsequent well-being awaits the results of longer-term follow-up. Studies in the 1980s of infants born before 29 weeks found approximately one-third to be profoundly disabled; more recently a figure of 10 per cent has been reported (Tin *et al.* 1997). 🖳 The level of disability increases with lowering of gestational age at birth. The clinical, psychological, social, economic, and ethical aspects of extending care to infants of increasingly low gestational age must be addressed.

While conditions associated with prematurity account for the greatest proportion of neonatal deaths, 25 per cent of infants who die in the post neonatal period do so suddenly and unexpectedly, and postmortem may fail to reveal an explanation.

14.5 **Sudden Unexpected Death in Infancy**

The term 'sudden infant death syndrome' (SIDS) was first used in 1969 and refers to 'the sudden death of a baby that is clinically unexpected and in whom a thorough post-mortem examination fails to demonstrate an adequate cause of death'.

Up to this such deaths were usually termed 'cot death' or were attributed, often on flimsy pathological grounds, to respiratory conditions of uncertain specificity, for example interstitial pneumonia. It is by definition a diagnosis of exclusion; therefore variations in the degree of care or detail with which the post-mortem is conducted, in the interpretation of findings by different pathologists, or in the range of other investigations undertaken, will have considerable influence on the published figures. Comparisons of rates of SIDS should be made with caution unless the evidence for this final diagnosis is clear.

In the mid-1990s incidences ranging from 0.1 to 2.5 per 1000 live births were reported. A detailed study in five NHS regions with just under half a million births between 1993 and 1996, with appropriate epidemiological and pathological resources reported the incidence of SIDS to be 0.768 per 1000 live births (Fleming *et al.* 2000). 🖳 It is the leading cause of post neonatal mortality.

Deaths from SIDS are uncommon in the first month of life, rise to a peak at about 10 weeks and then fall more gradually, being infrequent after 6 months and, by definition, should not occur beyond one year. Boys are more vulnerable than girls, and some ethnic groups are less vulnerable than others. Other epidemiological features of a high-risk population include babies who are premature, of low birthweight or from multiple births, and those whose mothers are young, poorly educated, live in poor conditions, smoke, leave little interval between pregnancies, and whose fathers are absent or unemployed (Table 14.3).

A review of SIDS by Sullivan and Barlow (2001) 🖳 suggested that affected infants are not completely normal in development but have some inherent weakness, which may become obvious only when the infant is subject to some stress such as minor infection. Epidemiological confirmation of this hypothesis from human studies may be difficult.

Evidence from epidemiological studies in the 1980s had indicated that a prone sleeping position of infants was a factor in the causation of SIDS; in 1991 a national 'Back to Sleep' campaign was introduced in the UK. This had a demonstrable effect in reducing the number of deaths from SIDS though a biological explanation for this is obscure. Although sleeping position is important, the sleeping arrangements (for example bed sharing, sleeping elsewhere) are now also recognized as risk

TABLE 14.3 Putative risk factors for Sudden Infant Death Syndrome

Maternal characteristics	Birth characteristics	Pregnancy characteristics	Family characteristics	Postnatal characteristics	Time of death
Lower socio-economic status	First born	Younger age of mother at first pregnancy	Larger family size	Use of prone sleeping position	Age 1–6 months
Teenage mother	Multiple birth	Late attendance at antenatal clinic	School age sibling(s)	Use of side sleeping position	Winter
Unmarried mother	Low birthweight	Non-attendance at antenatal classes		Infection Maternal and paternal smoking	Weekends
Younger school-leaving age	Male infant	Higher parity		Bed sharing	Between midnight and 6.00 a.m.
Less formal education		Short inter-pregnancy interval		Not room sharing with adult(s)	Prone position
Depression		Short gestation		Not breast feeding	Non-use of pacifier
Illegal drug use		Intrauterine growth retardation		Overheating	Covers over face/head
Race/ethnicity		Maternal smoking		Overwrapping/overdressing. Non-attendance for postnatal health check. Admission to a special baby care unit	

Source: Sullivan, F. M. and Barlow, S. M. (2001). 'Review of Risk Factors for Sudden Infant Death Syndrome'. *Paediatric and Perinatal Epidemiology*, **15**: 144–200.

factors (Carpenter *et al.* 2004), 🖳 along with several other features of the postnatal environment. An updated national advice leaflet for parents is now available to ensure that these risk factors are known and the scope for further reduction in deaths is widely recognized (Department of Health 2005). 🖳

In low-risk families the likelihood of SIDS is estimated to be one in 8500 (Craft and Hall 2004). 🖳 More than one unexplained death in the same family is rare. Hill (2004) 🖳 has reported the probability of SIDS occurring two or three times in a family. In the UK (1996) 🖳 it was estimated that around 10 per cent of all otherwise unexplained infant deaths may be caused by deliberate suffocation, though this probably varies over time and between populations, and unequivocal evidence of such action is often absent. The level of professional and public concern about infant deaths that are sudden and unexpected has been heightened recently by several highly publicized murder trials of mothers who have had more than one such death in their family. Statements about the statistical probability of such occurrences, and of demonstrable shortcomings in the way some of these deaths have been investigated, have been highlighted during some of these trials, or subsequent appeal hearings.

Parents have a right to expect that their baby's sudden and unexpected death will be thoroughly investigated by a paediatric pathologist and other medical professionals. Professionals have a duty to work to strengthen the reliability of research findings, to seek clinical evidence of possible causes, and to justify their interpretation of their findings. It is now a matter of some urgency to ensure that effective multiagency protocols are adopted nationwide so that a standard, detailed, thorough examination of all genetic, social, environmental, and pathological factors that may be relevant to the death is conducted in all cases (Fleming *et al.* 2004). 🖳

Q2(a) How are sudden infant deaths currently investigated?

Q2(b) What should the investigation protocol include?

Q2(c) Who coordinates the investigation?

14.6 Congenital Anomalies

How frequent are congenital anomalies?

Two to four per cent of babies are diagnosed with one or more major malformations or chromosomal anomalies, with serious medical, functional, or cosmetic consequences. The exact prevalence found in any

TABLE 14.4 Total prevalence (per 10 000 births) of selected congenital anomalies in Europe 1999–2002	
Central nervous system	21.5
Neural tube defects	10.0
Cardiovascular anomalies	61.4
Cleft palate and cleft lip	15.5
Limb defects	35.5
Urinary system	27.4
Musculoskeletal	20.9
Chromosomal anomalies	33.4
Down syndrome	19.1

Source: EUROCAT (2004). Database of population registries, www.eurocat.ulster.ac.uk/pubdata/tables.html.

survey of births depends crucially on the rather arbitrary division between 'major' and 'minor' anomalies; 'minor' anomalies are generally much more common, and **ascertainment** may be incomplete or vary between reporting centres. Population-based registries that access multiple sources of health information and clinical specialties, and which cover (at the least) diagnoses made in the first year of life, provide the most reliable data sets. Estimates of prevalence have increased during the past few decades because of the increasing frequency of ultrasound screening for internal, hidden anomalies such as urinary tract and cardiac defects, some of which might not otherwise be revealed until later life. The most common group of anomalies is cardiac (Table 14.4).

Q3 What does 'population-based' mean and why is it important for a registry to be population-based (see Chapter 2)?

Because congenital anomalies, particularly chromosomal ones, are selectively lost as spontaneous abortions (Vogel and Motulsky 2002), 🖳 the term **prevalence** (rather than **incidence**) is the most appropriate for the number of cases diagnosed (surviving) in a given population. The *numerator* is the number of babies born (live- and stillbirths) with congenital anomalies; the *denominator* is the number of births (live and still) in the population. It should be remembered that differences in prevalence between populations, or between groups with different environmental exposures, may reflect differences in survival of affected foetuses during pregnancy, rather than differences in incidence.

In the past few decades in Europe, the practice of prenatal screening, often followed by termination of a severely affected pregnancy, has become widespread.

For example, in 32 European regions from 1995 to 1999, 53 per cent of spina bifida cases and 33 per cent of Down syndrome cases were prenatally diagnosed, leading to termination of pregnancy. These are averages in a range from 0 per cent (in regions where termination is illegal) to over 75 per cent, for both of these conditions. To compare prevalence rates between populations for possible environmental causes without differences due to prenatal screening, it is now common to calculate a **total** or **adjusted prevalence rate**, which includes terminations of pregnancy for congenital anomaly in the numerator. Most of these terminations would have been live- or stillborn, rather than result in spontaneous abortion, if the congenital anomaly had not been diagnosed prenatally. Increasing termination rates for congenital anomaly are one factor that has led to decreases in perinatal mortality in European countries.

What causes congenital anomalies?

Approximately 15 per cent of cases of congenital anomaly recorded by European registries have a chromosomal anomaly (Table 14.4). It has been estimated that 7–8 per cent of cases have a single gene defect with autosomal dominant, autosomal recessive, or X-linked inheritance (Mueller and Young 2001); ▯ and the number of recognized single gene syndromes is growing. Several malformations, including neural tube defects (NTDs), certain cardiac defects, hypospadias, cleft lip and cleft palate, renal agenesis, congenital dislocation of hips and talipes are attributed to a **multifactorial** aetiology, where the diffuse pattern of recurrence within families suggests that many genetic factors are involved, potentially in combination with environmental factors. Environmental factors, such as folic acid (see below), are known to be important contributors to this aetiology and perhaps to the large proportion of cases currently classified as 'of unknown aetiology'. Few cases (less than 10 per cent) can be wholly attributed to a single environmental exposure with known **teratogenic** effects (Greek: *teras*, monster) such as maternal illnesses, infections, drugs and chemicals, radiation or alcohol (Table 14.5). Even in many of these apparently environmentally caused cases, genetic factors may play a role in determining susceptibility to the exposure, because not all exposed foetuses (at relevant dose and time of pregnancy) are affected.

An environmental cause generally has a *preconceptional* mutagenic action (maternal or paternal) or *postconceptional* teratogenic action. Postconceptional action is generally during the first trimester of pregnancy when most **organogenesis** occurs, although relevant exposures may have occurred earlier if their effects are indirect (for example effects on endocrine function) or if a chemical has a long biological half-life in the body (for example polychlorinated biphenyls (PCBs)). The development of the brain remains subject to adverse influences well into the second trimester and beyond.

A **teratogen** is a chemical or agent that can cause a congenital malformation. However, whether an agent acts as a teratogen is crucially dependent on dose. Animal experiments show that a vast array of chemicals, if given in high enough doses early in pregnancy, will cause foetal malformation. The agent will be considered teratogenic if it causes malformation without significant maternal toxicity. For practical purposes, each agent can be considered to have a threshold dose above which it starts to cause foetal malformation, and below which the developing foetus is unaffected, or is able to self-regulate or repair damage. For the protection of humans, it is important to determine whether the highest exposures experienced in the population are anywhere near the estimated threshold (taking into account also the likely variation of individual thresholds).

The thalidomide tragedy first brought the world's notice to the potential for drugs to profoundly affect the developing foetus, and since then testing regimes have been instituted to improve drug safety for pregnant women. These are far from perfect, and post-marketing drug surveillance and epidemiological research aim to detect any increase in congenital malformations associated with maternal drug intake. Pregnancy is often a contraindication to drug prescription, whether based on direct evidence of a teratogenic effect, or on the lack of relevant evidence. However, the period after conception but before the pregnancy is recognized and confirmed, is a particularly important time for all measures to prevent congenital anomalies to be applied. A busy medical practitioner should consider the possibility of pregnancy before prescribing any drug not established as non-teratogenic.

> **Q4** The epidemiological approach (for example a case–control study) can be contrasted to case reports in which a mother or mothers took a certain drug and had a child(ren) with a birth defect. Why is the interpretation of case reports limited?

When dealing with *cause*, we do not simply have a horizontal array of different biological, chemical, or physical agents, but also vertical causal pathways and networks which determine exposure to these proximate agents. For example, maternal rubella infection and rubella

TABLE 14.5 Risk factors for congenital anomalies: some examples

Risk factor	Comment
Sociodemographic	
Older maternal age	Chromosomal anomalies; little or no effect for non-chromosomal
Young maternal age (<20)	Fivefold excess of gastroschisis, not a strong risk factor for other anomalies
Low socioeconomic status	Higher risk of non-chromosomal anomalies; lower risk of chromosomal anomalies due to lower average maternal age associated with low socioeconomic status
Maternal disease, infection, and drug exposure	
Epilepsy	2-fold risk, probably mainly due to anticonvulsant drugs
Diabetes	If sufficient glycaemic control not achieved
Rubella, cytomegalovirus, toxoplasmosis	Well established risk factors for congenital anomalies
Fever	Controversial
Thalidomide	Caused many babies to be born with limb and other defects in the 1960s, when prescribed for nausea in pregnancy
Retinoic acid	Central nervous system, cardiac and ear defects. Particular concern over use in acne drugs
Nutrition and related	
Low folic acid status	See text (neural tube defects)
High Vitamin A intake	Threshold unclear
Alcohol	Threshold unclear; microcephaly, heart defects, dysmorphic facial features, learning disabilities
Obesity	Recent evidence mainly for neural tube defects
Physical agents	
Radiation	Central nervous system malformations, mainly microcephaly
Hyperthermia	Most evidence relates to maternal fever, but still controversial

vaccination policy are at different levels in the causal network leading to congenital rubella syndrome (characterized by eye defects, heart defects, and deafness); folic acid intake (see below) and social class or economic prosperity are all strands of the causal network for NTDs. Non-conformity with best clinical practice is also part of the causal network leading to malformations caused by maternal epilepsy and diabetes (Table 14.5). Preventive strategies use knowledge at more than one level in these causal networks.

Folic acid and neural tube defects

Periconceptional folic acid is now well established as preventing NTDs, and possibly a range of other congenital anomalies. During the 1970s and 1980s, the main evidence for a protective effect was from case–control and non-randomized intervention studies. Many of these studies were performed in the UK and Ireland, where, at that time, the total prevalence of NTDs

was three to four times higher than in other European countries, although the difference is now very small.

> **Q5** One of the criticisms of case–control studies is the possibility of 'maternal recall bias'. How do you think this might apply to case–control studies of maternal nutrition in pregnancy?

In 1991, the results of a randomized trial were published which confirmed the evidence from previous studies that periconceptional folic acid supplementation could prevent NTDs (MRC Vitamin Research Group 1991). ⌨ The trial was conducted in women who already had a child with NTD and therefore were at high risk of having another affected child. There is now other evidence that the results of this trial are also applicable to women without a previously affected child; homozygotes for variants of the gene for the MTHFR enzyme involved in folate metabolism are at greater risk of NTDs (Brody *et al.* 2002). 🖳

Unfortunately, more than ten years later, epidemiological studies show that disappointing progress has been made converting research into practice. Most pregnant women either do not take supplements at all, or do not start preconceptionally as is necessary; and as a result the prevalence of NTDs has not fallen markedly in Europe as a whole. It is particularly hard to reach women who do not plan a pregnancy, and there is evidence that differences in access to health promotion messages and pregnancy planning may be increasing socioeconomic inequalities in the prevalence of NTD affected pregnancies (De Walle *et al.* 1998). 🖳 Women may assume that healthy eating leads to sufficient folic acid intake, but studies have suggested that even 'healthy diets' are inadequate in folic acid. Many countries of the world, including the USA and Canada, but not yet European countries, have therefore introduced fortification of staple foods with folic acid as the most effective preventive strategy. More recently, research has suggested a role for folic acid in protecting against cardiovascular disease, an additional argument for fortification (Wald *et al.* 2002). 🖳

Environmental pollution

Environmental contaminants that have been the focus of recent research include by-products of chlorination of drinking water, endocrine-disrupting chemicals, particularly in relation to hypospadias and cryptorchidism, unspecified releases from landfill sites, and pesticides, particularly when used occupationally. There is still no consensus about the level of relative risk associated with these exposures. A particular problem for epidemiological studies is the difficulty in estimating individual exposure to environmental contaminants, leading to considerable **exposure misclassification**.

> **Q6** What would you imagine to be sources of exposure misclassification when studying the risks associated with contaminants of drinking water? How would you expect misclassification of exposure to affect the estimates of risk obtained in the study (see Chapter 3)?

Reports in the media of a *cluster* of birth defects, often associated with suspected local contamination of air or water, are relatively frequent. A random distribution of cases in space and time is not a regular distribution, and there will be patches of a denser concentration of cases. A community may become aware of an aggregation of cases in their area, and blame the 'obvious' reason such

as a waste site or power line. The problem has been likened to the 'Texan sharpshooter' who draws his gun and fires at the barn door, and only afterwards goes and draws the target in the middle of the densest cluster of bullet holes. Investigating clusters to distinguish *random* clusters from clusters where there is a single cause is a difficult task for public-health practitioners. Most of the well-documented instances in the literature where a cluster was subsequently established as being due to environmental contaminants have been related to food exposures (Dolk and Vrijheid 2003); 🖳 these have involved both high numbers of cases and high relative risk, and include the Minnamata incident in Japan where fish and shellfish were contaminated with methylmercury, incidents of PCB contamination of cooking oil in Taiwan and Japan, and pesticide over-use at a fish farm in Hungary.

Continuous epidemiological surveillance of pregnancy outcomes, fertility, infant, and child health, and improved detection of environmental hazards, are required to maintain and improve current levels of maternal and child health.

Web Addresses

Confidential Enquiry into Maternal and Child Health (CEMACH 2005), www.cemach.org.uk.

Department of Health (2005). SIDS: Advice for parents, www.dh.gov.uk/publications.

EUROCAT (2004). Database of population registries, www.eurocat.ulster.ac.uk/pubdata/tables/html.

Human Fertilisation and Embryology Authority, www.hfea.gov.uk.

Office of National Statistics, www.statistics.gov.uk.

PatientPlus (contraception), www.patient.co.uk/Health Information for Doctors (for model answer on contraception (Q1)).

US Census Bureau (2005). International database, summary statistics available at www.census/gov/ipc/idbsum.html.

References

References for this chapter can be found at www.oxfordtextbooks.co.uk/orc/yarnell. Where possible, these are presented as *active links* which direct you to an electronic version of the work. If you are a subscriber to that work (either individually or through an institution), and depending on your level of access, you may be able to peruse an abstract or the full article if available. 🖳

Model answers

Q1 Legally available methods of birth control appear to be culturally determined in most countries, but culture would include social, religious, and economic aspects of each society. What appears inescapable is that birth control is popular with women as it allows control over the size of family achieved, or indeed, in well-developed countries in which gender equality is socially and legally the norm, whether any children are desirable. Methods of birth control are discussed in detail elsewhere (see www.patient.co.uk/Health Information for Doctors).

Q2(a) Sudden Infant Deaths are currently investigated by the Coroner's Officer, who is usually a specially trained police officer. It is a requirement that any medical practitioner called to the scene of a sudden unexpected death should inform the Coroner's Office, whatever the age of the patient.

Q2(b) For full details of the protocol see Fleming *et al.* (2004). 💻

Q2(c) Coordination is by the Coroner's Office.

Q3 Population-based means relating to a population defined by geographical area of residence, as opposed to hospital-based, which defines the study population according to the hospital of delivery or diagnosis. A hospital-based study can give biased estimates of prevalence as high-risk pregnancies may be referred to certain hospitals, resulting in higher rates of congenital anomaly in those hospital populations.

Q4 In case reports, selective factors may operate which predispose a mother to take a particular drug and this group includes women at particularly high risk of a poor pregnancy outcome. A control population is essential to monitor the possibility of selecting mothers unrepresentatively from the general population of those exposed to risk.

Q5 Mothers taking part in retrospective case–control studies who have experienced a poor pregnancy outcome may be particularly likely to link coincidental events in pregnancy with their poor outcome or may be more motivated than other mothers to remember all the possibly relevant exposures during their pregnancy.

Q6 Variability in amounts of tap water drunk and variability in levels of contaminants in tap water, consumption of tap water outside the home, and moving house between early pregnancy and birth when the water source is recorded, are all potential sources of misclassification of exposure. Exposure misclassification would be most likely to reduce the size of the estimates of risk obtained in a study.

Neoplasms

This chapter briefly reviews the pathology of cancer and how information on cancer incidence is collected (cancer registration). The epidemiology of selected cancers is reviewed. These include: skin cancers, the hormone-related cancers (breast, prostate, ovary) and haematopoietic cancers. Finally genetic, lifestyle, environmental, occupational, and dietary risk factors, and the prospects for cancer prevention, are discussed. Respiratory cancers (Chapter 7) and gastrointestinal cancers (Chapter 9) are discussed elsewhere.

Introduction

What is cancer?

Cancer is the result of a breakdown in the normal growth of body cells. It is ultimately a disease of the genetic material that regulates cell growth, is very common in human populations, and can be induced also in laboratory animals. It has been estimated that one in two men will develop an invasive cancer in their lifetime and one in three women (estimates for the USA). Almost every type of cell in the human body is capable of malignant change and over 100 forms of cancer have been described. There is ongoing debate about the exact mechanisms by which this transformation occurs, but it is agreed that cancer is the result of cumulative mutations in genes that regulate cell growth, the expression of other genes, and cell death. Two principal kinds of cancer genes contribute to the successful malignant transformation of a pre-cancerous cell:

(i) **Tumour suppressor genes** restrict the ability of cells to divide, and have an important regulatory role in the normal cell. Mutations that permanently disable these genes, or reduce their capacity to regulate cell division, contribute to malignant change.

(ii) **Proto-oncogenes** also have roles in growth regulation but mutations leading to the development of oncogenes characteristically enhance the usual function of the gene.

By 2002 over 20 tumour suppressor genes and over 75 oncogenes had been described. DNA-repair genes have also been described, and further classes of cancer genes may be revealed in future research. All cancer genes require a minimum of two mutations in the most strongly inherited forms of cancer, such as retinoblastoma, but several mutations or 'hits' are required in the case of most cancers, which show only weak familial aggregation.

Somatic cells in the body each derive from genetic material from both parents. It has been shown that mutations in both alleles at the gene locus for a tumour suppressor gene are required to promote cancer whereas, in the case of proto-oncogenes, a mutation in only one allele is required. Some general properties of malignant cells are shown in Box 15.1.

It has been estimated that for most normal cells this number of mutations would not occur naturally during the lifetime of a human being, but many agents present in the environment are known to promote carcinogenesis (malignant transformation) by causing mutations in relevant genes. These agents include many chemicals, viruses, reproductive hormones, and ionizing radiation, among others. Industrial carcinogens, including

those found in food and drink, are classified according to their known or suspected toxicity in humans or other animals. All agents are discussed further in section 15.5.

15.1 Cancer Registration

Epidemiological information on cancer in various countries is available from mortality data; but these records do not count people cured from their cancer or in long-term remission, or those who die of other causes, and may not give an accurate idea of cancer burden. For example, epithelial skin cancers, which are the commonest cancers in most countries, tend not to be invasive and can be readily treated. Thus the high incidence rates for these cancers are not reflected at all in mortality data. Therefore, cancer registration, the systematic recording of details on cancer cases, provides an estimate of incidence and often provides additional information such as histological and clinical data which allow the separation of primary and secondary tumours. The latter occur by metastatic spread in the lymphatic or capillary systems. The most common secondary sites are liver, bone, lung, and brain. Such information is used for 'staging' of tumours at diagnosis and during treatment.

Two types of cancer registry are common: (1) hospital-based, which are selective in nature and of limited representativeness; and (ii) community-based, which record all cancer cases arising in a defined population. The latter are an invaluable part of any rational programme of cancer control. They assist in planning services and in evaluating treatment and prevention for the population concerned. They provide a data resource for aetiological studies, and are used for monitoring cancer risk in occupational groups and other cohorts of individuals exposed to various carcinogens.

All relevant epidemiological disease measures can be made from cancer registries which can provide reliable population-based data with follow up (see Chapter 2). These include **incidence (rate)**, **cumulative incidence**, **prevalence**, **mortality**, **case-fatality**, **survival** (five-year survival rates are the standard measure used by registries globally), **life-years lost**, and **disability-adjusted life-years (DALYs)**. The last two measures require population-based life tables, usually available only for large geographical regions and countries.

The ability of cancer registration to provide accurate incidence and survival statistics is related to the quality of data and the completeness of the database. Cancer registration is required by law in many countries

---

BOX 15.1 PROPERTIES OF CANCER CELLS

- They continue dividing in situations in which normal cells would wait for a chemical signal, for example in response to injury.
- They do not respond to signals to stop dividing.
- Normally damaged cells self-destruct (a process termed apoptosis), but this does not happen in cancer cells despite significant DNA damage.
- Cancer cells have the ability to promote the growth of blood vessels (angiogenesis) to provide nutrients for tumour growth.
- Cancer cells, unlike normal cells, are not limited in the number of times they can divide.
- Cancer cells invade nearby tissue and then metastasize to distant parts of the body.

including the USA, Denmark, Canada, New Zealand, and Finland. In some countries, concerns about individual privacy have led to the requirement of informed consent for cancer registration. This has reduced the completeness of cancer registration and its utility in these countries. The first population-based cancer registry was started in Hamburg 1929, although in Germany the move to achieving informed consent for all patient-based data to protect patient confidentiality in the mid-1980s has resulted in a breakdown in the system; by 1993 results for this registry were no longer of a standard suitable for publication.

In England and Wales legislation in 2001 provided a mechanism whereby cancer registries could continue to receive confidential, named patient data without explicit patient consent because individual identification details are necessary to eliminate multiple registrations.

Registration data for cancers, collected to international standards, have allowed comparison of cancer survival between countries (Berrino *et al.* 1995). 💻 This variation in survival promoted a radical change in the delivery of cancer care in the UK (Department of Health 1995) 💻 by providing a more patient-centred centralized service, with specialists working in multidisciplinary teams. Services are being concentrated in cancer units, with regional cancer centres providing expertise in rarer cancers. Five-year survival rates for European countries for the common cancers are shown in Table 15.1.

TABLE 15.1 European cancer survival: patients diagnosed 1990–1994 and followed up to end of 1999

			Percentage of patients alive five years after diagnosis							
	Prostate	Breast	Skin* (F)	Colon (F)	Colon (M)	Lung (F)	Lung (M)	Ovary	All (M)	All (F)
England	53.8	73.6	85.6	46.2	45.7	7.7	7.4	31.5	37.1	50.8
Scotland	53.6	72.3	90.1	47.2	45.3	6.8	7.0	30.1	35.6	49.5
Austria	83.6	75.4	88.2	58.4	N/A	16.0	13.4	49.3	47.5	57.9
Czech Republic	50.1	64	78.1	36.4	38.1	8.2	6.3	31.7	32.3	46
Denmark	41.5	74.9	88	47.6	43.2	5.9	6.1	30.9	33.5	51.2
Finland	66.5	81.4	84	52.7	54	10.9	7.8	35.4	41.4	55.8
France	75.2	81.3	85.3	58.7	55.9	15.9	13.1	38.5	44.5	57.9
Germany	75.9	75.4	89.9	54.5	50.5	10.5	10.8	40.8	44.1	55.6
Italy	63.9	80.6	82.5	52.1	51.2	10.5	9.8	37.2	41.2	55.6
The Netherlands	68.4	78.2	87.7	54	51.9	12.4	11.7	36.7	42.7	55.7
Norway	62.1	77.2	88.4	53.6	51.4	10.5	8.0	39.8	40	54.9
Poland	38.6	63.1	57.9	28.7	26.3	6.8	6.1	30.2	25.2	40.5
Portugal	44	71.9	68.9	43.5	49			45.9	N/A	N/A
Slovenia	48.8	67.4	70	38.8	34.8	9.3	8.0	36.4	31.2	47
Spain	65.5	78	89.8	55.8	55	12.8	12.4	43.2	43.9	57.1
Sweden	67.4	82.6	90.6	54.4	52.2	11.5	8.5	41.3	42.5	57.6
Switzerland	67	80	91	56.3	55	16.2	9.7	36.6	43.5	56.7
Europe	**65.4**	**76.1**	**84.3**	**51.0**	**49.2**	**9.6**	**9.7**	**36.7**	**40.5**	**53.6**

*Melanoma skin cancer.

Source: Sant, M., Aareleid, T., Berrino, F. *et al.* (2003) 'EUROCARE-3: Survival of Cancer Patients Diagnosed 1990–94 – Results and Commentary'. *Annals of Oncology*, **14**: 61–118.

15.2 **Common Cancers**

Cancer is a major cause of morbidity and mortality. As noted earlier, up to a half of all men and a third of all women in developed countries can expect to develop an invasive cancer during their lifetime. Cancer is the second commonest cause of death after cardiovascular disease. Worldwide, in the year 2000, at least 5.3 million men and 4.7 million women developed a malignant tumour and 6.2 million died from the disease. The number of new cases is expected to reach 15 million per year by 2020. Cancer mortality in developed countries is twice that of developing countries, and this has been attributed to the impact of tobacco, diet, and lifestyle (Stewart and Kleiheus 2003). 🖥

> **Q1** What other information would you need before you could agree with the statement above?

Figure 15.1 shows the incidence of common cancers in developed and developing countries. The data were compiled by the International Agency for Research on Cancer (IARC) and were compiled from reliable registries. These data tend to support the comment of Stewart and Kleiheus (2003) 🖥 (see above) about cancer mortality, but also point to the potential value of ecological research in generating hypotheses on aetiological factors in the environment. Many of these research opportunities remain to be fully exploited.

In the UK, cancer causes 23 per cent of deaths while more than 270 000 new cases of cancer were registered in 2000. There are more than 100 different varieties of cancer but the four major sites, lung, breast, prostate, and colorectal, account for over half of the cases diagnosed (Cancer Research UK 2004). 🖥 Non-melanoma skin cancer, which is easily treated, usually by surgery, accounts for another 25 per cent of cases but a very small proportion of deaths. The relative incidence, mortality, and major risk factors for the common cancers in England and Wales are shown in Table 15.2.

Cancer trends

Crude mortality rates suggest that cancer incidence has increased during the twentieth century. Increased life expectancy with an ageing population is a major factor contributing to the increase. Age-standardization (see Chapter 14) is important when comparing different time periods or countries with different population structures, and allows us to detect differences in mortality or incidence that are not due to changes in the age structure of the population. Other reasons for the upward trend in cancer incidence include: improved diagnosis, control of competing causes such as infections and heart disease, and the effect of changing lifestyle and exposure to risk factors. Risk factors include tobacco, increased exposure to the sun for melanoma, human papilloma virus for cervical cancer, and HIV infection for lymphoma. Obesity is an emerging risk factor that is linked to endometrial, breast, colon, and possibly renal and prostate cancers. Cancer rates may also increase substantially for a limited period during the '**prevalence round**' if a new screening test is introduced when more cancers will be detected at an earlier stage (see Chapter 5).

Skin cancers

Skin cancers are most common in White populations across the globe, with rates several-fold higher in Whites than in races with all other shades of skin pigmentation. Most skin cancers appear to be caused by excessive exposure to the sun. Within countries rates vary with latitude, which support this view, but tar and arsenic are also risk factors. **Basal cell cancer (rodent ulcer)** is the most common type of skin cancer, accounting for 50 per cent of cases. It grows slowly, mainly affecting

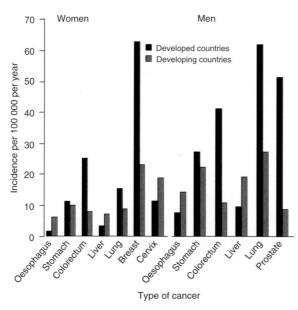

Fig. 15.1 Cancer incidence in developed and in developing countries.
Source: Key, T. J., Allen, N. E., Spencer, E. A. and Travis, R. C. (2002). 'The Effect of Diet on Risk of Cancer'. *The Lancet*, **360**: 861–8.

TABLE 15.2 Common cancers: proportion of all cancers, proportion of cancer deaths and risk factors (England and Wales, 1994)

Cancer	Proportion of cancers (%)	Proportion of cancer deaths (%)	Risk factors (strength of relationship)*
Lung	13.6	22.2	Tobacco smoke +++
Skin (non-melanoma)	14.1	0.3	Solar radiation, occupational carcinogens +++
Breast	12.2	8.6	Hormone replacement therapy+, obesity+, nulliparity ++
Colorectal	11.1	11.0	Fat/meat consumption ++, sedentary behaviour ++, obesity +
Prostate	7.4	6.3	Black race ++
Bladder	4.5	3.3	Tobacco smoke, occupational carcinogens +
Stomach	3.7	4.7	H. pylori ++, diet deficient in fruit & vegetables ++, salty foods +++
Ovary	2.0	2.9	Nulliparity +
Skin (melanoma)	1.8	1.0	Solar radiation +++
Cervix	1.2	1.1	Multiple sexual partners +++, Human papilloma virus +++

Source: Doll, R. and Peto, R. (2003). 'Epidemiology of Cancer', in D. A. Warrell, T. M. Cox, J. D. Firth and E. J. Benz Jr (eds.), *Oxford Textbook of Medicine*. Oxford: Oxford University Press, 193–218.

*+, weak: ++, moderate: +++, strong.

people over 60 years of age, usually appearing on the face or ears. It rarely metastasizes but can cause local damage and so warrants treatment. A quarter of skin cancers are squamous cell tumours, which may spread but can be treated successfully by surgery. **Melanoma** of the skin accounts for only 2 per cent of male and 3 per cent of female cancers, but unlike non-melanoma skin cancer, which very rarely causes death, it accounts for about 1 per cent of cancer deaths despite the fact that five-year survival in Europe approaches 90 per cent in many countries (see Table 15.1). The median age at diagnosis, 57 years, is relatively young for cancer. Rates have increased, probably because of increased exposure to ultraviolet radiation, both of duration and pattern. Prevention by taking care in the sun, avoiding sunbed use, and early detection are key public-health strategies. In Australia, stabilization of the incidence rates for melanoma in White Australians attests to the success of a national public-health campaign to reduce exposure to solar radiation.

Cancers at several sites are related to hormones that affect local tissue as part of normal physiological functioning. Not all cancers at these sites are hormone-dependent for their growth but, for those that are, this provides a valuable opportunity for therapy. Sites that have such cancers include the breast, prostate, and ovary.

Breast cancer

Breast cancer is the most common cancer in women after non-melanoma skin cancer but about 1 per cent of cases occur in men. In the UK, and in most European countries, screening by mammography is offered to all women aged 50–64 years and detects tumours earlier than they would present clinically. Plans are underway to extend screening to older age groups. Breast cancer, like most cancers, increases with age and over 50 per cent of cases are diagnosed over the age of 60 years. Other risk factors include a family history of breast or ovarian cancer, although only 2 per cent of all breast cancers are inherited through breast cancer genes (e.g. *BRCA1/BRCA2*) (Peto 2001). Another 15 per cent of breast cancers are known to cluster in families. Early menarche, late menopause, nulliparity, or first birth after age 30 years, and lack of breast feeding of offspring, are all risk factors, as is exposure to oestrogen through hormone replacement therapy of more than five years duration. Other risk factors are a previous history of breast cancer and exposure to ionizing radiation. There is some evidence that obesity and habitual alcohol consumption increase risk, whereas exercise of four or five hours per week reduces risk. Breast cancer is more common in affluent populations, which may reflect lower levels of parity and delayed age at first pregnancy. The outlook in breast cancer is good, with average survival relative to the general population of more than 70 per cent at five years (see Table 15.1). Most breast tumours are sensitive to the effects of oestrogen (oestrogen-receptor positive) and respond to oestrogen antagonists such as tamoxifen.

Trends in breast cancer: period and cohort effects

Age adjustment will take account of changes in the age structure of the population over time but changes in trends may be also due to **period** and **cohort effects**. A period effect influences disease rates in all ages at a single point in time. A good example occurred in America when, in 1974, Betty Ford, the wife of the President, was diagnosed with breast cancer. This resulted in more openness about breast cancer and an increase in breast cancer rates in all age groups. This may reflect over-diagnosis at that point of time and under-diagnosis in other periods. An initial increase in breast cancer incidence may also be predicted on the introduction of population-wide screening programmes (see Chapter 5).

A cohort effect relates to specific birth cohorts. For example, women born 1900–1930 in the USA had higher rates of non-parity than women born from 1930 to 1945. Non-parity (nulliparity) is an independent risk factor for breast cancer, and the effect may be amplified by the absence of the protective effect on breast

cancer of breast-feeding. We can predict a future cohort effect with current levels of non-parity, late age at first pregnancy and low breast-feeding levels, leading to increased levels of breast cancer in the current cohort of women.

Prostate cancer

This is the third most common cancer in males after non-melanoma skin cancer and lung cancer. It accounts for one in eight cancers diagnosed in men. Age is a risk factor and over half the cases are over 74 years at diagnosis. The average age at diagnosis is falling due to the use of prostate-specific antigen (PSA) testing in younger men, which has resulted in an increase in the detection of this cancer. The rates of prostate cancer vary widely internationally with the highest rates in the USA and Canada, and the lowest in Korea and Japan (Figure 15.2). High rates are found in black populations and the lowest in Japanese, but both Japanese Americans and Black Americans have higher rates than men in their native countries. Some of this variation may be due to access to PSA testing as there is less variation in deaths from prostate cancer, but this is unlikely to explain the excess in Black rather than White Americans. The variation may also reflect an environmental aetiology possibly related to diet. See Chapter 5 for discussion on evaluating the use of PSA testing and on the natural history of this cancer.

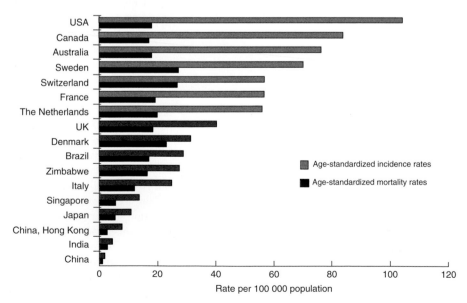

Fig. 15.2 World age-standardized incidence and mortality rates for prostate cancer for selected countries: estimates for the year 2002. Source: CRC CancerStats (2002).

Prostate cancer may also be hormone-dependent as the prostate gland is dependent on androgens for its growth and function. Bilateral orchidectomy and chemical forms of anti-androgenic treatments are used to treat prostate cancer and can produce significant remission in many cases, although five-year survival is lower than that for breast cancer (Table 15.1).

> **Q2** The mortality rates from prostate cancer shown in Figure 15.2 are similar in the USA, France, and UK but incidence rates are five times, three times, and twice the rates for mortality. List the possible explanations for this observation and suggest which is the most likely explanation.

Ovarian cancer

This is the fifth most common cancer in females and the commonest gynaecological cancer. It often presents late as symptoms are vague. It is more common with increasing age and with affluence. A woman's ovulatory history plays an important role in the risk of developing the disease. As in the case of breast cancer, nulliparity is a risk factor. There is a decreasing risk with each pregnancy whereas oral contraception and premature menopause each have a protective effect. Epidemiological studies of risk factors for ovarian cancer tend to be case–control rather than cohort studies, because there are few established cohorts of women of sufficient size and length of follow up to give an adequate number of ovarian cancer cases. About 5 per cent of ovarian cancers are due to genetic factors associated with a faulty copy of the BRCA1 gene.

National screening is not yet recommended in the UK but a trial is underway to determine if the use of CA125 as an immunological marker for ovarian cancer, combined with ultrasound, has a role in population screening.

15.3 Haematological Malignancies

Haematological cancers account for 7 per cent of all cancers in England. They arise in haemopoietic tissue associated with blood, bone marrow, and lymphoid tissue, including the spleen. They comprise a broad range of diseases, with significant variation in their presentation, natural history, treatment, and prognosis. The main groupings are **acute and chronic leukaemias, Hodgkin's and Non-Hodgkin's lymphoma, myeloma**, and other **lymphoproliferative** conditions; the premalignant

states comprising **myeloproliferative** disorders, **myelodysplastic** syndromes, and **aplastic** conditions are usually also included in this group of diseases.

The diagnosis and classification of haematological malignancies has evolved in parallel with developments in laboratory techniques ranging from microscopy through cytochemical staining and antibody detection to DNA analysis. The ability to define subgroups is increasingly important as treatment is tailored, not only to specific types of leukaemia and lymphoma, but also on the basis of their prognostic group. Such changes in nomenclature pose problems both for registration systems and for epidemiologists interested in examining trends in the incidence of these diseases over time. In an attempt to produce more meaningful epidemiological data for this group of disorders, several specialist registries have been established (Cartwright *et al.* 1999). The relative frequency of the haematological malignancies is shown in Table 15.3.

Acute myeloid leukaemia

This is a leukaemia of the myeloid cells of the bone marrow and may occur de novo or following the development of a pre-leukaemic condition. The reported incidence varies widely throughout the world; the annual UK rate is estimated as 3.0 per 100 000 population. It is rare in children and young adults, but the incidence rises with increasing age. Below age 65 years, *de novo* acute myeloid leukaemia (AML) predominates. There is a slight male preponderance of cases and an apparent slow decline in numbers of cases over time, possibly because of a rise in cases presenting in the pre-leukaemic phase. Aetiological factors that have been suggested include smoking, and exposure to ionizing radiation, benzene, and chloramphenicol.

Acute lymphoblastic leukaemia

Acute lymphoblastic leukaemia (ALL) is a leukaemia of lymphoid precursor cells of either B- or T-cell origin and there are several subtypes. It is the commonest cancer of childhood and has a characteristic peak of incidence among 2- to 7-year-olds. Males are more often affected than females. Worldwide reported incidence varies widely, but is highest in developed countries. The current annual UK incidence rate is 1.0 per 100 000 population. Although reported childhood rates increased before the 1970s, probably owing to improved diagnosis, there is no convincing evidence of a change in reported rates for any age group in more recent years. The favoured aetiological hypothesis involves atypical responses to infection as a result of delayed antigenic

TABLE 15.3   Haematological cancers: proportion of all cancers, proportion of cancer deaths and risk factors (England & Wales 1994)

	Proportion of all cancers (%)	Proportion of cancer deaths (%)	Risk factors (Strength of relationship)*
Leukaemias	2.3	2.6	Ionizing radiation++
			Smoking+, some occupational carcinogens+
			(e.g. benzene)
Lymphoma:			
Hodgkins	0.5	0.2	Epstein–Barr virus+
Non-Hodgkins	2.8	2.9	Viral infections of lymphocytes++
Myelomatosis	1.5	1.6	Racial and ethnic factors+

Source: Doll, R. and Peto, R. (2003). 'Epidemiology of Cancer', in D. A. Warrell, T. M. Cox, J. D. Firth and E. J. Benz Jr (eds.), *Oxford Textbook of Medicine*. Oxford: Oxford University Press, 193–218.
*+, weak: ++, moderate: +++, strong.

exposure in childhood, but this has proved hard to test in epidemiological studies.

Chronic myeloid leukaemia

Chronic myeloid leukaemia (CML) is characterized by the presence of the Philadelphia chromosome resulting in the expression of the *BCR/ABL* fusion gene. This gene codes for an abnormal cell-signalling protein, tyrosine kinase, which mediates sustained cell proliferation. The reported worldwide incidence again varies (UK incidence is 1.0 per 100 000 population), but is consistently reported more often in males. It is rare in childhood, with the peak incidence occurring in the 40- to 50-year-old age group. Overall, there appears to be a steady decline in the number of cases over time.

Chronic lymphocytic leukaemia

Chronic lymphocytic leukaemia (CLL) is a malignant proliferation of mature lymphocytes which produces the most difficulty for epidemiologists because of an enormous variation in presentation (often asymptomatic), differences in diagnostic practice (blood film examination only), and advances in immunophenotypic subclassification. It is predominantly a disease of old age, but no reliable data exist for incidence or secular trends.

Myeloma

This is a malignant proliferation of plasma cells, and incidence increases with age. Similar diagnostic difficulties occur in the elderly as occur for CLL, leading to problems in interpretation of routine incidence data and secular trends. Worldwide, reported rates vary widely, but most show an increasing incidence. It is thought

that this represents improved diagnosis in the elderly, and more recent data suggest a levelling in incidence rates. Myeloma accounts for 1.5 per cent of all cancers and 1.6 per cent of cancer deaths (Doll and Peto 2002).

Hodgkin's disease

Hodgkin's disease (HD) is a lymphoma distinguished by the presence of the Reed–Sternberg cell, with subtypes recognized by the background cellular composition of involved lymph nodes. International rates vary widely, being lowest in the Far East and highest in Europe and America. The annual UK incidence is 2.2 per 100 000 population. In all areas there is a male excess. This disease has a typical age distribution, with a peak incidence in young adults, caused predominantly by the nodular sclerosing subtype. In the USA an increase in rates of HD in this young adult age group has been reported. In contrast, in the UK overall rates in males are reported to be declining, with no change in female rates over time. Some of this reduction may be due to changes in classification between HD and non-Hodgkin's lymphoma. The disparity in UK and USA trends has not been explained. Some cases have been linked to the Epstein–Barr virus, a ubiquitous herpes virus associated with glandular fever.

Non-Hodgkin's lymphoma

This is not a specific disorder but a collection of distinct disease entities characterized by a malignant proliferation of lymphocytes. Incidence rises with age, with a male excess in all age groups. The striking, on-going increase in incidence of this group of disorders, dating from the 1950s, is apparent in developed countries with less convincing increases in developing ones. The annual UK incidence is 10.9 per 100 000. Increases have been apparent at all ages apart from younger age groups in whom the condition is rare. A rise in the number of cases of both high- and low-grade lymphoma has been reported. However, not all subtypes show a consistent increase in incidence: greater rises have been shown for extra-nodal disease, in particular for gastric and small bowel lymphoma, for B cell skin lymphoma, and for CNS lymphoma.

Aetiological factors include infection, immunosuppression (incurred in tissue transplantation or infection with HIV, for example), antibiotic use, environmental exposure to agrichemicals, atmospheric pollution, and exposure to sunlight. Known risk factors for lymphoma do not account for the well-documented rise in incidence; to produce this consistent and universal increase, any alternative explanation would have to affect large numbers of people, which suggests that a ubiquitous environmental factor, such as exposure to sunlight, might be implicated.

15.4 Genetic and Environmental Factors

Many rare cancers such as polyposis coli, retinoblastoma, and Wilm's tumour, show clear evidence of Mendelian inheritance (see Chapter 18) but altogether contribute only a small percentage of total cancer cases (Peto 2001). 🖳 It has been suggested that cancer is a genetic disease in that it is ultimately caused by mutations in somatic cell lines. However, as discussed in the introduction, most cancers show only weak evidence of familial aggregation, but, despite this there is intense research interest in the study of genes such as *BRCA1* and *BRCA2* which has contributed greatly to our understanding of cellular mechanisms of carcinogenesis.

A growing list of genetic markers is under epidemiological investigation in large cohort studies, which will allow the examination of gene–environment interactions for major cancers. Meanwhile, however, studies of twins have been used to provide estimates of heritability (see Chapter 18). Collaborative studies in Twin Registries indicate that for prostate cancer 42 per cent (95% CI 29–50 per cent) of the risk could be explained by genetic factors. Significant heritability was also reported for colorectal cancer, 35 per cent (95 per cent CI 10–48 per cent) and breast cancer, 27 per cent (95% CI 4–41 per cent). Even in these cancers, however, environmental factors *not shared* between the twin pairs were estimated to account for between

58 per cent and 67 per cent of the risk (Lichtenstein *et al.* 2000). 🖳

Lifestyle and environmental risk factors

Tobacco

Smoking is a major risk factor for cancer, and is causally linked with cancer of the lung, larynx, mouth, oesophagus, kidney, bladder, pancreas, and cervix. In most developed countries tobacco accounts for as much as 30 per cent of all malignant tumours (Doll and Peto 2003). 🖳 It is causally linked with 80–90 per cent of lung tumours and causes a 70 per cent increased risk of pancreatic cancer. Half of all regular cigarette smokers will eventually be killed by their habit (Doll *et al.* 2004). 🖳 Stopping smoking reduces the risk of these cancers, but the risk does not return to that of a non-smoker for some years, and up to 30 years in the case of bladder cancer.

Global marketing of tobacco has resulted in an increase in the number of people in the developing world who are now smoking. Currently two out of three smokers live in developing countries where the number of smokers is predicted to rise further, from current levels of 1.25 billion to 1.64 billion by 2025; in China, where most men smoke, it is estimated that one-third of all men will die from lung cancer. Breathing other people's smoke has also been confirmed as a cause of lung cancer and other diseases; the excess risk for lung cancer of environmental tobacco smoke is 25 per cent (see Chapter 7). Although early detection of lung cancer would significantly improve outcome there is no evidence to show that screening can reduce lung cancer mortality (NHS Centre for Reviews in Dissemination 1998). 🖳 Survival from lung cancer is poor, with only 24 per cent of patients surviving at one year and fewer than 10 per cent at five years. Lung cancer trends reflect changing patterns in tobacco consumption, with falling rates in men and steadily rising rates in women. Prevention of lung cancer will be achieved by reducing tobacco use. The prevention of tobacco-related disease is further discussed in Chapters 7 and 17.

Alcohol

Heavy alcohol consumption is closely associated with cancer of the oral cavity, pharynx, larynx, and oesophagus, mainly acting synergistically with tobacco smoking. These cancers are rare in non-smokers and drinkers, but, as the habits are linked, assessment of the contribution of the individual risk factors poses difficulties. Nevertheless, the contribution of alcohol to risk of cancer can be assessed from well-designed cohort studies, and summary results for colon and breast cancer are shown in Chapter 17 (Table 17.1).

Alcohol also causes cancer of the liver, in combination with smoking. Liver cancer is the commonest cancer in China, where it causes 20 per cent of cancer deaths. The underlying risk factor is chronic active infection with hepatitis B virus, but heavy alcohol consumption is likely to be a major contributory factor.

It has been estimated that alcohol causes between 4–8 per cent of cancer deaths (Doll and Peto 2003). 🖳 Alcohol has a direct, but mild, carcinogenic action, although some alcoholic drinks may contain more potent carcinogenic contaminants such as nitrosoamines, polycystic aromatic hydrocarbons, mycotoxins, esters, and phenols from the raw material and the production processes (World Cancer Research Fund 1997). 🖳

Occupational carcinogens

Many occupations and some specific chemicals are associated with increased risk of cancer. Most occupational carcinogens have been eliminated from, or are closely controlled, in the workplace, but some past exposures carry a significant burden. For example, although the use of asbestos was banned in the 1990s, the incidence of mesothelioma is still increasing in the UK, and may not peak for some years to come (Peto 2001). 🖳 The lengthy incubation period or lag time (up to 40 years) from exposure to the clinical presentation of this cancer is characteristic of this tumour and several others associated with industrial exposures. It has been estimated that occupational exposures account for 2–3 per cent of fatal cancers in the UK, although in developing countries this figure may be higher (see also Chapter 7). The International Agency for Research on Cancer (IARC) classifies 95 agents as carcinogenic to humans, a further 66 as probably carcinogenic, and 241 as possibly carcinogenic. To date 900 agents, which include chemicals, mixtures, beverages, biological and physical agents, and cultural habits, have been evaluated. A detailed list is available (IARC 2005). 🖳

Radiation

Exposure to ionizing radiation, natural as well as that from industrial, medical, and other sources, can cause a variety of neoplasms including leukaemia, and breast and thyroid cancer. Much of the epidemiological information has been gleaned from studies of the survivors in the Japanese cities devastated by atomic explosions in 1945, and from patients given relatively high doses of radiotherapy several decades ago. A dose-dependent

linear relation with no threshold is observed for most cancers, but for leukaemia, at higher levels of radiation, the risk is associated with the square of the dose, a proportionately higher risk. A recent study of a large cohort of airline pilots from Nordic countries, who are exposed to higher-than-average levels of cosmic radiation, showed higher levels of skin cancers but no overall increase in cancer incidence. Radon, a radioactive gas associated with granite, may contribute to up to 6 per cent of all lung cancer cases in the UK and 12 per cent in the USA (Doll and Peto 2003). 🖳

Infections

Up to 21 per cent of all cancers in developing countries may be due to infectious agents: these are predominantly viral, with the exception of *Helicobacter pylori* and some tropical parasitic infections such as liver fluke and schistosomiasis. In developed countries the proportion is less, estimated to be about 9 per cent (Pisani *et al.* 1997). 🖳 Four DNA viruses and five RNA viruses are associated with common cancers (see Box 15.2).

With the exception of the hepatitis C virus, the other cancer-associated RNA viruses are retroviruses, and the two human immunodeficiency viruses (HIV-1 and HIV-2) are the most widely known. They cause gradual destruction of T-lymphocytes. DNA viruses often persist in human cells, with normal immune function, but are contained: in immunodeficiency or in immunosuppression three DNA viruses (Epstein–Barr virus (EBV), human herpes virus 8, and human papilloma virus) spread more widely through body tissues and cause cancers opportunistically.

EBV is associated with Hodgkin's disease, and in Africa, with Burkitt's lymphoma where the disease is endemic. In many African countries the immune system is weakened by poor nutrition and malarial infection and EBV is facilitated to promote the growth of this lymphoma. EBV is also implicated in the pathogenesis of nasopharyngeal cancer (Kieff *et al.* 1995) 🖳 (see also Chapter 16).

Hepatitis B viral infection is closely associated with hepatocellular carcinoma, and is a particular health problem in developing countries and in China, where hepatitis B is endemic. In these countries liver cancer is the third most common type of cancer. Hepatitis C is also closely associated with hepatocellular carcinoma, but in Japan and southern Europe rather than in the developing regions. Sixty per cent of liver cancers are reported to be due to hepatitis B and 24 per cent to hepatitis C (Pisani *et al.* 1997). 🖳 Vaccination for the hepatitis B virus is now recommended by the World Health

BOX 15.2 VIRUSES THAT CAUSE CANCER IN HUMANS	
Virus	**Disease**
RNA viruses	
Human T-cell leukemia virus type 1 (HTLV-I)	Adult T-cell leukemia
Human T-cell leukemia virus type II (HTLV-II)	Hairy cell leukemia
Human immunodeficiency virus types 1 and 2 (HIV-1,2)	Acquired immune deficiency syndrome
Hepatitis C virus	Primary liver cancer
DNA viruses	
Hepatitis B virus	Primary liver cancer
Human papilloma viruses types 16, 18, etc.	Cervical cancer
Epstein–Barr virus	Burkitt's lymphoma; nasopharyngeal carcinoma
Human herpes virus 8	Kaposi's sarcoma

Organization (WHO) for inclusion in routine childhood immunization schedules, to reduce the global burden of this cancer.

Diet and nutrition

Based on differences in the incidence of cancer in different countries with widely varying diets and availability of nutrients, it has been estimated that dietary factors may account for up to 30 per cent of cancers (World Cancer Research Fund 1997). 🖳 In developed countries the contribution may be less at 20 per cent (Key *et al.* 2002). 🖳 These estimates are based largely on ecological studies in which there is a possibility of confounding: (see Chapter 3); more secure evidence comes from cohort studies, and this is strongest for over-nutrition (overweight and obesity).

Diet and nutrition play a very complex role in the modification of cancer risk and, although the mechanisms of action may not be fully understood, there is sufficient evidence, largely from observational epidemiological studies, to identify and recommend dietary practices that decrease cancer risk. These recommendations, if fully implemented, would also reduce risk of other major chronic disease, such as cardiovascular diseases and diabetes. Dietary factors that have been studied most frequently include: energy intake (overweight and obesity), fruit, vegetable, and fibre consumption, and the intake of micronutrients and bioactive compounds. This body of literature has been reviewed by a Working Group of the UK Committee of Medical Aspects of Food and Nutrition Policy (COMA: Working Group on Diet and Cancer 1998). 🖳 It assessed the strength of the evidence for causal relations between these dietary factors and increased risk of cancer, applying criteria for causality similar to those established by Bradford and Hill (see Chapter 1). Their main findings are shown in Table 15.4.

Overweight and obesity

There is strong evidence from observational studies (six cohort and five case-control) for a causal relation between overweight and endometrial cancer (World Cancer Research Fund 1997). 🖳 Risk increases threefold in the range of body mass index 20 to 35kg/m². There is also a consistent but weaker association between overweight and postmenopausal breast cancer. These effects are probably mediated by increased serum concentrations of bioavailable oestrogens. There is weaker evidence supporting a causal relation between overweight and colorectal cancer, and some evidence for increased risk of kidney and prostate cancer in people who are overweight or obese. Evidence is increasing that obesity is a risk factor for oesophageal adenocarcinoma, and population trends in obesity may be contributing to recent rapid increases in the incidence of this cancer in developed countries.

Physical activity

A moderate-to-high level of physical activity has been shown consistently to be associated with a reduced risk of colon cancer (by 40–50 per cent) (Colditz *et al.* 1997). 🖳 Physical activity helps prevent obesity and cancers related to it; in addition, moderate physical activity bolsters the immune system and reduces bowel transit time. This may help to explain the association between physical activity, colon cancer, and some other cancers, although the extent of the contribution remains to be established.

TABLE 15.4   Summary of the strength of the evidence for causal relationships between dietary factors (excluding alcohol) and increased risk of cancer

Cancer site	Strong evidence	Moderate evidence	Weak evidence	Inconsistent/insufficient evidence
Breast cancer	Obesity, especially central obesity (post menopausal only)		Low fruit and vegetable consumption High consumption of red and fried meat	Low dietary fibre consumption Low antioxidant vitamin intake
Lung cancer			High meat consumption	Low fruit and vegetable consumption Low antioxidant vitamin consumption
Colorectal cancer		High red and processed meat consumption Low dietary fibre consumption Low vegetable consumption	High fat consumption Overweight and obesity	Low antioxidant vitamin (C, E, and carotenoids) consumption
Prostate cancer			High meat consumption	Overweight and obesity Low fruit and vegetable consumption Low antioxidant vitamin consumption High fat consumption
Stomach cancer		Low fruit and vegetable consumption		High meat consumption High fat consumption Low antioxidant vitamin consumption
Bladder cancer				Low fruit and vegetable consumption Low antioxidant vitamin consumption High meat consumption
Cervix				Low fruit and vegetable consumption Low intakes of vitamins A, C, E, and carotenoids High consumptions of meat and fat
Endometrium	Overweight and obesity			
Pancreatic cancer		Low dietary fibre consumption	High meat consumption	High fat consumption Low fruit and vegetable consumption Obesity
Oesophagus				Low antioxidant vitamin intake High meat consumption Low fruit and vegetable consumption High fat consumption
Cancer of the mouth, larynx, and pharynx				High meat consumption

Adapted from: Bingham, S. (1999). *Nutritional Aspects of the Development of Cancer*. London: Health Education Authority.

Fruit and vegetable consumption

There is weak-to-moderate evidence for a protective effect of fruit and vegetable consumption against colorectal, stomach, and breast cancers (World Cancer Research Fund 1997). 🖥 Diets that are high in fruit and vegetables may protect against these cancers because they are rich in fibre and antioxidants or other metabolically active compounds, or because people with diets high in fruit and vegetables also tend to consume less meat and fat, and may be leaner.

Micronutrients and bioactive compounds

Oxidative DNA damage by free radicals may predispose to cancer. Therefore, high intakes of antioxidants, such as vitamins C and E, carotenoids, and selenium, can be expected to reduce cancer risk. There is evidence from observational studies that higher intake of antioxidants is associated with reduced risk of breast, colorectal, lung, stomach, oesophageal, and cervical cancers. However, intervention studies showed that dietary supplementation with carotenoids increased the risk of lung cancer (Bowen *et al.* 2003) 🖳 especially in individuals who continued to smoke. Dietary supplementation with antioxidants is not recommended as a means of reducing cancer risk; instead dietary intake of these micronutrients should be increased by greater consumption of fruit and vegetables.

Folate plays an important role in DNA methylation, synthesis, and repair, and several prospective studies have shown low folate consumption to be associated with increased risk of colorectal cancer (Key *et al.* 2002). 🖳 High intakes of calcium and vitamin D may also protect against colorectal cancers. There are many other bioactive compounds that are naturally present in plants that may offer protection against cancer. These include phyto-oestrogens (isoflavones, lignans), flavonoids, resveratrol, lycopene, and organosulphur compounds (Kris-Etherton *et al.* 2002). 🖳 Much research is ongoing into the biological activities of these compounds and foods, such as those shown in Box 15.3, which have the potential for cancer prevention.

BOX 15.3 FOODS WITH POTENTIAL CANCER PREVENTION ACTIVITY

Mode of action

I Drug detoxification:
   broccoli, cucumber, squash, parsley, carrots, lemon oil, peaches, apples, cranberry, garlic, beets

III Anti-inflammatory effects:
   melon, shitake mushrooms, oats, liquorice, ginseng, parsley, fish

IV Antibacterial/antifungal effects:
   garlic, onions, cranberry, green tea, black tea, chocolate

V Anti-oestrogenic effects:
   soybean, fennel, anise, carrots

Meat consumption

Evidence for an association between meat consumption and cancer is most convincing for colorectal cancer; a large, recently reported cohort study found that consumption of red and processed meats was associated with higher risk, and that consumption of poultry and fish was protective (Chao *et al.* 2005). 🖳 Meat consumption may increase colorectal cancer risk by increasing the levels of carcinogens within the bowel. These carcinogens include dietary haem found in red meat, nitrosamines and salt in processed foods, and compounds produced in smoked meats. There is also weak evidence supporting a causal relation between meat consumption and pancreatic, breast, and prostatic cancers.

Fibre consumption

Data from the large European Prospective Investigation into Cancer and Nutrition (the EPIC Study) have confirmed a substantial reduction in the risk of colorectal cancer among people who have a high fibre intake (Bingham *et al.* 2003). 🖳 Fibre may decrease colorectal cancer by bulking stools and decreasing transit time, allowing carcinogens in faeces less contact time with colonic mucosa. High fibre consumption may also increase fermentation in the bowel, with higher production of butyric acid, which appears to have antimitotic effects. There is also inconsistent evidence of a protective effect of a high fibre diet against breast cancer.

Dietary recommendations for reducing cancer risk

The COMA Working Group's recommendations on dietary practices to reduce cancer risk are shown in Box 15.4.

These recommendations are broadly consistent with those from other bodies such as the World Cancer Research Fund and the American Institute for Cancer Research (WCRF 1997). 🖳 Between 30 per cent and 40 per cent of cancer may be preventable by adhering to such recommendations.

15.5 Prevention of Cancer

It represents a challenge for epidemiologists to achieve for cancer prevention what seems to have been accomplished for cardiovascular disease in the past few decades (see Chapter 6). Major opportunities exist for the primary prevention of some cancers, such as respiratory cancers, where the attributable fraction for tobacco smoking is close to 90 per cent in developed

BOX 15.4 RECOMMENDATIONS OF THE UK WORKING GROUP ON DIET AND CANCER

- Increase the consumption of a wide variety of fruits and vegetables.
- Increase intakes of dietary fibre from bread and other cereals (particularly wholegrain varieties), potatoes, fruit, and vegetables.
- Maintain a healthy body weight (within the BMI range 20–25) and avoiding an increase during adult life.
- Avoid an increase in the average consumption of red and processed meat, current intakes of which are about 90 g/day.
- Avoid the use of beta-carotene supplements to protect against cancer and being cautious in using high doses of purified supplements of other nutrients.

Source: Department of Health (1998). 'Nutritional aspects of the development of cancer: report of the Working Group Cancer of the Committee on Medical Aspects of Food and Nutrition Policy'. London: The Stationery Office.

countries (see Chapter 7). As noted above in section 15.4 smoking may account for about 30 per cent of all cancers, alcohol for 4–8 per cent, occupational exposures for 2–3 per cent of fatal cancers, and domestic radon for 6 per cent of lung cancer in the UK. Effective childhood immunization programmes with Hepatitis B vaccine may eventually reduce the global burden of liver cancer, but HIV infection, and much cervical cancer, could be eliminated by improvements in sexual hygiene. Reduction in population levels of overweight, obesity, and sedentary behaviour could also decrease the incidence of certain cancers, such as colorectal and breast cancers, but the public-health reality is that the obesity epidemic is likely to get worse before it gets better. Opportunities also exist for research into specific foods and micronutrients, but with the current levels of evidence, the COMA Working Group recommendations (see Box 15.3) to reduce the population levels of cancer risk, seem uncontroversial. Some major trials of dietary intervention in cancer prevention may help establish the utility of these proposals within a few years. It has been estimated from the Global Burden of Disease project (Ezzati *et al.* 2003) 🖳 that implementing the proposals for fruit and vegetable consumption (to increase the average consumption to 600 g per day for adults, or five portions per day) would lower the Global Burden of Disease by 1.8 per cent compared with 2.3 per cent for the reduction of obesity (see Chapter 17, Table 17.2). Both risk factors contribute significantly to the risk of cardiovascular disease, in addition to selected cancers.

Early detection of cancers by the use of population or selective screening programmes may offer future prospects for cancer prevention (secondary prevention), particularly in the development of molecular assays for biomarkers in clinical samples such as saliva, sputum, urine or faeces (Caldas 1998). 🖳 As noted in Chapter 5, however, these programmes require careful evaluation by large-scale controlled trials before their introduction into routine practice.

Finally, improvements have been made, and are likely to continue to be made, in the treatment of cancer, improvements both in five-year survival and quality of life. Updated evidence on the effectiveness of cancer treatments is available from web sources such as the National Cancer Institute (US) (2005) 🖳 and Cancer Back Up (UK) (2005). 🖳

In conclusion, it is clear that both epidemiological and basic research are required in parallel, to improve our understanding of the causes of cancer. Large-scale follow-up studies of tumour markers, in particular, should assist in detecting important gene–environment interactions, and enhance the prospects for cancer control.

Further Reading

Adami, H.-O., Hunter, D. and Trichopoulos, D. (eds.) (2002). *Textbook of Cancer Epidemiology*. New York, NY: Oxford University Press.

Coop, A. and Ellis, M. J. (2003). 'The Nature and Development of Cancer', in D. A. Warrell, T. M. Cox, J. D. Firth and E. J. Benz Jr (eds.), *Oxford Textbook of Medicine*. Oxford: Oxford University Press, 219–28.

Doll, R. and Peto, R. (2003). 'Epidemiology of Cancer', in D. A. Warrell, T. M. Cox, J. D. Firth and E. J. Benz Jr (eds.), *Oxford Textbook of Medicine*. Oxford: Oxford University Press, 193–218.

Nasca, P. C. and Pastides, H. (2001). *Fundamentals of Cancer Epidemiology*. Gaithersburg, MD: Aspen Publishers.

World Cancer Research Fund (1997). *Food, Nutrition and the Prevention of Cancer: A Global Perspective*. World Cancer Research Fund/American Institute for Cancer Research, Washington, USA.

Web Addresses

Cancer Research UK Factsheets, www.cancerresearchuk. org/aboutcancer/statistics/factsheets.

Cancer BackUp (2005). Information source for cancer patients (and professionals), cancerbackup. org.uk/Home.

International Agency for Research on Cancer (2005). Monographs on the evaluation of carcinogenic risks to humans, www-cie.iarc.fr/monoeval/cie.html.

National Cancer Institute (2005). Website: www.nci. nih.gov/.

References

References for this chapter can be found at www.oxfordtextbooks.co.uk/orc/yarnell. Where possible, these are presented as *active links* which direct you to an electronic version of the work. If you are a subscriber to that work (either individually or through an institution), and depending on your level of access, you may be able to peruse an abstract or the full article if available. 🖳

Model answers

Q1

- Information should be obtained on the reliability of cancer diagnoses in developing countries. In Figure 15.1 information from developing countries was obtained using only reliable cancer registries which would ensure that ascertainment of cancer diagnoses would be reasonably complete.

- Risk of cancer increases with length of exposure to tobacco products, and adverse dietary and lifestyle factors. In the absence of competing causes of death, exposures would be more likely to be prolonged in developed countries in which relative life expectancy is extended, leading to prolonged exposure times.

Q2

- One possibility is that incidence rates are truly different in each country and the similarities in mortality rates are a reflection of the relative success of treatments in the USA, France, and UK.

- The alternative explanation is that the incidence rates in the USA and France are inflated by the inclusion of slow-growing or innocuous cancers which are detected by higher levels of screening practice in these countries compared with that in the UK.

- The most likely explanation is that less malignant tumours are being detected in the screening programmes in the USA and France compared with those detected opportunistically in the UK. This can be checked by the number or rates of PSA testing in each country in men over the age of 50 years, for example.

Infectious diseases

This chapter reviews the epidemiology of infectious disease, immunization, surveillance, the emergence of new diseases, and the control of outbreaks. Three examples of epidemiological studies during outbreaks are provided at the end of the chapter.

Introduction

Understanding infectious diseases and their control requires an encompassing and increasingly global perspective, one in which individuals and populations interact with each other and with broader ecosystems. Three aspects of these systems conspire to produce epidemics of disease: the agent, the host, and the environment. In most countries, the pace of environmental change is such as to promote the spread of old infections and to encourage agents to evolve into human environments. This dynamic global situation requires continuous surveillance and responsive international control measures.

16.1 Epidemiology of Infectious Disease

For most of the 180 000 years of modern man's existence, it was only a minority of each generation that reached adulthood, if they managed to avoid or survive the physical hazards, starvation, or infection that prevailed upon the rest. Man's evolution after the exodus from Africa brought him into contact with many unfamiliar physical, dietary, and microbiological environments to which he was forced to adapt or perish. The rise of agriculture and the domestication of several animal species provided new opportunities for the formation of human settlements and exposure to a wider range of potentially pathogenic organisms.

Pathogens include protozoa, fungi, bacteria, and viruses; more recently 'slow viruses', more appropriately described as prions (proteinaceous particles) have passed from cattle to man (bovine spongiform encephalopathy), although the precise nature of the prion and its level of infectivity remains controversial (Cheeseboro 1998). ⌨ Detailed consideration of biological principles in human infectious disease is beyond the scope of this text but a basic understanding of the wide ranges of *infectivity, pathogenicity, modes of transmission, virulence, immunogenicity and antigenic variation* in infectious agents is important for an understanding of the principles of spread and control of epidemics (see Box 16.1).

The emergence of infections, such as smallpox, plague, cholera, measles, pertussis, meningococcal meningitis, gonorrhoea, and syphilis around 10 000 years ago, depended as much on population dynamics as on any inherent pathogenicity of the organisms themselves. The creation of villages, then towns, and finally cities, provided the opportunity for the emergence and spread of the major epidemic diseases. Box 16.2 shows the main modes of transmission of common communicable diseases.

The spread of communicable disease

Infection is considered directly transmitted when passed by direct contact with an infected person. In indirect transmission the agent has passed into the wider environment and may be passed on through water, air, food, insect, or animal vectors, or through the soil. Person-to-person transmission is governed by a factor known as the reproductive rate, which depends on host, agent, and population factors (see Box 16.3).

If each infected person infects only one other person on average the reproductive rate (Ro) is 1; the disease exists in a steady state and is said to be **endemic** in the population. If an infected individual infects more than one individual the number of cases builds up and the disease becomes **epidemic** ($Ro > 1$). Assuming the disease produces immunity then gradually the proportion of susceptibles in the population will fall; $Ro < 1$ and eventually the disease will die out. Artificial creation of this '**herd immunity**' is the aim of most immunization programmes. The recent outbreaks of measles and mumps in parts of the UK reflect decreasing herd

---

BOX 16.1 BIOLOGICAL DEFINITIONS IN INFECTIOUS DISEASE

Infectivity	The capacity of an organism to multiply in the host	Also defined as the proportion of exposures that results in infection
Pathogenicity	The capacity of an organism to cause disease in an infected host	Smallpox shows high pathogeneity: polio virus low pathogeneity (many infected individuals are asymptomatic)
Virulence	The degree of pathogeneity of an organism	Virulence may vary by strain, for example 'wild' strains of measles and polio Virulence may vary over time, for example streptococcus
Immunogenicity	The capacity of an organism to induce specific and lasting immunity in the host	Generalized systemic infections usually produce a strong, lasting immune response in contrast to localized infections
Antigenic variability	The capacity of an organism to exist or evolve different antigenic forms	Influenza is unstable and rhinoviruses exist in many antigenic forms
Host specificity	The lack of capacity of an organism to infect more than one animal species	Smallpox or measles specific to humans. TB and brucella in many animal species

Source: Modified from Farmer, R. D. T., Miller, D. and Lawrenson, R. (1996). *Lecture Notes on Epidemiology and Public Health* (4th edn). Oxford: Blackwell. Reproduced with permission from Blackwell Publishing.

BOX 16.2 DIRECTLY AND INDIRECTLY TRANSMITTED INFECTIONS

Direct

Droplets: influenza, coryza, measles, SARS

Blood: hepatitis B, C, HIV and other bodily fluids

Transplacental: toxoplasmosis

Epidermal: herpes type 1

Mucous membrane: STDs, HIV

Indirect

Water: hepatitis A and probably E, polio, cholera, typhoid, cryptosporidiosis

Air: chicken pox, anthrax, aspergillosis, legionella

Food: *Campylobacter*, *Salmonella*, *Staphylococcus* toxin, *E. coli* strains

Vectors: malaria, yellow fever, sleeping sickness, West Nile fever,

Soil: tetanus, anthrax

After: Giesecke, J. (2001). *Modern Infectious Disease Epidemiology* (2nd edn). Edinburgh: Arnold.

---

immunity because of poor uptake of combined measles, mumps, and rubella (MMR) vaccine. In the case of immunization against meningococcus type C, however, lower levels of herd immunity may be adequate, because the carriage rate in the nasopharynx in adolescents has been shown to have reduced from 0.45 per cent to 0.15 per cent (a fall of 67 per cent) resulting in lower transmission rates in those unvaccinated (Ramsay *et al.* 2003). 🖳

16.2 Immunization

Immunization and vaccination against an increasing range of bacteria, their toxins, and viruses have been a global public-health success and are among the most cost-effective health interventions. Through programmes coordinated by the World Health Organization (WHO) smallpox was declared eradicated in 1980; WHO has a current goal to eradicate poliomyelitis, a disease that once paralysed hundreds of thousands of children annually before the introduction of a suitable vaccine,

and which remains endemic in eight countries. While the incidence of vaccine-preventable infections has markedly decreased in many developed countries, globally WHO reports an estimated million deaths each year to such diseases of childhood, with 50–60 per cent of these deaths attributable to measles. In 2001 there were 30–40 million cases of measles worldwide. As noted in Chapter 8, many of these deaths can be attributed to decreased host resistance due to sub-optimal nutrition; nevertheless, measles vaccination campaigns in developing countries have been highly effective in preventing deaths.

The current immunization schedule for the UK is shown in Box 16.4 and since the introduction of MMR vaccine (1988) 🖳 two additional vaccines have been added: haemophilus influenza type b and meningococcus group C, each of which is active against a specific type of meningitis. Many other vaccines and immunizations are available for use by travellers to countries where several serious diseases remain endemic.

For some infections, such as tuberculosis (TB), the introduction of vaccination further accelerated a long-established downward trend in mortality rates (see Chapter 1, Figure 1.1) owing to improved housing and nutrition. Globally, TB remains a major cause of mortality and morbidity, with 2.4 million new cases reported in 2001. It disproportionately affects poorer nations, with human immunodeficiency virus (HIV) infection as a major factor driving the global TB pandemic. With 12 million people co-infected with HIV and TB, it is clear that control of TB cannot happen without control of HIV infection. Global control of TB cannot rely only on vaccination, which is contraindicated in those who

---

BOX 16.3 DETERMINANTS OF THE SPREAD OF INFECTION IN A POPULATION (REPRODUCTIVE RATE)

- Infectivity of agent
- Frequency and type of contacts in the population
- Period of infectivity in each infected individual
- Proportion immune in the population

After: Giesecke, J. (2001). *Modern Infectious Disease Epidemiology* (2nd edn). Edinburgh: Arnold.

BOX 16.4 UK CHILDHOOD VACCINATION SCHEDULE: MARCH 2004*

- 2 months: diphtheria, tetanus, pertussis, polio, haemophilus influenza type b (Hib), meningococcal group C (Men C)
- 3 months: diphtheria, tetanus, pertussis polio and Hib, Men C
- 4 months: diphtheria, tetanus, pertussis, polio and Hib, Men C
- 13 months: measles, mumps, rubella (MMR)
- by school entry: diphtheria, tetanus, pertussis and polio, MMR
- 10–14 years: BCG for those not immune to TB
- school leaver: tetanus, low dose diphtheria, polio

Source: http://www.immunisation.org.uk.
*Updated September 2006 (see above website).

---

are HIV positive, but must also address contributory social and environmental factors in addition to traditional public-health measures such as early detection and treatment of cases, and swift follow-up of contacts.

Benefits versus hazards of vaccination

Public-health immunization programmes in developed and developing countries need to retain public and professional confidence in both the efficacy of the programme and the perceived safety of the vaccines. Smallpox has been eradicated and routine vaccination was discontinued in the post-smallpox era when the hazards of continued vaccination were evaluated (Ada 2001). 🖳 For most vaccines, however, the infectious agents persist in the population, and continued immunization programmes are necessary. Public concern over pertussis immunization (Gangarosa et al. 1998), 🖳 and more recently MMR, has resulted in wider public debate of the issues and of the available data. All vaccines are fully tested in animal studies, human volunteers, and in field trials before being licensed for general use. Nevertheless, routine surveillance thereafter in the UK is dependent on the '**yellow card**' system of voluntary reporting by doctors, dentists, pharmacists, and others of suspected vaccine side effects or adverse reactions, to the UK Medicines and Healthcare Products Agency. In an epidemiological study based on the linkage of childhood immunization registers with hospital admissions in children (for febrile convulsions or similar conditions) it was estimated that 'yellow card'

reports underestimate the risk of complications by a factor of 50 per cent (Farrington et al. 1995). 🖳 The use of epidemiological methods in the evaluation and surveillance of immunization programmes is discussed in detail elsewhere (Chen and Orenstein 1996). 🖳

16.3 Surveillance of Communicable Disease

Communicable disease surveillance has been described as '… the continued watchfulness over the distribution and trends of incidence through the systematic collection, consolidation and evaluation of morbidity and mortality reports and other relevant data. Intrinsic in the concept is the regular dissemination of the basic data and interpretations to all who have contributed and to all others who need to know' (Langmuir 1963). 🖳 Surveillance is therefore information for action. Surveillance systems should ideally be: simple to use; flexible to adapt to changing circumstances; have complete and accurate data; acceptable to participants; sensitive with a high positive predictive value; representative of a population/event; timely, with a short interval between onset and report to the surveillance system, to facilitate early, appropriate action; and capable of being sustained over time (Klaucke et al. 1988). 🖳

Passive surveillance describes most routine systems in which doctors and others report diseases whereas **active surveillance** implies that a health authority or surveillance centre actively seeks out such reports, for example in an outbreak investigation. Surveillance systems should enable: the establishment of baseline trends in the incidence and demography of a disease or event; the early recognition of an outbreak or a new infection/syndrome; the identification of those at risk; the evaluation of controls and other interventions; and the development of policies, action plans, priority setting, and research. The two main components of routine surveillance in most advanced industrialized countries are (a) statutory infectious diseases notification, and (b) laboratory reporting of infectious agents.

Notifications

Most countries have a list of communicable diseases which doctors are legally required to report or notify to the appropriate authority. These notifications of infectious disease are the historical bedrock of surveillance having been in existence in the UK for over a century. There are currently 30 diseases notifiable in England under the Public Health (Infectious Diseases) Regulations, 1988.

Similar, though not identical, lists exist in the other parts of the UK. They comprise most of the vaccine-preventable infections whereas others such as cholera, plague, and yellow fever are included under WHO International Health Regulations.

Certain enforcement powers can be applied to an individual with a notifiable disease such as compulsory medical examination but treatment is not compulsory. Notifications can be used for:

◆ Baseline surveillance

◆ Assessing the efficacy of the childhood vaccination programme

◆ Initiating an investigation, for example food poisoning

◆ Initiating contact tracing to identify and protect others at risk, for example in tuberculosis and meningococcal infection.

Doctors are required to notify on the basis of clinical suspicion: laboratory confirmation is not required. However, although it is a legal requirement to notify (and a modest fee is paid) many doctors either fail to notify at all or do not notify in a timely manner to enable public-health action. This may reflect a lack of understanding of the purposes of notification, which also has no perceived benefit to their patient.

Laboratory surveillance

Laboratory reporting of organisms of public-health interest is now the cornerstone of communicable disease surveillance. This is undertaken on a voluntary basis though there are proposals to make it a requirement in the UK. Data on specific organisms can now be captured electronically from the laboratory computer system and forwarded to the public-health consultant for local surveillance and public-health action, as well as being forwarded electronically to regional and national surveillance centres.

However, even with complete laboratory reporting, the incidence of many infections remains underestimated. To be reported in the national database requires:

◆ The individual to seek medical attention. This will be influenced by the severity, nature and duration of symptoms.

◆ The doctor to initiate appropriate investigations. This will also be influenced by the patient's history and clinical examination, and the patient's willingness to provide a laboratory sample.

◆ The laboratory to perform the appropriate analysis. Laboratory practice using specific enrichment media or referral to a reference laboratory may depend on the clinical information on the request form.

◆ The laboratory to inform the national surveillance centre.

Some common infections of public-health concern may not be notifiable or not routinely subject to laboratory investigation; for example, influenza and viral gastroenteritis. Therefore alternative surveillance arrangements are required. Throughout the UK there are networks of **sentinel general practices** which report the number of consultations for influenza or influenza-like illness in the preceding week as a proportion of the practice population. Aggregation of these data provides age-specific consultation rates for a region which, combined with the laboratory analysis of nasopharyngeal swabs from such patients, can provide early warning of the emergence of influenza virus in the community before it would be normally noted from rises in hospital admission rates or positive laboratory reports from hospitalized patients.

Influenza

This is primarily a clinical diagnosis and it would be unusual for a general practitioner to seek laboratory confirmation. In addition, those with influenza or 'flu-like' illness are actively discouraged from visiting their general practitioner unless their symptoms are severe or prolonged. Therefore surveillance systems need to adapt to changes in health-service provision and the opportunities provided through the increased use of electronic datasets. For example, a study is underway to assess the potential of NHS Direct (nurse-led telephone helplines) to detect symptoms in the population that could be due to outbreaks or toxic environmental hazards (Baker *et al.* 2003). 🖳

Sexually transmitted diseases

These include infections such as syphilis, gonorrhoea, chlamydia, and HIV, which are not currently notifiable. However, genito-urinary (GU) medicine clinics throughout the UK are required to provide aggregate (anonymized) data on clinic attenders. This includes diagnosis, gender, age group, and sexual orientation, and these data are collected for selected conditions. HIV surveillance also includes confidential reporting by clinicians of diagnoses of HIV, acquired immune deficiency syndrome (AIDS), and HIV-related deaths to the national surveillance centres, and the unlinked anonymous surveys of attenders of GU clinics noted above, as well as injecting drug users attending specialist treatment/support services.

Q1 HIV infections can be passed from mother to baby before, during and after the birth. Breastfeeding can pass on HIV infection. What surveillance systems and control measures would be appropriate?

Nowadays air travel and the mass movement of people and foodstuffs mean that an infective source can readily transmit infection internationally, as illustrated in the worldwide outbreak of a new disease, severe acute respiratory syndrome (SARS). The WHO has a major role in coordinating international surveillance and outbreak response. Similarly, the European Community (EC) Communicable Diseases Network is progressively developing surveillance for a variety of communicable diseases including influenza, legionnaires' disease, tuberculosis, and enteric infections. It also operates an early warning and response system to alert public-health authorities, member states, and the European Commission on outbreaks with EC implications, to enable coordinated Community action. This will be further developed by the newly established European Centre for Disease Control in Stockholm. In the USA the Centers for Disease Control have two centres, each for the control of a specific group of infectious diseases (see Chapter 21, Box 21.3).

16.4 **Emergence of New Infections**

In the past three decades over 30 newly identified infections have emerged, some of major public-health importance such as HIV and hepatitis C. In the 1990s over two-thirds of emerging infections have been closely linked with animals, both wild and domestic. New strains of influenza virus have occurred in those farming geese, chickens, ducks, and pigs, and more recently the SARS virus originated in live animals in Asia markets (Webster 2004). Outbreaks of serious food-borne infections continue to be linked with faulty food-processing practices (*E. coli* 0157, bovine spongiform encephalopathy (BSE), and variant Creutzfeldt–Jacob disease). The continued emergence of such diseases emphasizes the need for an international surveillance network and a rapid and efficient outbreak investigation system. The biology of newly emerging organisms

and epidemics is discussed in detail elsewhere (Antia *et al.* 2003). In hospitals, infections are acquired by up to 10 per cent of patients in the UK (and up to 25 per cent in developing countries). Infections are commonest in the urinary and lower respiratory tracts (about 23 per cent) but are also common in surgical wounds (11 per cent), skin (10 per cent), and in the bloodstream (6 per cent). Some organisms such as *Staphylococcus aureus* and enterococci have acquired antibiotic resistance, for example methicillin-resistant *Staphylococcus aureus* (MRSA), and vancomycin-resistant *Staphylococcus aureus* (VRSA). If these become endemic in hospitals, they are difficult to eradicate and contribute significantly to morbidity in the hospital population. Appropriate control measures have been recommended (Ridwan *et al.* 2002).

16.5 **Outbreak Investigation**

An outbreak of infection is said to have occurred when the number of observed cases exceeds that which is expected in a particular population. There is no specific number of cases to constitute an outbreak. For example, a single case of a rare or highly virulent infection such as smallpox, diphtheria, or polio in the UK would be regarded as an outbreak with international consequences. Boxes 16.5 and 16.6 describe two large outbreaks and illustrate some of the key aspects of outbreak investigation.

In the UK the local Consultant in Communicable Disease Control (CCDC) may note, from routine surveillance of laboratory reports, an increase of a particular organism. A reference laboratory may note increasing cases nationwide as in the case of the *Salmonella agona* outbreak shown in Box 16.6. Clinicians may report seeing an unusually high number of patients with diseases such as acute gastroenteritis, severe flu-like illness, or an atypical clinical syndrome such as tetanus in injecting drug users. The public or media may contact the local environmental health department or CCDC directly to report illness after a particular event. The CCDC makes further enquiries to gather supporting evidence of a potential problem. This includes contacting neighbouring CCDCs and microbiologists, and often the regional and national surveillance centres. Checks are made to ensure no recent change in laboratory practice or catchment area, which could explain increased laboratory reporting. In the USA, HIV was first discovered by increased laboratory reports of atypical pneumonia.

BOX 16.5 A WATERBORNE OUTBREAK OF CRYPTOSPORIDIOSIS

Cryptosporidiosis is an acute gastrointestinal infection caused by the ingestion of cryptosporidial oocysts. It is characterized by diarrhoea which may last, on average, 14 days, abdominal pain, and fever. It can be acquired through faecal oral spread from other symptomatic individuals, animals (who are usually asymptomatic), and from food or water contaminated with cryptosporidial oocysts. Its public-health significance is that if oocysts enter the drinking water supply the normal chlorine concentration in the water is insufficient to kill them. There have been several water-borne outbreaks in the UK secondary to cryptosporidiosis. The largest reported outbreak in the world was in 1993 when an estimated 403 000 people in Milwaukee became ill (MacKenzie et al. 1994). 🖥

In early 1997 in North Thames there was a large waterborne outbreak with 345 confirmed cases of cryptosporidiosis associated with a borehole (Willocks et al. 1998). 🖥 A case was defined as an individual with microbiologically confirmed cryptosporidiosis and no recent history of travel abroad (person) who became ill between 1 February and 25 April 1997 (time) and who lived in any of the four health districts affected (place). To test the hypothesis that illness was associated with consumption of unboiled tap water, an unmatched case–control study was undertaken with controls of a similar age, sex, and area of residence randomly selected from the health authority databases or general practitioners' lists.

Drinking history in cases and controls

Risk factor	Case (n = 176)	Control (n = 75)	Total (n = 251)	Odds ratio (95% confidence interval)
Did not consume tap water	17	18	35	
Consumed tap water	156	57	213	2.90 (1.31–6.43)
Did not consume bottled water	152	53	205	
Consumed bottled water	18	21	39	0.30 (0.14–0.64)
Did not consume non-diluting soft drink	40	6	46	
Consumed non-diluting soft drink	85	54	139	0.24 (0.08–0.64)

This analytical study concluded that consumption of unboiled tap water was significantly associated with illness and consumption of bottled water and non-diluting soft drink were significantly associated with not being ill: the latter had a protective effect.

The investigators were also able to demonstrate a 'dose–response' relation between illness and the quantity of unboiled tap water consumed: the more water drunk the more likely an individual would be ill.

The preliminary enquiry can be quickly completed and, if initial suspicions of an outbreak are confirmed, a decision is required as to whether it should be investigated. Factors to consider include: initial information on morbidity and mortality; the vulnerability of the population at risk; association with a high-risk facility, for example a hospital or food premises; its transmissibility; the likelihood of continuing exposure to the suspected source; national and international implications through human travel or distribution of a particular food product; and potential media and political interest.

Usually the need for the CCDC to initiate an outbreak investigation is self-evident and a pre-prepared outbreak plan is activated. This initiates a sequence of events and may involve a large number and range of individuals and agencies, postponing routine work. An incident room may be required.

The CCDC will establish an outbreak control team (OCT) which: coordinates the investigation; ensures sufficient resources are made available to control the outbreak; ensures appropriate care for those who are ill; identifies the cause; initiates and evaluates the efficacy of control measures in preventing spread to others; and compiles a formal report.

Membership will reflect those agencies involved or likely to be involved in investigating and controlling

---

BOX 16.6 INTERNATIONAL OUTBREAK OF *SALMONELLA AGONA*: THE IMPORTANCE OF NATIONAL LABORATORY SURVEILLANCE AND INTERNATIONAL COOPERATION

Between 5 December 1994 and 30 January 1995, 27 isolates of *Salmonella agona* were identified in England and Wales by the Salmonella Reference Laboratory of the Public Health Laboratory Service (now the Health Protection Agency). This was in contrast to 12 isolates in the same period in the previous year. Many of the cases were children, there was geographical clustering, and many of the children had Jewish surnames. From initial interviews with eight primary cases, four had eaten a peanut-flavoured ready-to-eat snack made of maize and imported from Israel. Case finding was not restricted to the UK but included Europe using Salm-Net, a network for the surveillance of salmonella in Europe. Other countries including Israel, the USA, and Canada were also alerted (Killalea *et al.* 1996). 💻

A case–control study subsequently confirmed a strong association between infection with the outbreak strain of *S. agona* and consumption of the snack food. The outbreak strain was identified in 83 per cent (44/53) of packets obtained from retailers and manufactured on a certain day. Approximately 20 000 packets from this batch had been distributed throughout the UK. At the same time, Israeli authorities were investigating a large outbreak of *S. agona* and, with information from the UK, were able to ascertain that the savoury snack was the source of their outbreak (Shohat *et al.* 1996). 💻 Individuals with the outbreak strain were also identified in North America. However, none of the European members of Salm-Net reported any increase of *S. agona* isolates.

This study therefore highlights the role of national laboratory based surveillance and the benefits of international cooperation in outbreak investigation, particularly with a widely distributed food product.

Association between illness due to *Salmonella agona* phage type 15 and consumption of the kosher savoury snack

	Cases			Controls			Odds ratio (95% confidence interval)	P value (Fisher's exact test)
	Ate snack	Did not eat snack	Not sure	Ate snack	Did not eat snack	Not sure		
All cases	13	1	2	4	27	1	87.8 (7.5 to 2400)	<0.0001
Subset of cases*	6	0	2	4	27	1	∞ (14.6† to ∞)	0.0002

*Cases from preliminary inquiry excluded.
†Lower limit by profile likelihood approach.
British Medical Journal (1996), **313**: 1106, reproduced with permission from the BMJ Publishing Group.

---

the outbreak, including environmental health, the local microbiologist, a clinician, particularly if cases are hospitalized, and a public-relations officer. In zoonotic outbreaks, farm or animal investigations may be necessary and veterinary officers from the Department for Environment, Food and Rural Affairs (DEFRA), or an equivalent agency elsewhere, would attend. Similarly in an outbreak of legionnaire's disease involving industrial premises, officials from the Health and Safety Executive would be involved.

When appropriate, the OCT will initiate a **descriptive study** (see Chapter 3) to identify the characteristics of those affected, from which hypotheses are developed for testing in an **analytical study**. A case is defined in terms of time, place, and person (Box 16.5). The initial **case definition** may be relatively broad to identify as many potentially affected subjects as possible: that is, highly **sensitive** but not necessarily wholly **specific**. There may be a clinical case definition which is based on the presenting symptoms and signs found in the initial, reported cases. **Confirmed cases** will be those matching the case definition with subsequent laboratory confirmation (see Box 16.7).

A detailed interview of the initial cases is undertaken to ascertain the relevant symptoms, signs, and risk factors/exposure histories, namely: household and other contacts; travel history; occupational details; lifestyle factors; and knowledge of others similarly affected. In investigations of food poisoning, the history is usually confined to events or exposures in the 72 hours preceding illness. This period must reflect the incubation period of the anticipated organism. The initial interview is important and may take several hours of careful questioning to gather all relevant information. It may be possible, at this early stage, to identify a suspected location or exposure.

Based on these initial interviews a questionnaire is devised to capture details on all further reported cases. The investigators then need to identify other individuals who may have been infected (**case finding**). This includes alerting local general practitioners, accident and emergency departments, laboratories, CCDCs, and liaising with function organizers to obtain a guest list of those attending a particular event. If cases are suspected throughout the country, a national alert would be sent electronically from the Communicable Disease Surveillance Centre or Chief Medical Officer to clinicians and CCDCs advising how suspected cases should be reported; international liaison may also be required.

The questionnaires may be administered by telephone, face-to-face interview, or by post. Telephone interviews are quick, cheap, and usually associated with higher response rates. Data from completed questionnaires are coded and entered into an appropriate epidemiological software package such as EPIINFO, available from the Centers for Disease Control (USA) to enable the descriptive analysis. Tables are constructed classifying the cases by age, sex, date of onset of illness, and by exposure to the main risk factors. Graphs of the occurrence of cases over time (the **epidemic curve**) can provide valuable information on the incubation period and whether the outbreak is a **point source**, for example a food poisoning in a hotel outbreak with a short exposure period, or a **continuing source** indicating serial transfer from the infective source. The epidemic curve can also assist monitoring the impact of control measures. Box 16.7 describes the epidemic curve in the 2003 SARS outbreak; its shape is typical of a continuing source with person-to-person spread.

If salmonella is mainly in young children, it could suggest a food or drink usually consumed by this group. Mapping reports of cryptosporidiosis or legionnaires'

disease may reveal clusters in the distribution of a particular water supply or near a cooling tower, air-conditioning unit, or showers, taps, or other sources of water in hospitals or hotels.

If the preliminary, descriptive studies have revealed particular characteristics, or locations of affected individuals, further studies can be done to test particular hypotheses. A **cohort study** is typically undertaken when the population at risk can be readily identified. For example at a wedding reception, all on the guest list would be contacted and details sought on the food and drinks they consumed, and whether or not they had become ill. A table is constructed comparing the number (and proportion) of those who ate a particular food item and became ill (the **attack rate**) with the number of those who did not eat the food item but who also became ill. This allows comparison of the attack rates among different groups (Box 16.8).

A **case-control study** is performed when the population at risk is not known or it is impractical to follow up the whole population at risk. Controls, however, should have the same chance of being exposed to the risk factor as the case. Both examples shown in Boxes 16.5 and 16.6, respectively, are case–control studies.

All studies should be supported by an environmental investigation whenever relevant and practicable. In an outbreak of food poisoning this will include an inspection of the food preparation area, assessing kitchen practice, and hygiene. Environmental swabs and samples of remaining food items are taken; if the same pathogen is found in food as in the cases this would provide strong supporting evidence on the cause of the outbreak. In a legionnaire's investigation an environmental assessment would be made of large air-conditioning systems and processes generating water aerosols located in the vicinity of the outbreak, and appropriate water samples taken to detect the presence of legionella.

Control measures to prevent further cases should be introduced as soon as a suspect source is identified, often while awaiting the outcome of analytical studies. These include: withdrawing an infected food from sale; excluding a foodhandler with gastroenteritis from work; closure of a food premise pending refurbishment or deep cleaning; shut down and disinfection of an air-conditioning system; and issuing a 'boil water' notice.

Outbreaks increasingly attract public, political, and media interest and responding to this is an ongoing

BOX 16.7 SEVERE ACUTE RESPIRATORY SYNDROME (SARS): CASE DEFINITIONS

Clinical case

Fever of ≥38 °C (documented or reported)

And one or more symptoms of lower respiratory tract illness (cough, difficulty breathing, shortness of breath)

And radiographic evidence of lung infiltrates consistent with pneumonia or respiratory distress syndrome (RDS) or autopsy findings consistent with the pathology of pneumonia or RDS without an identifiable cause

And no alternative diagnosis to fully explain the illness

Possible case

Meets clinical case definition

And within 10 days of onset of illness travelled to a zone of potential SARS re-emergence (currently mainland China and Hong Kong)

Or within 10 days of onset of illness a history of exposure to laboratories or institutes which have retained SARS virus isolates and/or diagnostic specimens from SARS patients

Probable case

An individual with symptoms and signs consistent with clinical SARS (Possible case) and with preliminary laboratory evidence of SARS CoV infection based on the following:

Either Single positive antibody test for SARS CoV

Or Positive PCR for SARS CoV on a single clinical specimen and assay

Confirmed case

An individual with symptoms and signs consistent with clinical SARS (Possible case) and with preliminary laboratory evidence of SARS CoV infection based on one or more of the following:

a) PCR positive for SARS-CoV using a validated method from:

At least two different clinical specimens (e.g. nasopharyngeal and stool) Or

The same clinical specimen collected on two or more occasions during the course of the illness (for example sequential nasopharyngeal aspirates)

Or

Two different assays or repeat PCR using a new RNA extract from the original clinical sample on each occasion of testing

b) Seroconversion by ELISA or IFA

Negative antibody test on acute serum followed by positive antibody test on convalescent phase serum tested in parallel **Or**

Fourfold or greater rise in antibody titre between the acute and convalescent phase sera tested in parallel

Source: WHO consensus document on the epidemiology of SARS (2003), WHO, Geneva (http://www.hpa.org.uk/infections/topics_az/SARS/casedef.htm).

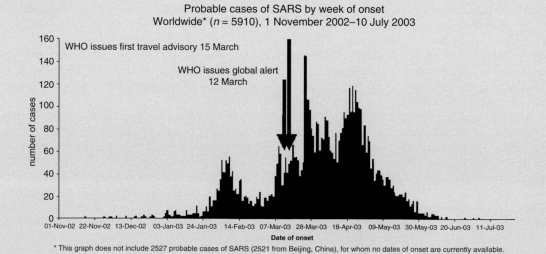

Probable cases of SARS by week of onset
Worldwide* (*n* = 5910), 1 November 2002–10 July 2003

* This graph does not include 2527 probable cases of SARS (2521 from Beijing, China), for whom no dates of onset are currently available.

BOX 16.8 COHORT STUDY OF FOOD POISONING INCIDENT (ANG 1998)

Nine out of 24 guests at a wedding party developed gastroenteritis between one and three days later. The menu consisted of a starter from a seafood platter or melon and strawberries. The main course consisted of duck or vegetable lasagne. A retrospective cohort study was undertaken of all the guests using a postal questionnaire containing the food items served at the party.

Twenty questionnaires were returned (87 per cent response rate). Analysis of food-specific attack rates showed that illness was significantly associated with eating items from the seafood platter. Nine of the 11 consuming raw oysters were ill compared with none of the nine who did not eat oysters. Small Round-Structured Virus (SRSV) infection was confirmed in two cases.

Raw oysters have been frequently associated with SRSV outbreaks. In this incident it is likely that those eating oysters consumed other types of seafood from the platter.

challenge to the outbreak investigators. In the midst of a large outbreak it is essential to have clear lines of communication between all agencies involved, ensuring that key stakeholders and local opinion makers are regularly briefed.

The outbreak may be followed by legal proceedings if patients seek financial compensation for their illness and loss of earnings. The investigators report is therefore an important document that should describe the outbreak chronology, investigations and results, control measures applied, and lessons learned, including how the outbreak occurred and how to prevent a recurrence.

Infectious diseases are a continuing challenge to the public health, particularly in an era of increasing global travel. Adequate control of these diseases, both old and new, requires the active partnership of many branches of medicine and biosciences, in addition to veterinary science and public health. Epidemiological research is needed to improve our understanding of many of these diseases and to provide adequate methods of control.

TABLE 16.1 Food-specific attack rates among wedding guests

Food	Ate food		Attack rate %	Did not eat		Attack rate %	p value*
	Ill	Not ill		Ill	Not ill		
First Course							
Oysters	9	2	82	0	9	0	0.0003
Smoked salmon	9	3	75	0	8	0	0.001
Crab sticks	9	3	75	0	7	0	0.001
Prawns	9	4	69	0	6	0	0.005
Lettuce garnish	8	4	69	0	6	0	0.005
Melon	0	2	0	9	56	0.47	
Raspberries	1	4	25	8	6	71	0.30
Main Course							
Duck with orange sauce	9	10	47	1	0	100	0.47
Mashed potato with spring onion ('champ')	5	5	50	1	5	57	0.31
Vegetable lasagne	1	0	100	8	10	44	0.47
Mixed vegetables	-	-	-	0	1	0	1.00

*Fisher's exact test.

Source: Ang, L. H. (1998). 'An Outbreak of Viral Gastroenteritis Associated with Eating Raw Oysters'. *Communicable Diseases and Public Health*, **1**: 38–40.

Model answer

Q1 In the UK, screening for HIV infection is available ante-natally. At the booking clinic (the initial antenatal appoint-ment), this will be done with the informed consent of the mother. In HIV-positive cases early treatment in pregnancy reduces the likelihood of the virus being passed to the foetus. In HIV-positive cases breast-feeding is contraindicated.

Further Reading

Damani, N. N. (2002). *Manual of Infection Control Procedures* (2nd edn). London: Greenwich Medical.

Farmer, R. D. T., Miller, D., Lawrenson, R. (1996). *Lecture Notes on Epidemiology and Public Health* (4th edn). Oxford: Blackwell.

Giesecke, J. (2001). *Modern Infectious Disease Epidemiology* (2nd edn). Edinburgh: Arnold.

Heymann, D. (2002). 'Infectious Agents', in R. Detels, J. McEwen, R. Beaglehole and H. Tanaka (eds.). *Oxford Textbook of Public Health* (4th edn). Oxford: Oxford University Press.

Web Addresses

Centers for Disease Controls (USA), www.cdc.gov.

European Commission. Communicable diseases net-works, www.europa.eu.int/.

Health Protection Agency (UK), www.hpa.org.uk.

World Health Organization (global reports), www.who.int/.

References

References for this chapter can be found at www.oxfordtextbooks.co.uk/orc/yarnell. Where possi-ble, these are presented as *active links* which direct you to an electronic version of the work. If you are a sub-scriber to that work (either individually or through an institution), and depending on your level of access, you may be able to peruse an abstract or the full article if available. 🖳

Social and behavioural factors in disease

In this chapter we examine social and behavioural factors as
causes of disease and how they may affect the effectiveness
of interventions to improve health at the population or
individual level. We discuss the extent to which 'lifestyle'
factors contribute to the major chronic diseases, the epidemiology of accidents, poisonings and violence, and social
inequalities in health.

Introduction

As noted in Chapter 1, social factors have been
implicated in the causes of disease since the time of
Hippocrates. Social class was introduced as an index in
the UK by the Registrar General in the early part of the
twentieth century to represent 'social position' in society; it was based on occupation and reflects both level
of education and income. It was constructed at that
time to correspond with the level of infant mortality
according to the occupation of the 'head of the household'; *Social Class I* representing professionally educated
families and *Social Class V* those of unskilled labourers.
Chapter 14 provides several examples of the relation
between infant mortality and social class in the UK.
Other European countries and the USA use different
indicators such as occupational group (white/blue
collar), home and car ownership, and length and type of
education to represent the socioeconomic strata. Each
stratum of society tends to live in particular neighbour-
hoods, and individuals generally absorb the culture and
behaviour of their own social group (the social norms),
which, in turn, can influence the general health of the
group. Section 17.5 discusses the inequalities in health
that can result from the 'accident of birth', but we

begin the chapter with the influence of some specific personal behaviours that can be addictive in nature and may have a profound influence on personal and population health, and on life expectancy.

17.1 **Addictive Behaviours**

The use of many substances for their pleasurable, mood-enhancing effects is well established in Western societies, but the pattern of use and types of substances commonly taken varies between social and cultural groups. Some psychologists make the distinction between 'physical' and 'psychological' dependence, or reliance on gratification through regular use of a particular substance, but the relative addictiveness of a particular substance is also relevant for therapeutic and preventive interventions. Nicotine, widely available through tobacco products, is one of the most highly addictive substances known, and simple questionnaires have been developed to evaluate the level of dependence (West 2004). 🖥 Dependencies on nicotine, alcohol, and illicit drugs are major public health problems in Western societies, each addiction or behavioural pattern having its distinct epidemiology but with some degree of overlap between them.

> **Q1** What problems do researchers face when assessing the proportion of individuals showing dependence on particular types of behaviour? For example, dependence on tobacco, alcohol, and illicit drugs.

Tobacco

At least one-third of the global adult population, or 1.1 billion people aged 15 years and older, smoke cigarettes. About 300 million of these smokers are in developed countries where twice as many men as women use tobacco. In developing countries the difference is greater, and about 48 per cent of men and 7 per cent of women smoke. In the UK, Europe, and the USA, tobacco smoking became a common habit in men at the beginning of the twentieth century with the advent of manufactured cigarettes, and was actively encouraged in soldiers in World War I with the result that about 80 per cent of men smoked at that time. It was not until the time of World War II that cigarette smoking began to increase rapidly in women. In the UK in the 1950s and 1960s almost 60 per cent of men and 40 per cent of women smoked. The prevalence of smoking started to decline in the 1970s in men but this was

delayed until the 1980s for women. Since 1994 the prevalence of smoking in the UK has been constant at about 28 per cent in both sexes, but this is evaluated only from data on manufactured cigarettes, which excludes hand-rolled cigarettes (Edwards 2004). 🖥 Globally, however, the tobacco epidemic is still expanding, especially in developing countries where seven out of every ten tobacco-related deaths occur. Tobacco is currently responsible for the death of one adult in ten worldwide (four to five million deaths each year). If current trends continue, by 2025 10 million deaths will be caused by smoking each year. Half the people that smoke today, about 650 million people, will eventually be killed by tobacco if major control measures are not introduced (see Chapter 7).

Alcohol

This is probably the oldest and most widely used drug. It is used in many situations and for many purposes: as a stimulant, a tranquilizer, an anaesthetic, as a social lubricant, a religious symbol, a food, and a fuel. Although alcohol is highly toxic in large quantities, it is a drug that is socially acceptable in many societies when used in moderation. Alcohol is a feature of many people's lives: 90 per cent of adults in the UK drink alcohol, starting in their teens; there is a huge industry involved in its production and sale worth £30 billion at current prices, which generates £7 billion in excise duty. But the cost of social and medical problems associated with alcohol abuse has been estimated at £20 billion (Cabinet Office, Prime Minister's Strategy Unit 2004). 🖥

Four levels of alcohol use have been described in Western societies: social drinking; 'at risk' consumption; problem drinking; and dependence and addiction (Peele 1997). 🖥 'At risk' consumption has been estimated by the UK Department of Health to be three to four units per day for men and two to three units per day for women (based on average weekly consumption and interspersed with alcohol-free days) (see Table 17.1 for units). Good evidence for defining these thresholds comes from a large prospective study of British doctors in which all-cause mortality increased steadily at an average consumption above three units per day (Doll *et al.* 1994). 🖥 However, surveys in the UK suggest that 5.9 million people, mainly under 25 years of age, exceed these guidelines. Binge drinking is a particular problem in this age group. In addition, 2.9 million (7 per cent of the population) are either problem drinkers (with social, legal, or work-related problems) or have some level of dependence on alcohol. The number of alcoholics (addicts) is estimated to be 200 000 in the UK

TABLE 17.1 Alcohol consumption levels and relative risk of mortality from key alcohol-related conditions

	Percentage of total deaths (England and Wales 2001)	Alcohol consumption					
		None	1–10 g/day*+	10–20 g/day	20–30 g/day	30–40 g/day	40–50 g/day
IHD men	23%	1	0.83	0.78	0.77	0.78	0.79
IHD women	17%	1	0.86	0.85	0.90	0.96	1.05
Colon cancer	2% (both sexes)	1	1.07	1.22	1.38	1.58	1.79
Breast cancer	4%	1	1.04	1.12	1.21	1.31	1.41
Haemorrhagic stroke	1% (both sexes)	1	1.08	1.25	1.46	1.69	1.96

IHD, ischaemic heart disease.

*Midpoint in each category used to calculate relative risks.

+8 g absolute alcohol ≡ 1 unit alcohol = (1/2 pint of beer, 227 ml) (1 glass of wine, 90 ml) (One measure of spirits, 25 ml).

Source: Modified after Britton, A. and McPherson, K. (2001). 'Mortality in England and Wales Attributable to Current Alcohol Consumption'. *Journal of Epidemiology and Community Health*, **55**: 383 8, reproduced with permission from the BMJ Publishing Group.

(about 1 in 200 or 0.5 per cent of the adult population) (Ashworth and Gerade 1997). 🖥

Heavy alcohol consumption is associated with liver cirrhosis, pancreatitis, cancer, stroke, and premature death. The risk of death from major diseases associated with increasing levels of consumption of alcohol is summarized in Table 17.1.

Two points should be noted from the data shown in Table 17.1. Firstly, the data relate only to mortality and do not show morbidity associated with alcohol consumption. Secondly, they show the extent of the reduction in ischaemic heart disease mortality associated with moderate alcohol consumption reported in major prospective studies, which is more marked, and maintained at higher levels of consumption, in men.

Alcohol is responsible for 150 000 hospital admissions per annum in the UK and up to one-third of all accident and emergency attendances. Alcohol abuse is involved in 30–60 per cent of cases of child protection, significant numbers of incidents of domestic violence, and many fatal car crashes. Figure 17.1 summarizes the social and economic costs associated with alcohol abuse in the UK.

Illicit drugs

Accurate statistics on the use of illicit drugs are more difficult to obtain than for tobacco and alcohol, and are based on data sources such as crime surveys, accident statistics, and a range of lifestyle surveys. Increasingly, statistics are gathered from multiple sources using capture–recapture techniques (see Chapter 2). The total number of drug users includes recreational, regular, and problem users. In the UK, class A drugs are cocaine, crack, heroin, ecstasy, methadone, LSD, and 'magic mushrooms'. Class B drugs include substances such as strong stimulants (amphetamines), barbiturates, and non-injectable opiates including codeine. Cannabis was recently reclassified as a Class C drug whose group also includes benzodiazepines. Problem drug users are those whose drug use is not controlled, and such addiction frequently involves use of opiates and cocaine. Self-report surveys indicate that around one-third of those aged 16–59 years have tried at least one illicit drug in their lifetime. All sources confirm that the use of drugs is common among younger people, and that the average age of first drug use is dropping: one in 12 of UK 12-year-olds have tried drugs at least once, as have one in three of 14-year-olds and two in five of 16-year-olds. These sources also confirm that most people have never taken drugs (Aust *et al.* 2002). 🖥 Community psychiatrists have noted an excess of drug and alcohol problems among patients with schizophrenia, but it remains to be established whether drug use predisposes to the development of schizophrenia (see also Chapter 12).

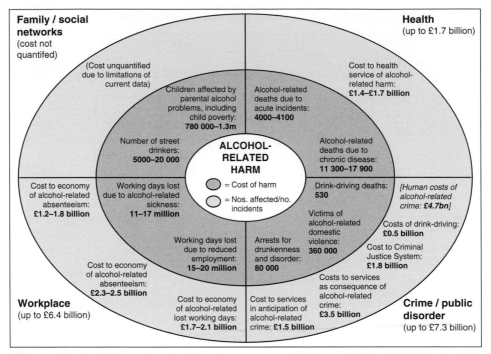

All figures are annualized. *Human costs are those incurred as a consequence of the human and emotional impact suffered by victims of crime (for example attending victim-support services); because of the lack of research in the field, equivalent costs have not been estimated for other alcohol-related harms. For this reason, human costs are not included in the crime/public disorder total figure.

Fig. 17.1 Aspects of alcohol-related harm and their costs.
Source: Cabinet Office, Prime Minister's Strategy Chair (2004). Alcohol Harm Reduction Strategy for England. London: Cabinet Office.

Drug experimentation, even a single episode of drug use, can result in harm to self or to others or serve as a *gateway* to additional use of alcohol and other drugs. **Social use of drugs** in social situations, or for social reasons, may reflect more consistent regular use in a particular setting. **Substance abuse** is a recognized disorder in ICD-10 and is classified according to both the substance and type of abuse, for example intoxication, dependence, etc. Abuse may, or may not, involve physical or psychological dependence or tolerance. Addiction, however, is a disorder in which a substance or substances have caused changes in a person's body, mind, and behaviour. This may be chronic and relapsing, and in due course, abstinence becomes more difficult. The degree of addiction experienced by an individual can probably be best assessed by the level of perceived and actual control exercised by that individual over his or her use of a drug, whether it be nicotine, alcohol, or illicit.

In a report from Canada (Single *et al.* 1999), ▢ substance abuse (tobacco, alcohol, and illicit drugs) was calculated to account for 21 per cent of all deaths, 23 per cent of the total years of potential life lost, and 8 per cent of hospital admissions. Tobacco and alcohol are responsible for most of this excess mortality and morbidity, which is also shown for all well-developed countries (Figure 17.2).

17.2 Health Education and Promotion

The complex interplay between historical, cultural, economic, medical, ethical, and legal factors in the social epidemiology of addictive behaviours perhaps best explains the failure of public health and other legislative measures to adequately control the social and personal harm caused by legal and illegal drugs. Education, imparting knowledge on the risks alone,

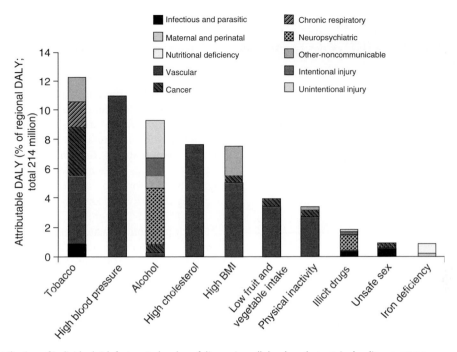

Fig. 17.2 Contribution of individual risk factors to burden of disease in well developed countries by disease category.
Source: Ezzati, M., Lopez, A. D., Rodgers, A., Vander Hoorn, S., and Murray, C. J. L. (2002). 'Comparative Risk Assessment Collaborative Group: Selected Major Risk Factors and Global and Regional Burden of Diseases'. *The Lancet*, **360**: 1347–60.

has largely failed for these disorders, perhaps insufficient in itself to stimulate a change of behaviour. Similar comments may also apply to the control of cultural factors and behaviours responsible for the rising epidemic of obesity (Chapter 8) and the worldwide spread of AIDS. The promotion of health implies taking more active steps to improve the population's health and is discussed below.

What is health? Can we measure it? What are the main causes of poor health?

Health has had, and continues to have, many definitions, from an early definition by the World Health Organization (WHO), 'an ideal state of complete physical, social and mental wellbeing', to the 'absence of illness'. More recent and broader definitions see health as 'a personal asset – the ability to adapt successfully to change, or as a resource to help us cope with challenges and processes of daily living' (Tones and Green 2004). 🖳

As discussed in Chapter 1, epidemiological tools are used to measure the health status of populations.

Indices such as mortality and morbidity are two of the usual measures used to compare the health of different populations. Composite indices such as **quality-adjusted life-years (QALYs)** and **disability-adjusted life-years (DALYs)** are discussed elsewhere (Chapters 12, 13, and 21), but both have limitations applied as objective indices (Dasbach and Teutsch 2003). 🖳

A primary purpose of epidemiology is to examine the causes of disease; but causes exist on different levels. Epidemiology has the tools to examine the question 'does smoking cause disease?' but is poorly equipped to answer such questions as 'why do people smoke or become alcoholics or drug addicts?'. Tools to fully examine these questions may one day be developed using qualitative methods described in Chapter 1, in the context of a sociological or anthropological framework.

Although clear answers to all these questions have not been obtained, distinct social and cultural patterns of disease can be seen in many societies. Theoreticians have proposed frameworks to assist the development of public-health policies. One report suggested that health was not simply a function of medical care;

> ### BOX 17.1 **THE OTTAWA CHARTER IMPROVING THE HEALTH OF THE POPULATION: PRIORITY AREAS FOR ACTION**
>
> 1 Building healthy public policy.
> 2 Creating supportive environments.
> 3 Strengthening community action.
> 4 Developing personal skills.
> 5 Reorienting health services towards health promotion and disease prevention.
>
> Source: World Health Organization (1986). *The Ottawa Charter for Health Promotion*. Ottawa: World Health Organization.

instead individuals could assume some responsibility for their own health through 'lifestyle' choices, but the importance of the social environment, personal competence, power and control, coping skills, social justice, housing, education, and civil society in promoting health is also recognized (Lalonde 1974). ▢ The acceptance of health as an outcome of many interacting factors led to proposals for action to develop and maintain good health. These proposals were formalized in the Ottawa Charter of 1986, which identified five priority areas for action (see Box 17.1).

The Charter recognized that there is a need to target behavioural change at the individual level as well as the need to affect social influences upon health, and to change organization and institutional structures. Changes in health behaviour occur in stages. In favourable environments, in the absence of adverse factors, individuals, families, small groups, and communities can be taught to assume responsibility for their health, which in turn changes their health behaviours and lifestyles. Change in health behaviour is usually a process, not an event. There is a range of theories to explain how health decisions are made and how people can be influenced to change their health attitudes, choices, and behaviours (see Tones and Green 2004). ▢

Early childhood has a profound impact on biological development through language development and learning capacity. Behaviours can be learnt through imitation and become, eventually, 'embedded' with lifelong effects on health. Epidemiological research suggests that children who have a healthy, stimulating start in life have fewer health and social problems later in life (Wadsworth 1997). ▢ Appropriate public health policies should invest in children (through early childhood education, nutrition) and in parents (through support for expectant mothers, parenting skills, including financial and emotional support) to bring health benefits for children and families.

Material conditions have a major effect on educational and social attainment, independent of disease. Gradients in health status are linked to gradients of socioeconomic status, and relative material wealth seems to have a substantial influence on an individual's overall health status. Government and social programmes such as economic development and wealth redistribution through taxation can be effective in reducing disparity and thereby improving health (see section 17.5 and Chapter 21).

Health promotion, which seeks to actively promote healthy behaviours, requires the cooperation of many sectors of society. Chapter 7 gave the example of tobacco control. More recently for alcohol, the evidence of medical and social harm has come under increasing scrutiny in the UK. Proposed actions and their consequences should be agreed by politicians with the participation of **stakeholders** in the public, voluntary, and private sectors. An example of two alternative strategies – high risk versus population based – to curb the rise in alcohol abuse are described below.

A 'high-risk' approach to alcohol harm reduction

The Alcohol Harm Reduction Strategy published by the Prime Minister's Strategy Unit (Cabinet Office, Prime Minister's Strategy Unit 2004) ▢ emphasizes the need to target problem drinking including binge drinking, long-term heavy drinking, under-age drinking, and drinking associated with crimes, for example violence and drink-driving. The report focuses on four areas:

- Education and communication. The report emphasizes individual responsibility for behaviour and concludes that controlling average consumption through the mechanism of raising the price and limiting access would have unwanted side effects and was not a viable option. Instead, the report recommended that the public should be better informed regarding the risks associated with alcohol, leading, hopefully, to more responsible drinking behaviour.

- Identification and treatment. Individuals with problems associated with alcohol should be identified earlier and have a ready access to appropriate treatment.

- Crime and disorder. Targeting of crime caused by excess alcohol with greater police powers was recommended.

◆ Alcohol industry. The industry, on a voluntary basis, should be encouraged to manufacture and market alcohol in a responsible fashion, for example not using young-looking actors or encouraging drunkenness.

A 'population-based' approach to alcohol harm reduction

In contrast, the report from a leading medical organization, the Academy of Medical Sciences, notes that public-health measures such as education and advertising have not been shown to have any discernible benefit, and that targeting problem drinkers alone will not be sufficient to address the national public health problem. The report suggested the following.

◆ Reducing consumption: (i) raising excise on alcohol to restore 1970s equivalent cost of alcohol; this should be particularly effective for under-age and chronic heavy drinkers; (ii) reducing the EU traveller's alcohol allowance to 10 litres of table wine or equivalent in beer or spirits (compared with 90 litres at present); and (iii) controlling advertising by the alcohol industry, especially that targeted to the young.

◆ Alcohol and driving. The acceptable blood alcohol level for driving should be reduced from 80 mg/dl to 50 mg/dl (and to 0 mg/dl for drivers under the age of 21 years).

◆ Public debate and Government response. There should be a debate started within society about public opinion towards alcohol and appropriate drinking levels. Government departments and researchers in the field of alcohol should develop a combined approach to alcohol harm.

In conclusion, it is clear that alcohol-related harm is a major and increasing problem in the UK. Eminent experts have reached two different conclusions on how to address this problem, based on the same evidence, suggesting that there is no single best solution and that possibly both strategies should be implemented concurrently.

17.3 Common Lifestyle Determinants of Major Chronic Diseases

In other chapters we have shown to what extent behavioural, 'lifestyle', factors contribute to specific major diseases. The **attributable fraction** of tobacco smoking for lung cancer is about 90 per cent in Western countries (Chapter 7); for cardiovascular disease this is around 30 per cent (Chapter 6). For type 2 diabetes mellitus in women the attributable fraction of obesity (body mass index at least 30 kg/m²) is estimated to be 61 per cent (Chapter 8). Thus the epidemiological evidence suggests that some of these diseases can be almost eliminated, and others cut substantially by the reduction of behaviours such as tobacco smoking or those leading to overweight and obesity. However, it seems clear that society and governments share a responsibility to develop policies of 'harm-minimization' because both tobacco and alcohol are legally available to adults. Table 17.2 shows some of the 'lifestyle' factors that have been investigated as potential determinants of chronic disease, along with the level of evidence and the extent of the preventive advice or policies adopted by major European and Western governments.

In a series of papers, and with the support of WHO, Ezzati *et al.* (2002) 🖥 have published several reports on the contribution of major risk factors (shown in Table 17.2) to the global burden of disease. In developed countries, they estimated that removal of these risks would increase healthy life expectancy by a minimum of 4.4 years (6 per cent). In the poorest region of the world (parts of sub-Saharan Africa), the mixture of risk factors also includes childhood and maternal undernutrition, and, in this region, it is estimated that removal of all risk factors would increase healthy life expectancy by over 16.1 years (43 per cent). The contributions to the global burden of disease shown in Table 17.2 should be used for comparative and illustrative purposes only, but they reflect global rather than regional levels of disease. In contrast, Figure 17.2 shows the contribution of each risk factor to the burden of disease in developed countries only, and illustrates the considerable scope for reduction of this burden. Tobacco and alcohol contribute to several different types of disease, whereas hypertension and high blood cholesterol contribute only to cardiovascular disease, although a major reduction in levels would have a significant impact on this burden.

17.4 Accidents, Poisonings, and Violence

An accident can be defined as 'an unusual event which proceeds from some unknown cause'. Accidents project an image of random events, 'acts of God', etc., but this is incorrect. Most accidents present characteristic patterns and are, therefore, predictable and potentially preventable. Particular patterns may be caused by

TABLE 17.2	Lifestyle factors and chronic disease: evidence and preventive measures		
Factor	**Evidence**	**Preventive measures**	**Contributions to global burden of disease***
Tobacco smoking	Strong evidence from observational studies that it is a major risk factor for respiratory cancers (Chapter 7), other cancers (Chapter 15), cardiovascular disease (Chapter 6) and osteoporosis (Chapter 13). Maternal smoking strongly associated with risk of miscarriage, prematurity, and SIDS (Chapter 14). Environmental tobacco smoke associated with excess risk of lung cancer in non-smokers (Chapter 7).	Health warnings on cigarette packets since 1970s, taxation used to limit demand. EU-led ban on tobacco advertising introduced in UK in 2003. Ban on smoking in many workplaces and public places.	4.1%
'Unhealthy' nutrition	Strong evidence from observational and some experimental studies on role of excess calories in overweight and obesity, salt and hypertension, saturated fats, and raised blood cholesterol (Chapters 6 and 8). Some evidence that fruit and vegetables protect against some cancers and cardiovascular disease (Chapter 15 and 16). Important area for future research	Nutritional recommendations made by the USA, UK and European agencies with updates. Involvement of food manufacturers and pharmaceutical industry.	Hypertension 4.4% High blood cholesterol 2.8% High BMI 2.3% Low fruit and vegetable intake 1.8%
Alcohol consumption above 'safe' limits	Evidence of J- or U-shaped relationship with mortality and cardiovascular disease, but major association with co-morbidity and social dysfunction and accidents; premature mortality at higher levels of consumption.	Limited availability to minors. General health promotion on 'safe limits' with limited effectiveness.	4.0%
Sedentary behaviour	Strong evidence on role of sedentary behaviour in overweight and obesity, type 2 diabetes, and cardiovascular disease (Chapters 6 and 8).	Report by US Surgeon General, UK Department of Health, etc., but only general health promotion and limited strategies so far.	1.3%
Psychological stress	Limited evidence from observational studies on job stress (control and working hours) (cardiovascular disease and hypertension). Improved epidemiological indicators are needed.	Health and safety and work legislation.	Not known

TABLE 17.2 Lifestyle factors and chronic disease: evidence and preventive measures *(continued)*			
Factor	Evidence	Preventive measures	Contributions to global burden of disease*
Illicit drug use	Class A drug use associated with premature mortality and co-morbidity.	Legal control of drugs. Drug addiction clinics. Health promotion directed at young people.	0.8%
Unsafe sex (HIV) Lack of contraception	High prevalence of HIV in developing countries. Strong association between abortion and maternal mortality in developing countries.	Extensive educational campaigns in western countries.	HIV 6.3% Lack of contraception 0.6%

*Estimates taken from: Ezzati, M., Lopez, A. D., Rodgers, A., Vander Hoorn, S. and Murray, C. J. L. (2002). 'Comparative Risk Assessment Collaborative Group: Selected Major Risk Factors and Global and Regional Burden of Disease'. *The Lancet*, **360**: 1347–60.

social, behavioural, or environmental factors, and identification of risk factors is a prerequisite for preventive measures. The phrase 'injury' is often preferred, as this relates to damage or hurt to the body produced by an external cause. This definition applies to both intentional and unintentional injuries. In ICD-10 '**accidents, poisonings and violence**' are classified according to their **external cause** in the interests of strategic planning of preventive policies. This classification also includes suicide and self-harm but, because of the mental health implications of these categories, they are discussed in Chapter 12.

Burden on public health

Quantifying the true burden of accidents and injuries is difficult as information is collated by different agencies for different purposes and using different definitions; for example, the police only count deaths within 30 days of an accident whereas the Registrars General for the UK regions include all deaths registered for the whole year. Many of the accidents leading to minor injury are not reported, and reporting systems based on only medical records invariably produce an underestimate. Box 17.2 gives examples of some agencies that hold data about accidents.

There were approximately 800 000 deaths due to injury throughout the WHO European Region in the year 2002, with twice as many male as female deaths (Figure 17.3). Half of all the deaths due to road traffic accidents (RTAs), fire, and self-harm, and two-thirds of the deaths due to violence occur between the ages of 15 and 44 years. Over half of the deaths due to falls are in people aged over 60 years and nearly one quarter are in the over 80s. The male excess is particularly noted for deaths due to violence and war but also for RTAs where, at younger ages, the male to female ratio is about 4:1. The male excess is attributed to greater exposure and more risk-taking behaviour.

BOX 17.2 SOME SOURCES OF DATA ON ACCIDENTS AND INJURY IN THE UK

Mortality data: generally very robust information source but delays in registration owing to legal proceedings and reluctance to declare suicide as cause of death may cause some difficulties.

- Hospital statistics (including A&E departments): presentation to health services is dependent on severity of injury and proximity to services.
- HASS and LASS (Home and Leisure Accident Surveillance Surveys): in the UK one of the few reliable sources of information on home and leisure accidents but dependent on data from A&E departments.
- Health and Safety Executive: gathers data on the more serious employment-related injuries and accidents. Dependence on compliance with guidelines.
- Police services: collate data on violence, RTAs, and causes such as speeding, alcohol, etc. However, many cases are not reported to police.
- Surveys such as the General Household Survey or Labour Force Survey.

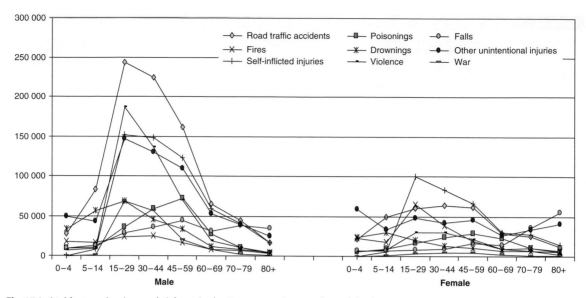

Fig. 17.3 Accidents, poisonings and violence in the European region: numbers of deaths per year.
Source: WHO European Health for All database (2002). *Health 21. The Health for All Policy Framework for the WHO European Region.* European Health for All Series No. 6. World Health Organization.

It is argued that counting deaths underestimates the burden on public health and importance of injuries because (i) it ignores concomitant disability and (ii) that, unlike chronic diseases and cancers, it is predominantly younger people who are affected. DALYs are often used as an alternative measurement tool. DALYs take account of the potential years of life lost (PYLL) and adjust the quality of the years lived for any persistent morbidity arising from the injury. Worldwide, injuries account for 11.6 per cent of male deaths but 19.6 per cent of all male DALYs. If the current trends continue it is estimated that RTAs, self-inflicted injuries, interpersonal violence, and war-related injuries will be among the highest-ranking causes of death and burden of disease in the world by 2020. Without appropriate action RTAs, which were ranked ninth in 1990, will become the third leading contributor to the burden of disease by 2020, with over two-thirds of the deaths, and 90 per cent of the DALYs, arising in low- and middle-income countries. In the UK the financial cost of RTAs amounts to approximately 0.5 per cent of the GNP and that of home accident injuries to £25 000 million annually.

Causes of injury

Haddon, the first director of the National Traffic Safety Bureau in the USA, proposed that standard public-health approaches could be applied to RTAs; they could be thought of as the action of various **host** (human), **vector** (vehicle), and **environmental** (road network) factors operating before, during, and after the accident. This approach has been successfully extended to other types of accident. For RTAs (Box 17.3) the three phases are: (i) pre-crash – crash prevention; (ii) crash – injury limitation and (iii) post-crash – health improvement.

Role of alcohol in injuries

Alcohol, because it impairs attention, coordination, and judgement, significantly increases both the *risk* of injury and the relative *severity* of the injury. Heavy drinkers are up to four times as likely to report an accident in the previous year compared with non-drinkers and a large proportion of all accidents, both road traffic and domestic, which arrive in accident and emergency (A&E) departments, involve alcohol. Alcohol is also an important antecedent for suicides and attempted suicides, deaths due to violence, fires, falls, and accidental drowning. The strength of the relationship seems stronger for males and in northern European countries and Russia where drinking patterns are characterized by episodes of heavy drinking (Skog 2001). 💻

BOX 17.3 THE HADDON MATRIX APPLIED TO ROAD TRAFFIC ACCIDENTS

	Host factors (human)	Vector factors (vehicle)	Environmental factors (road network)
Pre-crash	Education Attitudes Alcohol, drugs, fatigue Enforcement of traffic laws Reflective clothing for cyclists and pedestrians	Road worthiness Daytime lights on motorcycles Speed limitation systems	Road design including separation of car, pedestrians and cyclists Provision of transport alternatives Speed limitation Better road marking, lighting
Crash	Alcohol Use of seat belts	Car design Seat belts, air bags Child restraints Use of helmets	Crash barriers Centre isle barriers
Post-crash	First aid and resuscitation Access to medical and rehabilitation services	Fire risk	CCTV at danger points Access for rescue services

Source: Centers for Disease Control and Prevention (1999). 'Motor Vehicle Safety: A 20th Century Public Health Achievement'. *Morbidity and Mortality Weekly Report*, **48**: 369–74.

Prevention

Many injuries, such as RTAs and falls in the elderly, should be considered alongside heart disease, cancer, and stroke as public-health problems that respond well to preventive interventions. In the USA the reduction in the rate of deaths attributable to motor vehicle crashes has been hailed as one of the top public-health interventions of the twentieth century (Centers for Disease Control 1999). More recently, systematic reviews have suggested that it is possible to reduce by one-third the number of falls among older people (Gillespie 2004).

Haddon's matrix (Box 17.3) gives a good indication of opportunities for primary, secondary, and tertiary prevention. Others have emphasized the three underlying principles of education, engineering, and enforcement.

Education about the potential dangers around the home is now part of the national UK curriculum for schoolchildren; and new drivers are examined about road safety before they are allowed onto the road. Health promotional campaigns encourage the use of seat belts and avoidance of alcohol and drugs when driving. Induction periods make new employees aware of safe working practices.

One of the best ways to reduce the number of accidents is to 'engineer' the solutions. This is more likely to succeed because it requires no active intervention or thought on the part of the individual. Examples include better house design, use of safety glass and the fitting of smoke alarms (though many still need the battery to be periodically checked), child-proof medicine containers, safer play environments and cycle lanes.

It is also important that legislation to reduce accidents is enforced. This will ensure better compliance with speed limits and drink-driving laws. The higher levels of homicide and suicide in the USA than in the UK are primarily due to the availability of guns, and legislation to restrict access to firearms may lead to a reduced rate of suicides even if the underlying rate of attempted suicides is stable. Within the UK, restricting the sale of alcohol in teenagers under 18-years-old should reduce alcohol-related accidents in this age group.

Evaluation and monitoring are important, though often neglected, aspects of injury prevention. Evaluation will identify which aspects of the intervention worked and which groups or sub-populations were most affected, and this may influence the implementation of prevention strategies or indicate the likely success in other situations. Ongoing monitoring or surveillance complements and informs the evaluative process as well as detecting emergent threats to public health.

17.5 **Inequalities in Health**

Introduction

Even though most of this section relates to socioeconomic differences, a more complete discussion of inequalities in health extends beyond this, and would include variations by age, sex, and ethnicity, in rural and urban dwellers, and also in socially excluded people such as immigrants, homeless people, and travellers.

Records show that inequalities in health have been evident in populations throughout Europe since at least the eighteenth century, when absolute death rates were at much higher levels. Today, inequalities in health are an almost universal feature of most western countries including more egalitarian societies like those in Scandinavia. All strata in society are affected and no threshold is evident; at all levels, those higher in the hierarchy enjoy better health than those below (Marmot 2004). 🖥

Importance in terms of health

In the UK men in social class IV/V have a life expectancy at birth that is five years less than their peers in social class I/II; the difference for women is about three years. Men and women living in the most deprived inner city areas in the UK (such as those of Glasgow and Manchester) have life expectancies that are respectively 10.6 and 7.2 years lower than those in the more affluent and more rural areas (such as Dorset and Somerset). There exists throughout the UK a north/south, east/west gradient (Figure 17.4) in mortality that is almost entirely explained by differing levels of material deprivation, which is a proxy for income (Figure 17.5).

Socioeconomic differences in health are seen at all ages but are most pronounced for younger and middle-aged adults, and are more evident for men than for women. Mortality rates are higher in the lower social classes for most causes of death, with the current exception of breast cancer. Socioeconomic gradients are most evident for accidents, lung and stomach cancer, chronic respiratory disease, ischaemic heart disease (IHD), and strokes.

Steeper gradients are more usual for morbidity than for mortality, especially for self-reported ill health, so that differences in disability-free life expectancy are about twice those of life expectancy. Thus, the more affluent members of society not only tend to live longer, but also enjoy a better quality of life.

Dental health exhibits some of the most marked socioeconomic gradients. Children in lower social class households are much more likely to have decayed,

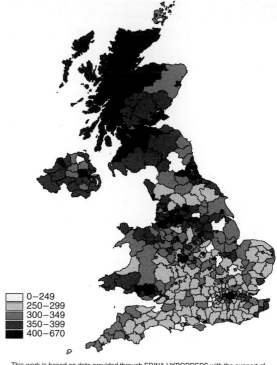

☐	0–249
▨	250–299
▩	300–349
▦	350–399
■	400–670

This work is based on data provided through EDINA UKBORDERS with the support of the ESRC and JISC and uses boundary material which is copyright of the Crown and the Post Office. Data relating to the base populations and mortality have been supplied by ONS (England and Wales), GRO (Scotland) and NISRA (Northern Ireland).

Fig. 17.4 Standardized mortality rates (0–74 years) by local authority (based on deaths between 2000 and 2002).

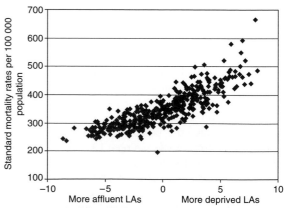

*Deprivation based on a combination of people in each LA who were renting, unemployed, of low social class, or who did not have access to a car.

Fig. 17.5 Association between deprivation* and mortality rates (0–74 years) by local authority in the UK source.
Source: As in Figure 17.4.

filled or missing teeth, and by middle age there is a fifteen-fold differential in the proportion of professional and unskilled groups with no natural teeth. Of those with teeth, professional groups are almost twice as likely to undergo regular dental attendance.

Causes of inequalities in health

It is perhaps rather surprising that despite all the research into inequalities in health, the pathways whereby socioeconomic standing affects health are not clearly understood, and a variety of mechanisms have been proposed. Health selection, which posits that health status determines socioeconomic status, rather than vice versa, has been shown to play only a minor role in shaping the socioeconomic gradients in health.

The type of disease exhibiting marked socioeconomic gradients suggests that health-related behaviours, such as smoking, may be important aetiologically; health surveys that are periodically undertaken in many countries invariably demonstrate the social patterns of many lifestyle and health-related behaviours. In most Northern and Western European countries, the proportions of the population smoking have been falling over the past 20 years; but this decline has been most evident among the more affluent groups, so that there is now a two- to three-fold difference in the prevalence of cigarette smoking between professional and unskilled groups for both men and women. In southern Europe, the prevalence may be higher among the more affluent groups owing to the later arrival of the smoking epidemic.

Data from the UK indicate that lower income households tend to have higher consumption of fats and sugars in the diet and lower intake of fresh fruit and vegetables, though there is no clear relation between socioeconomic status and fat intake. Those in the lower socioeconomic groups are more likely to be overweight or obese, particularly women, who are also less likely to participate in leisure-time physical activity. Whether this is balanced by increased activity during working hours is not known. The clustering of adverse lifestyle factors in the lower income groups, coupled with their known synergism, will lead to an amplified risk for these populations.

That the variation in classical risk factors such as cholesterol, cigarette smoking, and raised blood pressure explains less than half of the socioeconomic gradient in heart disease has prompted the search for other factors, including those related to psycho-social wellbeing. It has been shown that people in lower social groups are exposed to a greater variety and intensity of chronic stresses in their lives, with lower levels of social support to help buffer and offset these challenges. These stressors include jobs with high demand and low levels of control that have been shown to explain some of the social gradient in health (Marmot et al. 1997). 🖳

The lifecourse theory of health inequalities suggests that the social gradients in chronic disease evident in middle and later life are the product of accumulated effects of socioeconomic status throughout the lifecycle (Kuh and Ben Shlomo 2004). 🖳 With this approach it is easy to see how inter-generational patterns of health inequalities could arise, and that youth pathways may be particularly important. It also demonstrates the interrelationship between materialist/structural explanations (that is, less favourable material circumstances) and behavioural explanations (such as higher prevalence of health-damaging behaviours).

Figure 17.6 shows the hypothetical timeline of a child as (s)he progress to old age, and illustrates some of the many socioeconomic effects on health. Maternal smoking and diet are socially patterned and will influence the birthweight of the child and, together with breast feeding, subsequent growth and development in the first year of life. In turn, this pattern, according to the Barker hypothesis (Lucas et al. 1999), 🖳 influences the propensity towards diseases such as diabetes, obesity, raised blood pressure, and heart disease. The socioeconomic status of parents will directly influence the type and quality of the family's housing as well as the wider physical and social environment in which a child grows up. The educational attainment of every child is strongly associated with the parental socioeconomic status and this, in turn, will directly influence employment and career opportunities in later life. The health behaviours of the adolescent, such as smoking, drinking, and exercise, which are the antecedents of chronic disease, will, to a large extent, be shaped by their social and home environments. The type of job will determine income levels, but may also bring its own occupationally-related health risks and work-related stresses. Poor health in middle years may mean early retirement, limit earning potential, and act as a harbinger of a sharper decline at older ages. The living standards of retired people are related to the size of the pension, which is dependent on employment history, and will have a significant bearing on health status in later years.

A few years ago a new hypothesis emerged which proposed that the *relative distribution* of income within a country was also important for the health of

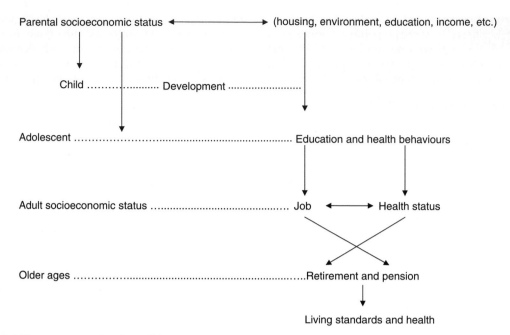

Fig. 17.6 A life course approach to inequalities.

the whole population, and not just those on the lowest incomes (that is, that countries with a greater range of income inequality fared worse than those where wealth was more evenly distributed). However, more recent studies have not supported this hypothesis, but have re-emphasized the powerful impact of individual income on health.

Policies to reduce inequalities in health

Reducing inequalities in health is now a priority for most European countries, and the WHO Health 21 Strategy (Target 2) states that by the year 2020, the gap between socioeconomic groups within European countries should be reduced by at least 25 per cent (WHO 1999). 🖳 This is a rather ambitious target given:

- the current trend in most countries is of increasing inequalities in health;

- the lack of a credible evidence-base to guide policy (Mackenbach and Bakker 2003); 🖳

- the multifaceted nature of the interventions needed to effect a change (for example fiscal policy, education, housing, transport, etc.);

- that many of these policy areas are outside the usual sphere of influence of those working in the health sector;

- the usually significant lag-time between intervention and measurable outcomes especially for 'upstream' interventions;

- that, in practice, it is difficult to target interventions: policies concentrating mainly on deprived areas tend to miss most people in need, who live outside these areas.

There is an ongoing debate around the extent to which health inequalities arise as a consequence of the life choices made by individuals, or as a result of the way in which society is organized and operates. Society's stance on this debate is likely to shape the direction of the policy initiatives. With this in mind, the reader may wish to compare two sets of top ten tips on how to obtain better health (Box 17.4). The first was suggested by the Chief Medical Officer for England (Professor Donaldson) and puts the emphasis squarely on the individual (Secretary of State 2002). 🖳 It assumes that each person is in control of the most important factors that determine their health. The second was proposed by Dr Gordon, from the Townsend Centre for International Poverty Research at the University of Bristol (quoted in Ness *et al.* 2002), 🖳 which takes a more sociological perspective, and assumes that the most important determinants of health are generally outside the control of individuals. Mackenbach and Bakker (2003) 🖳 have

BOX 17.4 OFFICIAL AND ALTERNATIVE TOP 10 TIPS FOR BETTER HEALTH

The official tips are:

1 Don't smoke if you can stop. If you can't, cut down.
2 Follow a balanced diet with plenty of fruit and vegetables.
3 Keep physically active.
4 Manage stress by, for example, talking things through and making time to relax.
5 If you drink alcohol, do so in moderation.
6 Cover up in the sun, and protect children from sunburn.
7 Practice safer sex.
8. Take up cancer screening opportunities.
9 Be safe on the roads: follow the Highway Code.
10 Learn the first aid ABC: airways, breathing, circulation.

(Professor Donaldson)

The alternative tips are:

1 Don't be poor. If you are poor, try not to be poor for long.
2 Don't have poor parents.
3 Don't live in a deprived area. If you do, move.
4 Own a car.
5 Don't work in a stressful, low-paid manual job.
6 Practise not losing your job and don't become unemployed.
7 Don't live in low quality housing or be home-less.
8 Be able to afford to pay for social activities and annual holidays.
9 Learn how to fill in the complex housing bene-fit/asylum application forms before you become homeless or destitute.
10 Use education as an opportunity to improve your socioeconomic position.

(Dr Gordon)

Sources: Chief Medical Officer (2004) and Townsend Centre for International Poverty Research, University of Bristol.
Chief Medical Officer (2004). Chief Medical Officer's top ten tips for better health, http://www.dh.gov.uk/Publications AndStatistics/PressReleases/PressReleasesNotices/fs/en? CONTENT_ID=4099742&chk=DI6Lfo

summarized policies in the UK, The Netherlands, and Sweden aimed at reducing inequalities in health.

Role of the health services

Though health services may have only a minor role to play in reducing inequalities in health they do have the advantage that they fall within the remit of health policy makers. Horizontal equity (that is, equality of access to health care for individuals in equal need) is one of the central tenets of the health services in most countries (see Chapter 21). However, the balance of research evidence suggests that this ideal still has some way to go before being achieved in practice. Most secondary level or specialist-led services throughout Europe are thought to favour the rich. Compared with their level of need, patients in lower socioeconomic classes are less likely to receive outpatient or inpatient treatment. On the other hand, the utilization of primary care services, in terms of the number of contacts, is now closely related to need. This does not necessarily constitute equity, as patients from more deprived areas tend to receive shorter consultations, are given less information during these consultations, are less likely to get a prescription or be referred for specialist care, and, overall, are less satisfied with their consultation. In the UK patients from deprived backgrounds are less likely to have access to good quality services, have a lower uptake of national vaccination and screening

Model answer

Q1 In adults, consumption of tobacco, alcohol, and illicit drugs are all likely to be significantly underestimated. However, in the case of tobacco validation studies, using bio-markers of nicotine suggests that consumption is not substantially underestimated by questionnaire data in population studies. However, in clinical studies, medical disapproval may be a factor in producing a more substantial underestimate or even denial of consumption. Similar comments can be made about alcohol consumption which has the additional problem of binge drinking, which can be difficult to define, and which may fall short of alcohol addiction or dependence. In the case of illicit drugs, clearly confidentiality is an issue, as fear of prosecution may produce a significant underestimate of usage.

In the case of children, questionnaires need to be designed particularly carefully as there may be a tendency towards overestimation, because it is not unknown for adolescents to claim behaviour that they believe to be fashionable but in which they have not actually participated.

programmes, and have significantly lower chances of surviving the most common types of cancer.

In conclusion, this chapter has demonstrated the profound influence of social and behavioural factors on individual and public health. Measures to improve health require a difficult balance between individual choice on the one hand, and social and governmental strategies promoting healthy lifestyles on the other. Equity in access to health-care services would seem to be an appropriate goal for all national health services. Further research is required to improve ways of reducing current health inequalities.

Further Reading

Academy of Medical Sciences (2004). *Calling Time: The Nation's Drinking as a Major Health Issue*. London: Academy of Medical Sciences.

Dasbach, E. J. and Teutsch, S. M. (2003). 'Quality of Life', in A. C. Haddix and S. M. Teusch (eds.), *Prevention Effectiveness. A Guide to Decision Analysis and Economic Evaluation* (2nd edn). New York, NY: Oxford University Press.

Kuh, D. and Ben Shlomo, Y. (eds.) (2004). *A Lifecourse Approach to Chronic Disease Epidemiology* (2nd edn). Oxford: Oxford University Press.

Marmot, M. (2004). *Status Syndrome*. London: Bloomsbury.

Tones, K. and Green, J. (2004). *Health Promotion. Planning and Strategies*. London: Sage.

Web Addresses

Centers for Disease Control, www.cdc.gov/.

Chief Medical Officer (2004). Chief Medical Officer's top ten tips for better health, http://www.dh.gov.uk/PublicationsAndStatistics/PressReleases/PressReleasesNotices/fs/en?CONTENT_ID=4099742&chk=DI6Lfo.

World Health Organization, www.who.int.

World Health Organization European Region, Injuries and violence in Europe. Why they matter and what can be done, www.euro.who.int/document/E87321.pdf.

References

References for this chapter can be found at www.oxfordtextbooks.co.uk/orc/yarnell. Where possible, these are presented as *active links* which direct you to an electronic version of the work. If you are a subscriber to that work (either individually or through an institution), and depending on your level of access, you may be able to peruse an abstract or the full article if available. ⌨

Genetic epidemiology

This chapter briefly introduces the molecular basis of genetic disease, and highlights differences between monogenic, polygenic, and multi-factorial diseases. A background understanding of basic genetics is assumed. Study designs used in genetic epidemiology will be discussed with methods for identifying candidate genes involved in specific diseases or biological pathways. Finally, pharmacogenetics and the complex ethical issues concerning genetic testing and screening will be briefly reviewed.

Introduction

Genetic epidemiology focuses upon the role of inherited factors in disease aetiology, with the aims of establishing: (i) whether a disease has a genetic contribution; (ii) the relative size of the genetic effect in relation to environmental effects; (iii) those genes which contribute to disease susceptibility; (iv) if the findings can be used to develop better tools for disease prediction, prevention, and treatment. It has been defined as 'the study of the joint actions of genes and environmental factors in causing disease in human populations and their patterns of inheritance in families' (Morton 1982). 🖳 It may further involve pinpointing the exact molecular pathways implicated in a disorder. It has been stated that 'except for some cases of trauma, it is fair to say that virtually every human illness has a hereditary component' (Collins 1999). 🖳 Thus it is clear that the scope of genetic epidemiological methods is extremely wide. Unlike traditional epidemiological analyses, genetic epidemiological methods often make use of available biological information. Much success in genetic epidemiology has been in studying **monogenic disorders**, which obey the laws of **Mendelian inheritance**, but currently there is an increasing focus on unravelling the interacting genetic and environmental aetiology of complex diseases such as diabetes mellitus, cardiovascular disease, and cancer. Some basic terms used in this chapter are summarized in Box 18.1.

18.1 Genetic Information: Understanding the Language

Understanding the role of genetics in disease causation requires an understanding of the principles of

---

BOX 18.1 GLOSSARY OF BASIC TERMS

allele Alternative forms of a gene, occupying the same position or locus on a chromosome. One allele is inherited from the father and the other from the mother.

bases Chemical building blocks of DNA: A (adenine), T (thymine), C (cytosine), G (guanine).

base-pairs The two strands of DNA in the double helix. Permitted pairings are AT and GC.

causal mutation A mutation which causes a disease or abnormality.

chromosome aberrations Typically a duplication of chromosomes or segments of chromosomes but can refer to any abnormality in chromosomal structure.

co-dominant Alleles that are both expressed in the heterozygote (for example ABO blood groups).

codon The sequence of nucleotides in DNA or RNA, which determines what specific amino acid will be inserted into a polypeptide chain.

concordance The degree of similarity between individuals for a particular trait.

crossing over Refers to the crossing over of genetic material from one chromosome to another during meiosis and gamete production.

dizygotic Twins arising from separate gametes.

dominant The allele which is expressed in the heterozygote genotype. By contrast the recessive allele is not expressed.

encoding In genetics used in the context of the structure of the genetic code which determines gene products.

epistasis The alteration of expression of a gene by the effect of an unrelated gene.

exon The protein-coding DNA sequence of a gene.

familial trait A characteristic or trait that occurs within families more often than expected by chance and which is suspected to be genetic in nature.

flanking region The DNA sequence extending on either side of a specific gene.

gene mapping Determining the position of genes or a particular gene along a chromosome. Several methods can be used to map genes.

gene–environment interaction Usually used in the sense of the postulated effects of genes which may differ in different environments.

gene–gene interactions Usually used in a sense of postulated effects of genes being modified by other genes.

genetic marker Any polymorphic variation at a locus which can be used to examine a chromosomal segment in a pedigree or population.

genotype A description of the chromosomal material and base pairs for a particular individual.

haplotype A particular group of alleles from two or more linked loci usually inherited as a unit, for example HLA complex. It may provide a more appropriate unit for investigating disease associations rather than single genes.

heritability The proportion of a disease or trait which can be attributed to genetic causes by regression/correlation analysis among twins or other close family members.

imprinting The phenomenon of differential expression of genes according to whether they are inherited from the father or mother.

introns A segment of chromosome without currently obvious genetic products or function.

knock-out model An animal model in which a particular gene is inactivated within an otherwise intact nucleus.

linkage The association of genes on the same chromosome.

linkage analysis A statistical analysis which is used to estimate distances between genes along particular chromosomes following recombination.

linkage disequilibrium The observed frequencies of haplotypes in a population are not in agreement with haplotype frequencies predicted from the frequency of individual genetic markers in each haplotype.

BOX 18.1 *(continued)*

locus The position of a genetic marker on a chromosome.

monogenic disorder A disorder or trait caused by a single gene.

monozygotic A member of a twin pair or multiple birth group derived from the same fertilized ovum.

multifactorial When used in genetics, this usually refers to a trait or disorder which is caused by a combination of genetic and environmental factors.

mutation A permanent and heritable change in DNA sequence.

nucleotide A combination of a purine or pyramidine base with a sugar and phosphate forming the backbone of the DNA molecule.

oligogenic A trait that is determined by a small number of genes acting together.

pedigree A family tree which assists the detection of inherited traits and the mode of inheritance.

phenotype The observable biological characteristic or trait exhibited by an individual: the expression of the genotype for that individual.

pleiotropic Multiple and diverse characteristics resulting from a particular gene.

polygenic Several genes believed to be acting together to produce a particular disease or trait.

polymerase chain reaction (PCR) A technique for the rapid amplification or replication of a sequence of DNA.

polymorphism A term often used loosely to indicate genetic variation but strictly the occurrence of two or more allelic variants at a frequency of greater than 1 per cent in a population. SNPs are a specific class of polymorphism studied by molecular geneticists.

population stratification and admixture The existence of genetically different groups in a population.

quantitative trait loci (QTL) The location of a marker that affects a phenotype measured on a quantitative (linear) scale.

recessive An allele which is expressed only in homozygote and not in heterozygote.

recombination The formation of new combinations of alleles by breakage and rejoining of lengths of chromosomes during meiosis.

segregation analysis The general statistical methodology for determining the pattern of inheritance.

single nucleotide polymorphism (SNP) A class of polymorphism showing polymorphic variation at a single nucleotide: used in large-scale automated genetic analyses.

spliced out Separation of exon and intron.

transcription The formation of a strand of RNA from a DNA template.

transgenic (organism) A hybrid organism which incorporates new DNA applied externally into the germ cell line of the hybrid.

translation The process of producing protein from messenger RNA.

twin/adoption study Study based on monozygotic and dizygotic twins which aims to distinguish genetic and environmental causes of disease. Studies of adopted twins raised in different environments represent an extension of this approach.

VNTR Polymorphism (variable number of tandem repeats). Short DNA sequences that are tandemly repeated a variable number of times at many defined regions throughout the genome. This has been used for DNA fingerprinting.

X-linked A gene located on the X but not on the Y chromosome.

Mendelian inheritance. Genetic information is **encoded** by double-stranded deoxyribose nucleic acid (DNA) which is made up of a sugar, a phosphate and a base. The particular sequence in which the bases – adenine (A), guanine (G), cytosine (C), thymine (T) – align, determines the specific genetic information for an individual. **Base-pairs** are the bases paired across the two separate strands of the DNA molecule, and are often quoted as follows in molecular genetics (AT, GC). The fact that A can only pair with T, and G can only pair with C, means that DNA replication can result in perfect copies of a parent molecule because the sequences of the pre-existing strands dictate the sequences of the new strands. During cell division the entire DNA of the cell is copied: DNA strands separate, complementary strands are generated, and two exact duplicate DNA sequences are produced. During **transcription**, DNA is copied into single-stranded ribonucleic acid (RNA), which is similar to DNA, but T is replaced by U (uracil), after which three-base units, together with the sugar and phosphate component (**codons**) are **translated** into proteins (see Figure 18.2).

A gene is that part of DNA, usually encoding for a protein, which represents a fundamental unit of heredity.

Around 50 per cent of the genome is made up of repetitive and non-coding sequences. At present, the number of genes coded by the human genome is estimated to be less than 30 000 (Lander *et al.* 2001). 🖥 **Exons** are the parts of a gene translated into protein whereas **introns** are the parts that are removed (**spliced out**) during the process of 'translation' of messenger RNA (mRNA) to protein. **Mutation** denotes the general process of alteration of the DNA sequence of an organism. Mutations may be large-scale involving whole chromosomes or large segments of chromosomes, or of smaller scale involving smaller regions of single chromosomes. Smaller mutations can arise by base substitution, deletion, or insertion (of nucleotides) into a DNA sequence. Mutations that occur in exons and lead to a change in order of amino acids in a protein may be pathogenic owing to loss or gain in protein function. Although introns do not encode for proteins, mutations can affect intron splicing, subsequently changing the protein's structure

or synthesis. Simple mutations, defined as involving only a single DNA sequence, are due to errors in the replication and repair of DNA, and are frequent during man's lifetime. Figure 18.1(a), (b) shows the essential elements of genetic structure as the DNA double helix and a 'mapped' chromosome respectively. Figure 18.2 depicts the synthesis of insulin from a gene activated in the cellular tissue of the islets of Langerhans.

In mRNA a sequence of three **nucleotides** (the basic building blocks of DNA shown in Figure 18.1(a)) specifies the coding unit for a particular amino acid, and is termed a **codon**. Several triplet codons can code for the same amino acid and the genetic code is said to be **degenerate**. Mutations arising from this process can be silent, apparently unexpressed, and may be dispersed throughout the population. Thus, at one particular **locus** in the human genome, several forms or variants may exist. These are called **polymorphisms**. Mutation is also used in a restricted sense in population

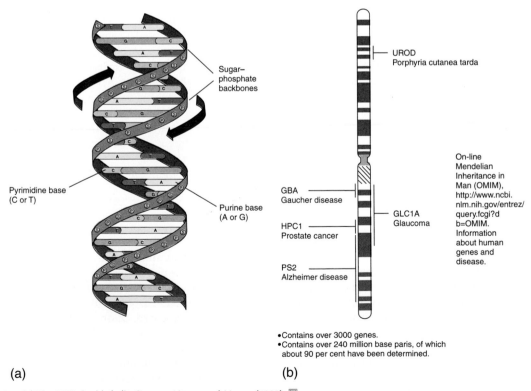

(a)   (b)

Fig. 18.1 (a) The DNA double helix. Source : Mange and Mange (1999). 🖥
(b) Chromosome 1. Source : OMIM (2005). 🖥

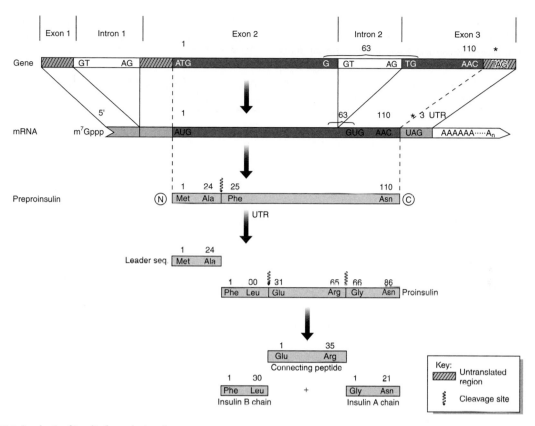

Fig. 18.2 Synthesis of insulin from the insulin gene.
Source: Strachan, T. and Read, A. P. *Human Molecular Genetics 3* (3rd edn). London: Garland Science.

genetics to indicate variants with a low frequency (less than 1 per cent), which may be highly pathogenic, whereas a 'common' polymorphism is arbitrarily defined as having a frequency of greater than 1 per cent in the general population. Common polymorphisms may be associated with only a modest increase in disease risk, or even be functionally unrelated to any disease. However, if they are common, disease-causing polymorphisms can have a significant population impact on disease burden, with a large **population attributable risk**. The human genome is extensively affected by sequence variation and it has been recently estimated that about 10 million polymorphisms exist in the human genome (Goldstein and Cavalleri 2005). ⌨ Certain regions of DNA are highly polymorphic because of the presence of **variable number tandem repeats**

(VNTRs), short DNA sequences that are repeated successively many times. The pattern of polymorphism in VNTRs is sufficiently distinctive to allow DNA fingerprinting. **Single nucleotide polymorphisms (SNPs)**, which arise as a result of change in only a single nucleotide, can occur as frequently as one in every 200 base pairs in the human genome. SNPs may be detected by microarrays or mass spectrometry and are widely used in studies of genetic susceptibility to diseases. Some SNPs can cause disease, for example by altering the regulation of transcription of a critical protein, but most do not. However, non-functional SNPs can still provide useful markers to fine-map disease-susceptibility genes (see below).

An **allele** is one of two or more alternative forms of a DNA sequence; for example, most persons have two functional (normal) alleles of the phenylalanine hydroxylase gene (one on each chromosome), whereas carriers of phenylketonuria have one functional allele and one mutant allele; patients with the disease have two mutant alleles. The **genotype** is the composition of alleles present in an individual at a given locus, while **phenotype** refers to a characteristic that is influenced by a specific genotype comprising one or more genes. This can be a trait such as eye colour, a physiological variable such as serum cholesterol or blood pressure, or a disease. Single-gene defects are rare, occurring in fewer than one in 200 births, and are typically associated with Mendelian inheritance. Some diseases formerly thought to follow Mendelian patterns are much more complicated, including diabetes, asthma, and fragile X syndrome (Chakravarti and Little 2003). 🖥 Incomplete penetrance of a single gene (variation in the extent of its expression in the phenotype) can complicate the interpretation of the pattern of inheritance; Mendelian disorders that are not completely penetrant may appear to be non-Mendelian when examined in a pedigree. Complex genetic diseases are caused by more than a single genetic variant and are characterized by interaction between the environment and the genome. The complexity of possible combinations of inherited and environmental factors is illustrated in Figure 18.3.

Mendelian and non-Mendelian disorders are discussed in the following two sections.

18.2 **Mendelian (Monogenic) Disorders**

The simplest genetic disorders are those that depend on the genotype at a single locus, which may be **necessary** and **sufficient** for the character or trait to be expressed. Such characters, traits, and diseases follow the patterns of inheritance first described for plants by Mendel. These diseases are usually rare, conferring a small population-attributable risk. The essential source of reference for these is the Online Mendelian Inheritance in Man (OMIM) database (see web addresses). Such diseases may have different **pedigree** patterns of inheritance. If the mutant allele results in the same phenotype irrespective of the second allele, the mutant allele is said to be **dominant** (for example Huntington's disease). If the mutant allele is required in both chromosomes (homozygosity) to yield the phenotype, then it is termed **recessive** (e.g cystic fibrosis). If the phenotype for the heterozygous genotype is intermediate, displaying characteristics of each allele, then the alleles are **co-dominant**

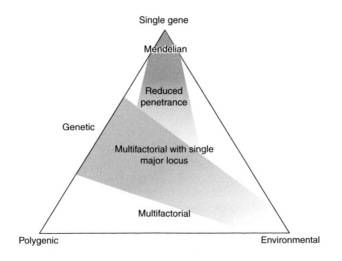

Traits or conditions associated with diseases are rarely due to single genes: reduced penetrance (the degree to which the gene is expressed in the phenotype) and interaction with environmental factors will disrupt typical Mendelian inheritance. In contrast many conditions (for example asthma, diabetes, ischaemic heart disease) probably lie towards the base and lower half of the triangle, indicating the contribution of several genes and a combination of environmental factors.

Fig. 18.3 The origin of human traits.
Source: Strachan T. and Read, A. P. (2004). *Human Molecular Genetics 3* (3rd edn.). London: Garland Science.

(for example ABO blood groups). **X-linked** disorders such as colour blindness, in which the mutation is carried on the X chromosome and not on the autosomes, also occur. Although these genes are mostly recessive, conferring carrier status in females, they display their effects in males, because men carry only one X chromosome.

18.3 Multifactorial Disorders

Oligogenic disorders are those in which a few different genes act to induce disease. An example is the effect of the methylenetetrahydrofolate reductase (MTHFR) and low-density lipoprotein (LDL) receptor genes jointly increasing the risk of coronary heart disease. If several or many loci act together then a disease is termed **polygenic**. For dichotomous traits (present/absent) the underlying loci are designated **susceptibility loci**, while for quantitative or continuous traits they are **quantitative trait loci (QTL)**.

For each of these types of genetic mechanism, if there are also important environmental factors contributing to risk, the disease is considered to be **multifactorial**. For many common diseases, for example hypertension, coronary heart disease, and most cancers, known genes appear to account for only a fraction of the estimated genetic component. This may be because simple genetic models do not explain several characteristics of 'genetic' diseases, including age of onset, sex-specific effects such as **imprinting** (in the child a gene originating from the father is expressed differently to the same gene coming from the mother), and secular trends in disease presentation. In addition, onset of these diseases is likely to be **multifactorial**, and may result from the combined small effects of multiple genes and modifier genes (which influence gene expression and genetic susceptibility), or from **gene–environment interactions**. Much remains to be understood about the mechanisms of gene interaction and expression. The substantial number of genes, their functional variants and genetic interactions indicate that extensive, multidisciplinary, collaborative research is required to unravel the biological complexity of human disease.

An example of multifactorial effects was observed in population-based **twin studies** in the Nordic countries in the 1990s which suggest that the **heritability** of asthma is around 70 per cent. This differs from the figure of 50 per cent, derived from studies carried out in the 1970s, and it is clear from epidemiological studies that asthma increased in prevalence over the intervening period. Although the prevalence of susceptibility genes for asthma cannot have changed in the population during one generation, their expression and interaction with environmental factors may have changed; this could be reversed if the appropriate environmental factors can be identified and eliminated.

In a large Swedish **twin study**, the association between a family history of premature coronary heart disease and risk of coronary heart disease was investigated. Among the men, the **relative hazard** of death from coronary heart disease when a twin died of coronary heart disease before the age of 55 years, compared with the hazard when a twin survived beyond 55 years, was 8.1 for **monozygotic** (MZ) and 3.8 for **dizygotic** (DZ) twins. Among the women, when a twin died of coronary heart disease before the age of 65 years, the relative hazard was 15.0 for MZ twins and 2.6 for DZ twins. The magnitude of the relative hazard decreased as the age at which the twin died increased; and the ratio of the relative hazard estimate for the MZ twins to that for the dizygotic twins, approached one with increasing age, although a small effect was apparent into ripe old age. This suggests that at younger ages, death from coronary heart disease is influenced by genetic factors, but that the genetic effects show a relative decrease with age (Marenberg *et al.* 1994).

Genes may also have multiple (**pleiotropic**) effects. A gene may convey an advantage early in life but may become a disadvantage in later life. However, the early advantage may result in a sustained frequency of the gene. An example of this is the polymorphism of *ApoE*, a gene with a modest effect on cholesterol levels. It has been suggested that lipids and lipoproteins could have a role as antiviral agents. If so, variation in a gene that affects cholesterol levels, such as *ApoE*, could have been selected for because of its antiviral effects. It is now clear that the specific *ApoE4* allele results in a greatly increased risk of Alzheimer's disease. Hence a gene whose primary effect is on lipid metabolism may have pleiotropic effects which result in pathological changes in the brain. Similarly, the mutations that lead to thalassaemia and sickle-cell disease are relatively common, and are believed to be selectively advantageous in evolutionary terms since they also confer protection against malaria, which kills vastly more people than either blood disorder. Even during the sixteenth and seventeenth centuries, when the slave traders were plying their lucrative trade, they found that West African slaves were best able to withstand the malaria-riven cotton fields of the southern states of North America.

18.4 **Methods in Genetic Epidemiology**

The major study designs currently used in genetic epidemiology are introduced in Box 18.2. Descriptive studies have tended to fall into the domain of classical epidemiology, whereas family studies have largely been conducted by geneticists. Population-based association studies have been conducted mainly by epidemiologists and biostatisticians specializing in genetics, and methodological advances may be expected to be greatest in this area.

Descriptive epidemiology

Clues to the contribution of genetic and environmental factors to disease aetiology can be gleaned from classical epidemiological studies. The pattern of international variation in disease, changes in risk among migrants, and also temporal, racial, and sociodemographic variations yield valuable insights. For example, the incidence of breast cancer varies 10-fold between countries, indicating that there must be a difference in genetic or environmental exposures, or both. Ecological comparisons of hormone levels among low-risk Chinese compared with (high-risk) Western populations, suggest that, given differences in the prevalence of polymorphisms in genes controlling hormone metabolism, a genetic component to breast cancer is probable. On the other hand, breast cancer incidence has been observed to increase in women migrating from relatively low-incidence countries to high-risk countries, confirming also the importance of environmental risk factors (Ziegler *et al.* 1993). 🖥 However, migrants take several generations to attain the risk of the host population.

Familial aggregation

If a possible genetic contribution to a particular disease has been shown, the next question is whether it is transmitted in families. In family studies, the disease risk (or strength of familial aggregation/degree of clustering) in relatives of a patient, is compared with the general risk of disease in the population. This risk is termed the recurrence risk or familial risk ratio (λ). Early examples of familial risk of some congenital malformations are shown in Table 18.1, and strongly suggest a genetic component. Familial aggregation may also indicate a shared environment, but the larger the gradient from identical twins to first- and second-degree relatives, the more likely the pattern is due to genetic factors. Malformations are further discussed in Chapter 14.

Case–control comparisons of family history or **twin/adoption studies** are most useful, but **cohort studies** can be informative for common diseases. Alternatively, a **familial trait** may be investigated by estimating **heritability** (h^2), the proportion of the total variance in a trait that can be explained by genetic effects. Heritability only applies to the population on

---

BOX 18.2 STUDY DESIGNS IN GENETIC EPIDEMIOLOGY OF COMPLEX DISORDERS

Design	Advantages	Limitations
Descriptive		
Ecological	Simple to conduct	Subject to confounding
Migrant	Simple to conduct	Migrant selection bias may operate
Familial aggregation		
Family	Relatively simple to conduct	Uncertain genotypic prediction
Twin	High level of genotypic accuracy if MZ/DZ correctly identified	Accurate twin registers required
Twin adoption	As above	Confidentiality and ethical issues restrict utility
Population-based association studies		
Case–control	Simple to conduct	Selection biases are likely
Cohort	Minimal selection bias; exposures examined prospectively	Expensive and difficult to mount

TABLE 18.1 Familial patterns in congenital malformation

Malformation	'Incidence' relative to the general population			
	Monozygotic twins	First-degree relatives	Second-degree relatives	Third-degree relatives
Cleft lip (± cleft palate)	×400	×40	×7	×3
Club foot	×300	×25	×5	×2
Neural tube defects		×8		×2
Congenital dislocation of hip (females)	×200	×25	×3	×2
Pyloric stenosis (males)	×80	×10	×5	×1.5

Sources: Carter (1968); Smith and Aase (1970).

Carter, C. O. (1969). 'Genetics of Common Disorders'. *British Medical Bulletin,* **25**: 52–7.

Smith, D. W. and Aase, J. M. (1970). 'Polygenic Inheritance of Certain Common Malformations'. *Journal of Pediatrics,* **76**: 653–9.

which observations are made and cannot be used to explain differences between populations, because populations may differ in allele frequencies and/or in the environmental exposures. Genetic differences in populations are termed **population stratification** and this is discussed in a subsequent section.

Twin studies play an important role in probing the genetic component of disease causation. A high **concordance** rate in MZ twins (whose genetic identities are the same, down to identical fingerprints) compared with that in DZ twins, (who share 50 per cent of their genes), provides evidence that genes contribute significantly to familial aggregation for a particular disease. Concordance, however, may be prone to **ascertainment bias** because symptomatic co-twins will be more likely to join a volunteer study. In addition, the twin design assumes that the degree of sharing of their environment is the same for both types of twin and, in general, an increased risk in family members does not necessarily indicate that the disease has an inherited component, but may be related to a shared environment which may include behavioural, biological and physical components (for example, smoking, diet, physical activity, infections, climate, and housing). MZ twins tend to select similar habits and microenvironments more commonly than DZ twins. However, as noted above, stratification of risk by degree of relatedness (first-degree versus second-degree relatives), and comparisons with unrelated individuals living in the same household (typically spouses), can assist in distinguishing genetic and non-genetic familial effects, whereas a detailed extended family history may provide crucial information about the level of genetic risk.

Among over 4000 twin pairs from six European countries and Australia, the heritabilities for systolic blood pressure were 52–66 per cent for systolic and 44–66 per cent for diastolic blood pressure, with little to no evidence of a significant contribution from a shared family environment. This suggests that the remainder of the contribution to these risk factors is due to individual or non-shared behaviours and/or environments (Evans *et al.* 2003) (see Table 18.2).

Twin studies, therefore, can assist in partitioning the three types of influence on a trait: genetic (**heritability**); shared environment (**family members**); non-shared environment (**individual**). However, in adoption studies correlation of a phenotype between adoptive siblings can only be due to shared environment. The correlation of a phenotype between adoptive and biological siblings can be used to estimate a genetic component, and shared and non-shared environmental components. Combinations of designs, such as the inclusion of parents and sibs in twin studies, can allow more incisive estimation of the role of genetic factors, particularly by extending the range of genetic stratification.

Segregation analysis

Before the advent of molecular genetics, evidence for a Mendelian genetic component to a particular disease was usually examined by **segregation analysis**. This determines whether the pattern of disease observed among relatives is compatible with one or more major genes or several minor genes. This was cumbersome

TABLE 18.2 Twin correlations (*r*) and heritability (*h²*) of blood pressure with 95% confidence intervals (95% CI), based on age and sex-adjusted data

	MZm	DZm	MZf	DZf	Heritability	
	r	*r*	*r*	*r*	*h²*	(95% CI)
SBP						
Australia	0.47	0.15	0.55	0.28	0.52	(0.44, 0.59)
Denmark	0.60	0.32	0.70	0.46	0.66	(0.60, 0.71)
Finland	0.45	0.33	0.50	0.43	0.53	(0.46, 0.60)
The Netherlands	0.50	0.25	0.47	0.36	0.54	(0.44, 0.62)
Sweden	0.51	0.28	0.51	0.28	0.54	(0.41, 0.65)
UK	—	—	0.56	0.27	0.53	(0.48, 0.58)
DBP						
Australia	0.47	0.23	0.53	0.39	0.51	(0.44, 0.58)
Denmark	0.63	0.31	0.71	0.43	0.66	(0.60, 0.71)
Finland	0.40	0.29	0.50	0.38	0.47	(0.39, 0.54)
The Netherlands	0.51	0.28	0.46	0.30	0.53	(0.44, 0.61)
Sweden	0.24	0.31	0.50	0.16	0.44	(0.29, 0.56)
UK	—	—	0.49	0.23	0.48	(0.42, 0.53)

MZm/f, monozygotic male/female; DZm/f, dizygotic male/female; SBP, systolic blood pressure; DBP, diastolic blood pressure.

Source: Evans, A., van Baal, G. C. M., McCarron, P. *et al.* (2003). 'The Genetics of Coronary Heart Disease: The Contribution of Twin Studies'. *Twin Research*, **6**: 432–41.

and has largely been replaced by direct **gene mapping** which has become more widely available for examining both Mendelian disorders and complex disorders involving several genes. Nevertheless, segregation analysis still has a role, particularly in focusing both **linkage** and **association** studies. In Figure 18.5 segregation analysis has been used to examine the possibility of genetic inheritance in 1500 families affected by breast cancer. This analysis indicated that 4–5 per cent of cases may be consistent with a dominant allele for disease susceptibility.

Identifying candidate genes

Animal studies can be used to help identify human candidate genes. Strains of various animals, typically rats and rabbits, have been widely used to study phenotypic traits such as hypertension or dyslipidaemias. In breeding experiments a particular phenotype is selectively bred. **Transgenic** or **knock-out models** in which the gene of interest is deleted (or another inserted,

or both) at the embryonic stage of development are widely used, and the resulting phenotype is examined. Such methods are clearly inappropriate in human studies. **Chromosome aberrations** in humans, such as translocation of most of chromosome 22 to the long arm of chromosome 9 (the Philadelphia chromosome), which is only found in tumour cells of chronic myeloid leukaemia, and trisomy of chromosome 21 (accounting for most cases of Down syndrome) serve as examples of (macro) genetic faults which can be easily identified.

Linkage analysis and genetic markers

Linkage aims to discover the approximate location of the gene relative to another DNA sequence, called a **genetic marker**, whose position is already known. This process is known as **gene mapping**. The principle of linkage analysis relies on the knowledge that although each pair of chromosomes contains the same genes in the same order, the sequences on the paternal

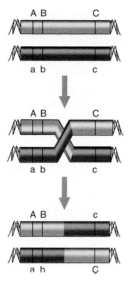

A B   C

Paternal (light shade) and maternal (dark shade) chromosomes aligned in a germ cell. Three paternal DNA sequences (alleles) are shown, A, B and C, (and maternal sequences a, b, and c).

a b   c

A B   C

Physical process of recombination: crossing over of DNA strands between the paired chromosomes.

a b   c

A B   c

What happens when the crossover is resolved? The maternal and paternal alleles are mixed (recombined) and these mixed chromosomes are passed to the germ cells. If A is the disease gene and B and C are genetic markers, recombination is likely to occur much more frequently between A and C than it is between A and B. This allows the disease gene to be mapped relative to the markers B and C.

a b   C

Fig. 18.4 Principle of linkage analysis.

and maternal chromosomes – **maternal and paternal alleles** – are non-identical at many loci. This establishes whether a particular sequence is paternal or maternal in origin and is illustrated in Figure 18.4.

This ability to determine the parental origin of a DNA sequence allows us to show whether **recombination** has taken place. Recombination occurs in the germ cells that make ova or sperm. During meiosis, maternal and paternal chromosomes pair up, breaks occur at several random positions allowing for exchange of **segments of chromosome** or **crossing over**. After recombination, the chromosomes contain a mixture of maternal and paternal alleles. If there is a large distance between two DNA sequences on a chromosome, it is highly probable that recombination will occur between them and both maternal and paternal alleles will occur. In contrast, if two DNA sequences are very close together, crossing over and hence recombination will be rare. It was believed this occurred randomly throughout the length of the chromosome but, more recently, 'hotspots' have been described where recombination is more likely to occur, and blocks between these hotspots are inherited with relatively little recombination. Such sets of alleles on the same

small segment of chromosome tend to be transmitted together, are termed **haplotypes**, and can be tracked through pedigrees and populations. In Table 18.3 the haplotype X, K_2 is strongly associated with cystic fibrosis in affected families.

TABLE 18.3 Distribution of two marker haplotypes in 114 British families with a child with cystic fibrosis

Marker alleles	Cystic fibrosis chromosomes	Normal chromosomes
X_1K_1	3	49
X_1K_2	147	19
X_2K_1	8	70
X_2K_2	8	25

Source: Strachan and Read (2004). Data from Ivinson et al. (1989).

Strachan, T. and Read, A. P. (2004) *Human Molecular Genetics* (3rd edn). London: Garland Science.

Ivinson, A. J., Read, A. P., Harris, R. et al. (1989). 'Testing for Cystic Fibrosis Using Allelic Association'. *Journal of Medical Genetics*, **26**: 426–30.

The results of linkage analyses are usually expressed in terms of a **lod score**, which utilizes logarithms to the base 10. The lod score is a function of the recombination fraction, θ; a lod score of three or more, which represents odds of 1000:1 or greater in favour of linkage, is used to indicate statistically significant linkage. A lod score of minus two or less indicates that linkage is unlikely. In the example shown for *BRCA1* in Figure 18.5 a significant range of values for the lod score was calculated.

In the search for a disease gene, the alternative alleles will be the normal allele and the disease allele, and they can be distinguished by looking for the disease expressed phenotypically in a family tree or pedigree. Genetic markers, used for the mapping of disease genes, need to show a degree of polymorphism (variations in size or sequence), which can be identified (**typed**) using techniques such as the **polymerase chain reaction** (**PCR**). Disease genes are mapped by measuring recombination against a panel of different markers spread over the entire genome. In most cases, recombination will occur frequently, indicating that the disease gene and marker are far apart. Some markers, however, owing to their proximity, will tend not to show recombination with the disease gene and these are said to be linked to it. Ideally, close markers are identified that flank the disease gene and define a candidate

region of the genome. The gene responsible for the disease lies somewhere in this region. In a genome-wide linkage analysis scan, markers at regular intervals covering the whole genome are typed. It is often the first approach when genetic information is lacking.

Linkage analysis can be carried out in affected pedigrees (parametric or model-centred approach) in which the mode of inheritance is defined and an example of this is given by the search for the *BRCA2* gene (Wooster *et al.* 1995). 💻 An alternative approach in which no assumptions are made about the mode of inheritance is to use affected sib-pairs (or further-extended groups of related individuals). A genome-wide search for genes linked with susceptibility to type 1 diabetes provides an example of this approach (Davies *et al.* 1994). 💻 A review of the relative merits and success of linkage studies in complex diseases is given elsewhere (Altmüller *et al.* 2001). 💻 Figure 18.5 shows the sequence of events leading to the discovery of the *BRCA1* gene.

A large-scale segregation analysis of 1500 families affected with early onset breast cancer carried out in 1988 suggested that about 4 per cent of breast cancer cases (especially those with early onset) could be attributed to inherited factors (top left and central panel, Figure 18.5). Some families showed a pattern of inheritance close to a Mendelian pattern. Subsequent linkage analysis showed that a susceptibility locus (designated

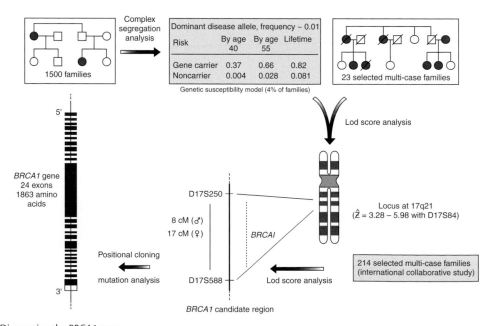

Fig. 18.5 Discovering the *BRCA1* gene.
Source: Strachan, T. and Read, A. P. (2004). *Human Molecular Genetics* (3rd edn.). London: Garland Science.

BRCA1) could be mapped to chromosome 17q. This was confirmed in a large-scale international study and the *BRCA1* gene was shortly afterwards isolated by positional cloning (see below).

Candidate gene association studies

Association studies are commonly used to map disease susceptibility genes in complex disorders in which several genes acting together are suspected to cause the disease. Narrowing the search region for candidate genes can be achieved by comparing population-based cases and controls on a more dense panel of markers

over the candidate region to look for associations that could indicate **linkage disequilibrium** (a statistical association between a marker and a suspected disease susceptibility gene) with the susceptibility gene (see Table 18.3 and the following section). This process is termed **fine mapping**.

Haplotypes can be constructed from a series of closely spaced markers. A haplotype map of the human genome has been published which will assist researchers worldwide (Goldstein and Cavalleri 2005). 🖳 A summary of genetic approaches leading to the identification of candidate genes in complex disorders is shown in Box 18.3.

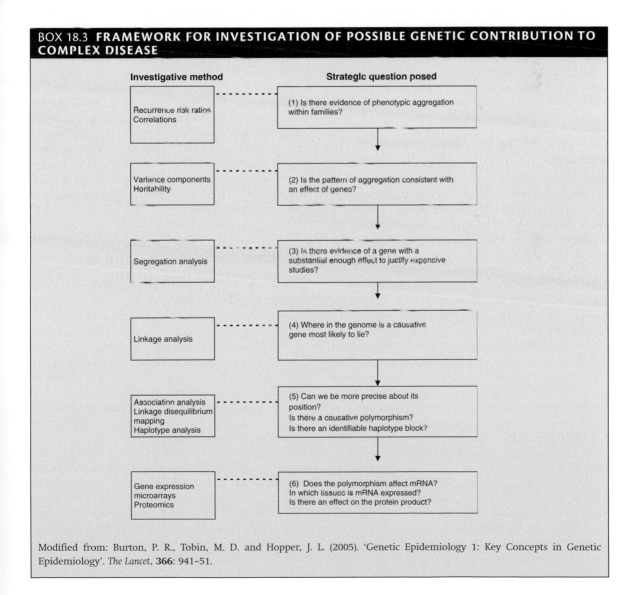

BOX 18.3 FRAMEWORK FOR INVESTIGATION OF POSSIBLE GENETIC CONTRIBUTION TO COMPLEX DISEASE

Investigative method	Strategic question posed
Recurrence risk ratios Correlations	(1) Is there evidence of phenotypic aggregation within families?
Variance components Heritability	(2) Is the pattern of aggregation consistent with an effect of genes?
Segregation analysis	(3) Is there evidence of a gene with a substantial enough effect to justify expensive studies?
Linkage analysis	(4) Where in the genome is a causative gene most likely to lie?
Association analysis Linkage disequilibrium mapping Haplotype analysis	(5) Can we be more precise about its position? Is there a causative polymorphism? Is there an identifiable haplotype block?
Gene expression microarrays Proteomics	(6) Does the polymorphism affect mRNA? In which tissues is mRNA expressed? Is there an effect on the protein product?

Modified from: Burton, P. R., Tobin, M. D. and Hopper, J. L. (2005). 'Genetic Epidemiology 1: Key Concepts in Genetic Epidemiology'. *The Lancet*, **366**: 941–51.

When a region linked to a disease has been identified, it is necessary to test whether it includes genes with known functions that might be implicated in the aetiology of the disease. By comparing the genotypes at these candidate loci between cases and controls (either population or family-based) it is possible to test the hypotheses that they are associated with the disease of interest. Association analysis in genetic epidemiology (a test of allelic association) tests whether a particular genetic exposure is consistently associated with a specific disease. Association, however, does not always signify causation as it may instead be a reflection of linkage disequilibrium. Two loci may be very tightly linked and tend to be inherited together; also the alleles may occur together only in subsections of the overall population, such as a particular ethnic group (ethnic stratification). Some populations exhibit a high level of linkage disequilibrium: for example genetically isolated populations such as those in Sardinia and in regions of Finland which have experienced little admixture from immigrant populations for several centuries.

Positional cloning and identifying disease mutations

Some authors refer to this as 'reverse genetics,' a strategy involving the isolation and cloning of a disease gene after determining its approximate physical location in the human genome using existing markers. When the candidate region is sufficiently narrow and no candidate gene has been found in that region, it can be searched for polymorphisms. Established sequence databases from the Human Genome Project, in combination with various molecular techniques, are used to identify coding sequences that can be screened for potential disease polymorphisms. Where such a polymorphism appears more frequently in cases than in controls, it is considered a possible **causal mutation**. Figure 18.6 shows the sequence of events leading to the association of the *ALOX5AP* gene with cardiovascular disease. HapA is a common haplotype defined by four SNP markers in the region of the gene. A summary of the relative risk of patients with cardiovascular disease having the HapA haplotype compared with controls is shown in Table 18.4.

Once a gene has been identified, it remains to characterize it by studying its structure, the function of each exon, regulatory elements and other features, using molecular methods. The magnitude of the effect of the various mutations in terms of relative and absolute risk can then be assessed; that is, the public-health importance of the mutation is investigated.

Proteins in a biological pathway leading to the phenotype of interest can be studied, which may lead to identification of related biological pathways relevant to the pathogenesis of the disease.

Study design

As noted previously, the rapid evolution and accessibility of genomic technology has created many published reports on genetic associations with disease, most of which have gone unreplicated by other investigators. A variety of study designs based on both epidemiological and genetic principles have been used and are summarized in Box 18.4. Cordell and Clayton (2005) 💻 have classified association studies into three main types: **direct** association studies in which the candidate gene has been designated and association is tested directly; **indirect** association studies where the candidate gene has not been identified but is linked to marker genes; **confounded** association in which the association is confounded by differences between allele and disease frequencies in different populations caused by racial or ethnic mixtures (population stratification and admixture). Family-based studies overcome this problem but may be too small to achieve adequate power to test genetic associations. Alternative methods for dealing with this problem in population studies are discussed elsewhere (Cordell and Clayton 2005). 💻

18.5 **Pharmacogenetics and the Future Practice of Medicine**

The clinical finding that drug dosages must be tailored for individual patients has been recognized for years. In many cases this was considered to be associated with the varying activity of drug-metabolizing enzymes in the liver: for example, slow and fast 'acetylators' of isoniazid (slow acetylators may be more susceptible to drug-induced peripheral neuropathy). Isoforms of such enzymes were known before the human genome was sequenced. Nevertheless, the potential for patients to be categorized as responders or non-responders, based on their unique genetic profile, has lent fresh momentum to arguments for pre-treatment genetic testing and for 'smarter' drug development. There is a real sense in which pharmacogenetics will not be so much about finding 'the right medicine for the right patient' but, through a process of molecular differential diagnosis, about finding 'the right medicine for the right disease' (Lindpainter 2001). 💻 However, the basic premise, that responsiveness to treatment may indicate a readily

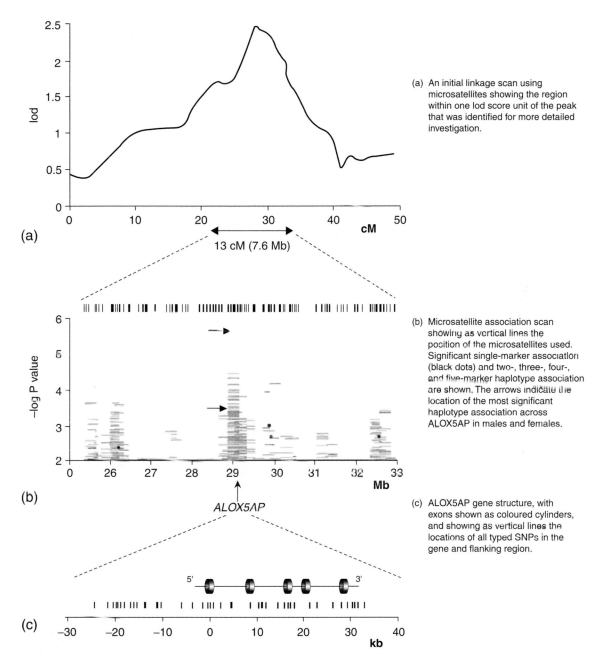

(a) An initial linkage scan using microsatellites showing the region within one lod score unit of the peak that was identified for more detailed investigation.

(b) Microsatellite association scan showing as vertical lines the position of the microsatellites used. Significant single-marker association (black dots) and two-, three-, four-, and five-marker haplotype association are shown. The arrows indicate the location of the most significant haplotype association across ALOX5AP in males and females.

(c) ALOX5AP gene structure, with exons shown as coloured cylinders, and showing as vertical lines the locations of all typed SNPs in the gene and flanking region.

Fig. 18.6 A disease-susceptibility gene for cardiovascular disease. Sequence of genetic analyses to locate a disease-susceptibility gene for myocardial infarction.
Source: Helgadottir, A., Manolescu, A., Thorleifsson, G., *et al.* (2004). 'The Gene Encoding 5-Lipooxygenase Activating Protein Confers Risk of Myocardial Infarction and Stroke'. *Nature Genetics*, **36**: 233–9.

TABLE 18.4 Association of HapA with myocardial infarction and stroke

	Frequency[1]	Relative risk[2]	Population attributable risk	P-value
Myocardial infarction ($n = 779$)	0.158	1.80	0.14	***
Stroke ($n = 702$)	0.149	1.67	0.12	***

***$P < 0.00009$.

[1]Frequency in control population = 0.095.

[2]Relative risk approximated from odds ratio.

Source: Adapted from: Helgadottir, A., Manolescu, A., Thorleifsson, G. *et al.* (2004). 'The Gene Encoding 5-Lipooxygenase Activating Protein Confers Risk of Myocardial Infarction and Stroke'. *Nature Genetics*, **36**: 233–9.

BOX 18.4 STUDY DESIGNS IN GENETIC ASSOCIATION STUDIES

	Details	Advantages	Disadvantages
Cross-sectional	Genotype and phenotype (that is, note disease status or quantitative trait value) a random sample from population	Inexpensive. Provides estimate of disease prevalence	Few affected individuals if disease rare
Cohort	Genotype subsection of population and follow disease incidence for specified time period	Provides estimate of disease incidence	Expensive to follow-up. Issues with drop-out
Case–control	Genotype specified number of affected (case) and unaffected (control) individuals. Cases usually obtained from family practitioners or disease registries, controls obtained from random population sample or convenience sample	No need for follow-up. Provides estimates of exposure effects	Requires careful selection of controls. Potential for confounding (for example population stratification)
Case–parent triads	Genotype affected individuals plus their parents (affected individuals determined from initial cross-sectional, cohort, or disease-outcome based sample)	Robust to population stratification. Can estimate maternal and imprinting effects	Less powerful than case–control design.
Case–parent–grandparent septets	Genotype affected individuals plus their parents and grandparents	Robust to population stratification. Can estimate maternal and imprinting effects	Grandparents rarely available.
General pedigrees	Genotype random sample or disease-outcome based sample of families from general population. Phenotype for disease trait or quantitative trait.	Higher power with large families. Sample may already exist from linkage studies.	Expensive to genotype. Many missing individuals.

BOX 18.4 *(continued)*			
	Details	**Advantages**	**Disadvantages**
Case only	Genotype only affected individuals, obtained from initial cross-sectional, cohort, or disease-outcome based sample	Most powerful design for detection of interaction effects	Requires assumption that genotype and exposure are unrelated in controls
DNA pooling	Applies to variety of above designs, but genotyping is of pools of anywhere between two and 100 individuals, rather than on an individual basis	Potentially inexpensive compared with individual genotyping (but technology still under development)	Hard to estimate different experimental sources of variance

Adapted from: Cordell, H. J. and Clayton, D. G. (2005). 'Genetic Epidemiology 3: Genetic Association Studies'. *The Lancet*, **366**: 1121–31.

detectable genetic trait that could result in better-targeted treatment, needs further examination.

Where have the data come from?

In many cases, the relevant data may have been generated from a clinical trial that has been subsequently analysed to show that treatment efficacy varies in subgroups of patients defined, either on clinical grounds alone, or on the basis of their genetic constitution. Increasingly, clinical trials will have collected DNA from participants as a matter of routine. Often, however, a precise a priori hypothesis will not have been specified. Thus, any sensible interpretation of subgroup results must consider whether the magnitude of the difference between responders and non-responders is clinically important, whether the hypothesis preceded rather than followed the analysis, and whether there was appropriate adjustment of the statistical tests for multiple comparisons, which may inevitably be involved in such studies.

There have been only a few concrete examples of proven pharmacogenetic strategies in action, such as testing for variants of Factors II and V before treatment for deep-vein thrombosis, and testing for rare alleles before treatment of acute lymphoblastic leukaemia in childhood (Khoury *et al.* 2004). 💻 Soon, it has been suggested, people will realize that the sequencing of the human genome will seem like the easiest thing biologists ever accomplished. Magic bullets may remain mythical for some time to come.

18.6 The Human Genome and Issues in Screening

Population-based genetic screening has, until very recently, focused on the identification of persons with certain Mendelian disorders before they develop symptoms, and thus on the prevention of disease (for example screening of newborns for phenylketonuria), or the testing of selected populations for carrier status (for example cystic fibrosis), to follow advice to be given to prospective parents, and the use of prenatal diagnosis to reduce the frequency of disease in subsequent generations (for example, screening to identify carriers of Tay–Sachs disease among Ashkenazi Jews).

However, genetic testing for clinical purposes, and screening, which identifies persons at a higher risk of a genetic disease or condition, are increasingly utilized in practice. Genetic screening is now a reality for an increasing number of disorders, and safeguards are required to ensure that its potential is fully realized. The availability of genetic tests at low cost should not lead to the systematic offer of screening tests without the appropriate medical environment for providing information before testing, and for subsequent counselling. The prevalence of genotype, laboratory quality, the magnitude of the association (consistently replicated) between genotype and disease, interaction with known modifiable risk factors, available interventions or prevention methods, must all be understood before embarking on screening programmes. In addition, the disease should fulfil most of the criteria for population screening discussed in Chapter 5 (Box 5.2). For example, Mendelian disorders such as Huntington's disease (autosomal dominant) and cystic fibrosis (autosomal recessive) do not fulfil some crucial criteria; Huntington's disease is untreatable and only develops in middle age; cystic fibrosis is treatable (and early treatment can improve life expectancy), but the need to test for several polymorphisms makes testing expensive. Each genetic disorder needs to be considered separately, therefore, and the potential benefits and harm carefully reviewed. These issues are further discussed elsewhere (UK National Screening Committee 2005). 🖳 Genetic testing and screening have the potential to improve public-health outcomes, but also involve significant ethical, legal, and social issues. Within the context of conflicting ethical values from the individual and public-health perspectives, individual values such as informed consent, privacy, and discrimination, must be respected.

Genetic epidemiology is seen by some to be the brightest future for epidemiology, perhaps reflecting a growing awareness of the limitations of observational epidemiology. Genetic epidemiology is concerned with understanding heritable aspects of disease risk, individual susceptibility to disease, and ultimately with contributing to a comprehensive molecular understanding of pathogenesis and better means of control. Major research collaborations are required to ensure efficient uses of resources and the sharing of genetic data. Practitioners, in clinical, public health, and basic science will need to ensure that the massive investment and expansion of human genetics is carefully integrated into their practice for the ultimate benefit of the whole population.

Further Reading

Khoury, M. J., Beaty, T. H. and Cohen, B. H. (1993). *Fundamentals of Genetic Epidemiology*. New York, NY: Oxford University Press.

Mange, E. J. and Mange, A. P. (1999). *Basic Human Genetics* (2nd edn). Sunderland, MA: Sinauer Associates.

Storm, B. (2000). *Pharmacoepidemiology*. Chichester: Wiley.

Strachan, T. and Read, A. P. (2004). *Human Molecular Genetics* (3rd edn). London: Garland Science.

Urquhart, J. (2004). 'Getting a Handle on Why Good Drugs Sometimes Don't Work'. *Journal of the Royal College of Physicians of Edinburgh*, **34**: 90–8.

Web Addresses

Human Genome Epidemiology (HuGE) Net, http://www.cdc.gov/genomics/hugenet/.

Cancer Genome Anatomy Project (CGAP), http://cgap.nci.nih.gov/.

National Centre for Biotechnology Information (NCBI) dbSNPs, http://www.ncbi.nlm.nih.gov/SNP/.

On-line Mendelian Inheritance in Man (OMIM), http://www.ncbi.nlm.nih.gov/entrez/query.fcgi?db=OMIM. Information about human genes and disease.

SNPs consortium, http://snp/cshl.org/.

UK National Screening Committee (2005), www.nsc.nhs.uk.

References

References for this chapter can be found at www.oxfordtextbooks.co.uk/orc/yarnell. Where possible, these are presented as *active links* which direct you to an electronic version of the work. If you are a subscriber to that work (either individually or through an institution), and depending on your level of access, you may be able to peruse an abstract or the full article if available. 🖳

Oral health

This chapter describes the epidemiology and aetiology of oral diseases. It examines the causation of dental caries and examines the influence of diet and fluoride on the prevention of tooth decay. Periodontal disease, neoplasia, and the primary prevention of oral diseases are also reviewed.

Introduction

With the rise of dental knowledge and the development of professional power of the barber surgeons, in the mid-nineteenth century, the mouth became dissociated from the rest of the body and gradually became a bodily entity in its own right (Nettleton 1992). 💻 So it became necessary to create the new profession of dentistry, which would provide all the health care and treatment for this unique bodily part. While the existence of the dental profession allowed for appropriate training, it also created a division between those who cared for the body (doctors) and those who cared for the mouth (dentists). Consequently, in the training of health professionals, other than dentists, knowledge about oral diseases was vanquished: only those caring for the mouth were empowered with oral health and disease knowledge. The aim of this chapter is to bridge this division and to introduce the subject of oral health. Many of the risk factors for poor oral health are common to those for other chronic disease; by promoting a healthy lifestyle, restricting the intake of cariogenic sugars, increasing the consumption of fruit and vegetables, moderating alcohol consumption, and avoiding smoking, significant amounts of tooth decay, periodontal disease, and oral cancer may be prevented.

19.1 Dental caries

Definition

Dental caries (Latin *caries*, decay of teeth or bone) evolve from the dynamic interplay between a disease process (demineralization of the enamel) and attempts at repair (remineralization of the enamel). It is the imbalance in the favour of demineralization that results in dental caries. Clinically the most obvious sign is a brown discolouration (caused by bacteria) indicating demineralization of the enamel and cavitation of the tooth (Figure 19.1). Pain is a late clinical sign after demineralization of the enamel and exposure of the dentine. Deeper penetration of the pulp cavity and inflammation of nerve endings is likely to cause persistent pain.

Epidemiology

Dental caries is a worldwide health problem. In a recent World Health Organization (WHO) report, 32 per cent of 12-year-old children were found to have three or more decayed teeth, and dental caries affected between 60–90 per cent of children and adults. For epidemiological surveys a standard measure summarizing the total number of decayed, missing, or filled teeth (DMFT) at a given age, is used (Box 19.1).

Figure 19.2 shows the prevalence of dental caries in 12-year-old children in world regions.

In the UK surveys have shown that the prevalence of childhood caries has reduced, and the proportion of young middle-aged adults (40–44 years) who were **edentulous** between 1988 and 1998 was only 1 per cent, also showing a decline from previous generations (Kelly *et al.* 2000). 🖳 This suggests that there have been

gains in oral health in the UK, but some areas show a different pattern. In Northern Ireland during the same time period, the average number of decayed, missing, and filled teeth for five- and nine-year-olds was more than double the average rate in the UK. Nearly 70 per cent

> ### BOX 19.1 EPIDEMIOLOGY OF DENTAL CARIES
>
> - Dental caries prevalence is measured using the DMFT[1] and dmft[2] indices.
> - 32 per cent of 12-year-old children worldwide have more than three decayed teeth.
> - 60–90 per cent of children, adolescents, and adults worldwide have had dental caries.
> - 70 per cent of adolescents in Northern Ireland have had dental caries.
> - Dental caries prevalence is an indicator of social inequality.
> - 20 per cent of a population have 80 per cent of the dental caries.
>
> [1]The DMFT Index is used in oral health epidemiological surveys to measure dental caries in the permanent dentition. The DMFT index is an arithmetic sum of the number of permanent teeth (T) that are decayed (D), missing (M), or filled (F).
> [2]The dmft index is used to assess decay experience in deciduous dentition.
> Data from: Petersen, P.-E. (2003). *The World Oral Health Report 2003. Continuous Improvement of Oral Health in the 21st Century – The Approach of the WHO Global Oral Health Programme.* Geneva: World Health Organization.

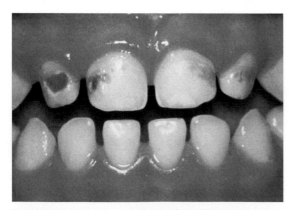

Fig. 19.1 Dental caries on the labial surfaces of the upper anterior deciduous teeth.
Source: http://www.dental.washington.edu.

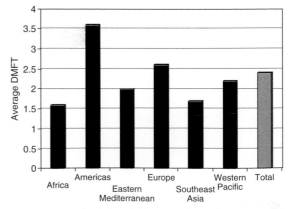

Fig. 19.2 Decayed, missing, or filled teeth (DMFT) in 12-year-olds in world regions.
Source: Petersen, P.-E. (2003). *The World Oral Health Report 2003. Continuous Improvement of Oral Health in the 21st Century – The Approach of the WHO Global Oral Health Programme.* Geneva: World Health Organization.

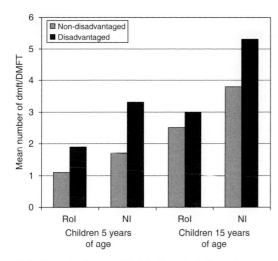

Dmft: Decayed, missing and filled deciduous teeth (5 years).
DMFT: Decayed, missing and filled permanent teeth (15 years)

Fig. 19.3 Mean number of decayed, missing, and filled teeth by disadvantage in Northern Ireland (NI) and in the Republic of Ireland (RoI).
Source: Whelton, H. P. (2003). *Children's Oral Health in Ireland 2002: A North–South study*. Cork: Oral Health Services Research Centre, University College. (With permission.)
Web reference: Whelton, H., Crowley, E., O'Mullane, D., Donaldson, M., Cronin, M., Kelleher, V. (2006). 'Dental Caries and Enamel Fluorosis among the Fluoridated Population in the Republic of Ireland and Non Fluoridated Population in Northern Ireland in 2002'. *Community Dental Health*, **23**: 37–43.

of 15-year-olds in Northern Ireland have caries, and children living in conditions of social disadvantage have the highest prevalence of decay. Data from a survey across the whole of Ireland (Figure 19.3) show the likely impact of fluoridation, because water supplies in the Republic of Ireland are fluoridated (71 per cent), and those in the North are mainly not.

These findings support the idea that dental caries is a disease of social deprivation and inequality. Generally surveys have found that 80 per cent of the disease is found in 20 per cent of the people (Pitts *et al.* 2003), 🖳 and this group is usually the most socioeconomically disadvantaged.

Aetiology

The carious process is initiated by the consumption of refined or fermentable sugars which are converted to lactic and other acids in the plaque (a biofilm of bacteria and food debris), which then attack the tooth structure. Lactic acid is the major metabolite of the

bacterial action on fermentable sugars, which are now termed, more specifically, **non-milk extrinsic sugars (NMES)** (see Box 19.2).

Lactic acid promotes demineralization of the enamel with loss of calcium and phosphates from the enamel structure (the hydroxyapatite crystal). For demineralization to occur lactic acid must be present for at least 20 minutes. This first stage in the carious process is observed clinically as 'white spot lesions', which are shown in Figure 19.4.

The enamel is breached by cariogenic bacteria, principally *Streptococcus mutans*, which enters the enamel and body of the tooth. The bacteria stream along the border between the enamel and the dentine (the amelo-dentinal junction) before assaulting the dentine. As the carious attack continues there is destruction of the structure of the dentine (dentinal tubules) but, at the same time, with attempts at repair in which secondary dentine is produced. Dental decay is characterized by a brown discolouration at this stage of the pathogenic process, as illustrated in Figure 19.1.

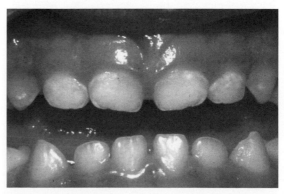

Fig. 19.4 'White spot lesions' on the upper anterior deciduous teeth.
Source: http://www.dental.washington.edu.

It has been estimated that eating less than 15 kg of sugar/person/year or 60 g of NMES/day is commensurate with good dental health providing the individual uses fluoride toothpaste (Sheiham 2001). ⌨ In practical terms, this means that sugar should be consumed only with meals as saliva, which contains bicarbonate, tends to counteract the effect of lactic acid.

Pits and fissures in a tooth which occur naturally, and with considerable variability from individual to individual, increase its susceptibility to decay. These parts of the tooth are impervious to cleaning with fluoride toothpaste and are the focus for caries. Tooth maturity has been highlighted as a factor in the carious attack, since the longer the tooth has erupted the greater its immunity to decay. Characteristically, middle-aged and older individuals experience a lower rate of dental decay than younger adults.

Restriction of consumption of NMES to meal times means that the fall in pH associated with the carious attack, which then lasts from 20 to 30 minutes, is time-limited. Consuming NMES with meals maximizes the saliva's protective actions. Saliva has a resting pH of 7.0 but, when the saliva flow increases, the pH rises to at least 8.0 buffering the local effect of lactic acid on a particular tooth and restoring the pH to 7.0. At pH 7.0 there is saturation of the saliva with calcium, phosphate, and hydroxyl ions, which maximizes the possibility of remineralization of the tooth. Furthermore, saliva washes food from the mouth thus physically reducing the time that food is in contact with the teeth (Box 19.3).

Prevention of dental caries

Dental caries can be prevented or reduced, therefore, by restricting consumption of NMES to mealtimes, and by using a fluoride toothpaste.

Fluoride can prevent dental caries both when applied topically and when absorbed systemically, and has both pre-eruptive and post-eruptive effects. Pre-eruptively the fluoride acts to replace the hydroxyl ion in the hydroxyapatite crystal, making the enamel less susceptible to caries. Post-eruptively fluoride assists remineralization of the enamel.

The best-known form of systemic fluoride is water fluoridation. When fluoride is added to the water supplies with levels below 0.5 parts per million (ppm) to produce levels of up to 1 ppm it becomes the most efficient and cost-effective way to prevent dental caries. Nevertheless, fluoridation of water supplies remains controversial to some pressure groups and some 'environmentalists'.

A recent systematic review of 214 studies from 1945 onwards (McDonagh *et al.* 2000) ⌨ found that 17 supported the evidence of benefit, 10 were inconclusive (with insufficient statistical power) and one showed no benefit. At a fluoride level of 1 ppm the authors estimated that 12.5 per cent (95% CI 7.0–21.5 per cent) of exposed people would have dental fluorosis (mottled discolouration and pitting of the tooth enamel), and that the proportion of the population with fluorosis is dose-dependent. The remaining studies were of possible adverse effects associated with disease outcomes, and were negative. The authors reviewed studies with several designs: 45 before-and-after, 102 cross-sectional,

---

BOX 19.3 **THE DENTAL CARIES PROCESS**

- Cariogenic, acidophilic bacteria (for example *Streptococcus mutans*) are present in plaque.
- Non-milk extrinsic sugars (fermentable carbohydrates) are consumed.
- Cariogenic bacteria produce lactic acid from ingested NMES and initiate the carious process.
- Immature teeth and pits and fissures in teeth are attacked.
- Saliva attempts to buffer the acid and restore health by aiding remineralization. It also helps remove food from the mouth.
- The time necessary for demineralization (dental caries) to occur is between 20 and 30 minutes.

BOX 19.4 **PREVENTION OF DENTAL CARIES**

- Reduce consumption of NMES to four times per day with meals.
- Consume no more than 60 g per day of NMES.
- Promote water fluoridation.
- In the absence of water fluoridation advise fluoride supplements for at risk children.
- Use fluoride toothpaste twice a day and avoid mouth rinsing after use.
- Advise the use of fluoride mouthwashes and professionally applied fluorides for those at high risk.
- Use fissure sealants to protect pits and fissures in those at high risk.

47 ecological, 13 cohort, and 7 case–control studies (McDonagh *et al.* 2000). 🖳

In the USA much of the ecological and interventional evidence on the role of fluoride was obtained from the 1930s onwards, and 67 per cent of the population, who are served by public water supplies, receive optimal levels of fluoride for preventing dental decay (US Surgeon General 2004). 🖳 In the UK, however, only 10 per cent of the population receive fluoridated water, but health authorities have now been given the power to recommend and implement water fluoridation, after local public consultation, under legislation introduced in 2003 (British Fluoridation Society 2003). 🖳

In the absence of water fluoridation in districts with levels below 0.3 ppm, children can be given daily fluoride supplements from six months of age (0.25 mg fluoride up to ten years, 0.5 mg from 3 to 6 years and 1.0 mg from six years onwards) (Holt *et al.* 2000). 🖳

Topical forms of fluoride include fluoride toothpaste, mouthwash, and professionally applied fluoride varnishes. These have a post-eruptive effect which assists remineralization of the enamel. Teeth should be brushed twice daily with a fluoride toothpaste on going to bed and at one other time of the day. Mouth rinsing with water after brushing must be discouraged. The concentration of fluoride used in toothpaste is determined by age (for example adult toothpaste contains 1450 ppm, compared with 500 ppm in children's toothpaste) and caries risk. People with moderate-to high risk of dental caries should rinse daily with fluoride mouthwashes, while professionally applied fluorides are for individuals with high risk of caries, for example those with a reduced salivary flow.

The use of fissure sealants to protect fissures and pits are a particularly cost-effective preventive intervention in children with a history of rampant caries, and for those where dental treatment may put their physical health at risk. However, a recent randomized controlled trial was inconclusive on the use of fissure sealants in the general population of pre-school children (Chadwick *et al.* 2005). 🖳 But Uribe, reviewing the evidence in the journal *Evidence-Based Dentistry*, has suggested that fissure sealing of the first permanent molar in a caries-active child will confer useful protection.

> **Q1** What elements should be included in an assessment of epidemiological needs to investigate whether fluoridation of the water supplies should be instigated in a particular health district?

19.2 Periodontal Disease

Definition

The periodontium (Greek *peri*, around; *odontos*, tooth) comprises the tissues that support the teeth and includes the gum, the periodontal ligament, and the alveolar bone. The main functions of the periodontal tissues are to attach the teeth to the bone of the jaws and to maintain the integrity of the surface of the masticatory mucosa of the mouth. Diseases of the periodontal tissues are among the most common to affect mankind.

Gingivitis represents the inflammatory response of the gum to the accumulation of dental plaque on the surface of the teeth. Those affected will often complain of bleeding gums, particularly while toothbrushing and after eating hard foods, but the condition is not usually painful. Gingivitis is a reversible disease process and removal of dental plaque and calculus (calcified plaque) will result in a return to gingival health. Gingivitis is a very common inflammatory process and is evident to some degree in virtually all adolescents at puberty. There is a reduction in the prevalence of gingivitis during teenage years before a gradual increase in adulthood.

Periodontitis is a chronic inflammatory condition which results in irreversible destruction of the periodontal ligament and the alveolar bone which supports the teeth. It is not usually painful and often does not become evident to affected individuals until they notice loosening, or a change in the position, of one or more of their teeth. Ultimately periodontitis can result in the loss of some, or all, the teeth.

Bacteria, principally Gram-negative anaerobes, which are to be found in most mouths, are required to cause periodontitis, but there must also be a susceptible host. Factors regulating susceptibility are still unclear, but include genetic variation between different individuals in immune or inflammatory responses to the bacteria that cause periodontal disease.

Periodontitis does not have a well-defined phenotype and there is currently no universally accepted 'gold standard' for the extent of changes in the tissues that should be present before an individual is classified as having periodontal disease. The situation is further complicated because, in individuals, different teeth may be affected to varying degrees. In the local lesion of periodontitis, as tissue damage progresses, gaps are formed between the gum tissue and the root surfaces of the teeth, termed periodontal pockets. In severe disease these pockets are several millimetres deep. There is also recession of the gum margin on to the root surface of teeth with increasing age; this complicates the assessment of periodontal disease, for example by leading to a reduction in the depth of periodontal pockets. However, where there is advanced disease the diagnosis is unequivocal.

Epidemiology

Various studies have used different clinical definitions of periodontal disease. The earliest epidemiological studies of periodontal disease in the 1950s and 1960s suggested that periodontal disease was a major global health problem with severe disease affecting most of the adult population. These studies used a scoring system known as the **Periodontal Index** (Russell 1956), 💻 which is now acknowledged to be flawed and to have overestimated the extent and severity of periodontal disease. Nevertheless, the early studies showed that, on a population basis, dental plaque and calculus were strongly correlated with the severity of periodontal disease. A classical longitudinal investigation of the natural history of periodontal disease was performed by Löe and his co-workers in the 1970s and 1980s. A group of Sri Lankan workers in two tea plantations was examined over a 15 year period between 1970 and 1985 (Löe *et al.* 1986). 💻 Three subpopulations were identified: a small high risk group (8 per cent) with rapid progression of periodontal disease who had lost virtually all their teeth by the age of 45 years; a large group (81 per cent) with moderate progression, who had lost on average seven teeth by the age of 45 years; and a group (11 per cent) with no progression beyond gingivitis and no tooth loss. All these individuals were free from dental decay and had no dental treatment; therefore, it was argued that tooth loss was due to terminal periodontal disease. This study provided a significant contribution to our understanding of the natural history of periodontal disease in man. It was acknowledged that this represented a unique population without dental intervention and, therefore, was very different from the situation in developed countries. However, the finding that sizeable variations in the progression of periodontal disease occurred in these circumstances was important. The concept of the existence of a high-risk group for severe periodontitis has been generally accepted.

Cross-sectional epidemiological studies of periodontal disease in the UK have been performed as integral parts of the national surveys of adult dental health which occur at ten-year intervals. In 1998 over 3500 adults had a dental examination in their home (Morris *et al.* 2001). 💻 Only 8 per cent of those aged 16 years or older had evidence of severe periodontal destruction;

however, this was much more prevalent with increasing age and affected 31 per cent of those aged 65 years and over. Advanced periodontal disease, even in older subjects, did not affect many teeth per person. A higher proportion (85 per cent) of those aged 65 years or over had moderate disease, and this affected 30 per cent of the remaining teeth. Thus low grade, slowly destructive, periodontal disease was the norm in the UK. In the third National Health and Nutrition Examination Survey (NHANES III) in the USA, 13 per cent of those aged 30 years or older had severe or moderate periodontal disease (Albandar *et al.* 1999), 💻 and 68 per cent of those aged 65 years or over had moderate periodontal destruction. Analysis of data from 45 European studies found that in 33–44 year-olds 14 per cent (95% CI 11–17 per cent) had evidence of deep periodontal pockets sufficient to warrant periodontal treatment (Sheiham and Netuveli 2002). 💻

There is an increase in the severity and extent of periodontal disease with increasing age. In NHANES III, males had a higher prevalence of periodontal disease than females regardless of age; this has been confirmed in other studies worldwide. There are racial differences in disease; for example, in NHANES III non-Hispanic Blacks had the highest, and the non-Hispanic Whites the lowest, prevalence. It is not clear whether this represents a true difference in susceptibility or is related to other factors that could promote the disease, such as poorer education, nutrition, and socioeconomic circumstances. There is general agreement that smoking is the principal environmental risk factor for periodontitis; this is particularly so in aggressive forms of periodontal disease which occur in young individuals. Data from NHANES III have shown that over 50 per cent of all periodontitis can be attributed to cigarette smoking. Other risk factors include nutritional deficiency, drug complications, psychological stress, acquired immune defects, and acquired endocrine diseases and disturbances.

The extent of periodontal disease is affected by the pattern of loss or retention of teeth; with the extraction of periodontally involved teeth the periodontal condition, as measured by any index, will improve. More people are retaining more teeth into later life. In the UK there has been the decrease in the proportion of the population who had no teeth from 37 per cent in 1968 to 13 per cent in 1998. This improvement is expected to continue with only 4 per cent projected to have no teeth in 2028 (Steele *et al.* 2000). 💻 In future years, therefore, more teeth will be placed at risk of developing periodontitis and this, coupled with increased numbers of older people in society, is likely to lead to higher levels of periodontal disease and an increasing treatment burden.

Prevention of periodontal disease

Periodontal disease consists of two major diseases: (1) gingivitis and (2) periodontitis in which there is destruction of the periodontal ligament and supporting bone. Whereas gingivitis is very common, and can be easily prevented, periodontitis affects 10 per cent of the adult dentate population in the UK (Kelly *et al.* 2000). 🖳 The prevention of periodontitis through screening programmes is difficult because the natural history of the disease is poorly understood. Although gingivitis is probably the natural precursor of periodontitis, the evidence remains inconclusive. Therefore Davies *et al.* (2003) 🖳 suggest that people must be assisted:

'to maintain a level of plaque control which ensures that the rate of tissue destruction is reduced sufficiently to ensure ... a comfortable and functional dentition'.

Regular toothbrushing is recommended to control plaque, as for preventing dental caries. A gentle scrubbing action and the use of dental floss or inter-dental aids will assist in removing plaque between the teeth. Toothpastes containing 'chemical plaque-suppressing agents' such as triclosan and zinc citrate antimicrobial mouthwashes may also be useful.

The cornerstone of primary prevention of periodontal disease is the provision and acquisition of oral hygiene skills, particularly in smokers who are at a higher level of risk. Equity in access to preventive dental care is required to reduce the future population burden of periodontal disease.

19.3 Oral Cancer

Definition

Oral cancers are predominantly squamous cell carcinomas occurring at most sites in the mouth, including the lip, tongue, or any mucosal surface. Pharyngeal and laryngeal cancers may also present in dental practice. A squamous cell carcinoma may be seen with the typical appearance of an ulcerated mass with raised, rolled, everted edges and an indurated base, or a non-healing ulcer; but, in the early stages, it may also present as a swelling or as a red or white patch(es). The latter are termed leukoplakia and are well-established as precursors of oral cancer, particularly of the tongue and cheeks.

Epidemiology

Oral cancer is one of the ten commonest cancers and is a major health problem in many parts of the world. On the Indian subcontinent, and in other parts of Asia, it remains one of the most common forms of cancer, particularly in men. In the UK, oral cancer constitutes 1–4 per cent of all malignant tumours, and approximately 3500 individuals are diagnosed each year with the disease. It is more common in men and this seems to be independent of tobacco use.

Oral, squamous-cell carcinomas metastasize early to regional lymph nodes in the neck. Detection of early, localized lesions has not improved significantly during the past three decades and, despite the ease with which the oral cavity can be examined, it is disappointing to note that the death rate for oral cancers is comparable to that for the cervix (Sasieni *et al.* 1995). 🖳 In recent years there has been no marked improvement in the five-year survival rates, particularly for those with metastases, which remain steady at about 50 per cent.

However, in those cases that have been successfully treated, there seems to be an increase in second primary tumours. It has been estimated that 20 years from the time of the first head and neck cancer, which include oral cancers, approximately 30 per cent of male patients and 20 per cent of female patients will have developed a second primary (Warnakulasuriya *et al.* 2003). 🖳 Furthermore, the relative risk for multiple primary cancer is higher in younger subjects.

Risk factors

Tobacco and alcohol

The major risk factors for oral cancer are tobacco use and alcohol consumption (Macfarlane *et al.* 1995). 🖳 Most individuals who develop oral cancer smoke cigarettes, but smoking cigars, pipes and using smokeless tobacco also poses significant risks (Rodu and Jansson 2004). 🖳 As shown in Chapter 7, the relative risk for laryngopharyageal cancers of smoking 25 cigarettes a day or more in British doctors recruited into a cohort study in the 1950s was 48, with an attributable risk of 98 per cent (see Table 7.2).

It is difficult to find evidence that alcohol is an independent risk factor for oral cancer as heavy users of alcohol also tend to be heavy smokers, and may have a poor diet. Among heavy drinkers, self-reported drinking levels may be unreliable, which may contribute to underestimation. There is a synergistic effect between smoking and alcohol which substantially increases the risk. For people who habitually smoke and drink, it has been estimated that their relative risk of oral cancer may be 30 times greater than that for non-smokers who drink occasionally (Levine and Stillman-Lowe 2004). 🖳 Other tobacco habits such as reverse smoking, seen in some developing countries (the lit end of a cigarette – usually hand rolled – smoked from inside the mouth), and the common practice for both sexes in Asian communities of chewing tobacco in 'betel nut quid', 'paan', or 'ghukta' significantly increases the risk of oral cancer (Balaram *et al.* 2002). 🖳

Nutrition

Diet also influences incidence rates of oral cancer. A diet that is poor in fresh fruit and vegetables may account for 10–15 per cent of cases of oral cancer in Europe (LaVecchia *et al.* 1997). 🖳 Evidence is mainly from case–control studies, but is inconsistent; the evidence generally supports the view that fruit and vegetable consumption protects against oral cancer, but individual foods that appear protective in some studies are not in others. The effects of diet appear to be modest when compared with those of smoking and alcohol consumption.

Infection

Human papillomavirus (HPV), a sexually transmitted virus, is established as a necessary cause for more than 95 per cent of cervical carcinomas; however, its association with oral squamous cell carcinoma is less certain. Early studies revealed the presence of HPV in a significant number of normal mucosal samples as well as cases of oral cancer, indicating that the virus may not be causal. However, HPV has been identified in 15 per cent of oral cancer cases compared with less than 5 per cent of controls; and it has also been shown that the risk of oral cancer associated with HPV infection is independent of tobacco and alcohol use. Recent studies have shown that a specific subset of oral cancers are highly associated with 'high risk' HPVs, particularly HPV 16 (Gillison and Lowy 2004). 🖳

Age

Oral cancer increases with age and those most affected are men in their sixth or seventh decade. Despite overall reductions for oral cancer in England and Wales during the twentieth century, significant increases in mortality and incidence have occurred in younger males during the past 30 years, possibly because of increased alcohol consumption, although some cases have never smoked or consumed alcohol. Recent work suggests that although oral cancer incidence continues to rise alarmingly, these increases have not been translated into higher mortality rates. This may indicate a changing natural history of oral cancers or a lower case-fatality rate due to improved treatments (Robinson and Macfarlane 2003). 🖳

Lip cancer

Lip cancer is a form of oral cancer with a distinctive global epidemiology, which supports the idea that the lip should be considered as a distinct cancer site rather than its inclusion with other forms of oral cancer. High rates of lip cancer in men (between 12.0 and 13.5 new cancers per 100 000 per annum) are reported for regions of Europe, North America, and Oceania whereas it is virtually unknown in much of Asia. Factors important in the aetiology of lip cancer include solar radiation, tobacco smoking, and viruses. Incidence rates of lip cancer are generally stable or falling among males worldwide; however, they are rising in many female populations (Moore *et al.* 1999). 🖳

Q2 Why might the rate of lip cancer be increasing in women?

Health promotion and prevention

Screening for oral cancer by visual examination is simple, inexpensive, and causes little discomfort, although there is insufficient evidence to recommend population screening for oral cancer in the UK (Rodrigues *et al.* 1998). 🖳 Measures aimed at primary prevention of the disease may be a more feasible form of disease control at present, although opportunistic screening is routinely conducted in dental practice.

Efforts designed to encourage smoking cessation in conjunction with programmes to discourage children from starting smoking could have a major impact in the future. There is a need also to provide information to people about the causes of oral cancer, as knowledge of risk factors is low. A lack of awareness of the signs and symptoms of oral cancer has been shown to be a factor in people who do not present early. Patient information leaflets have been shown to reduce patient anxiety while improving knowledge and willingness to be examined. The results from one randomized controlled trial suggest that people who benefit most from such campaigns are those at higher risk, especially smokers; smokers were 16 times more likely to believe that they are at risk from oral cancer (Humphris *et al.* 2004). 🖳

Smoking cessation is clearly an essential part of oral cancer prevention and people should be encouraged to adopt a healthier lifestyle with less alcohol, to increase their intake of fresh fruit and vegetables, and to attend for regular dental checkups.

This chapter has reviewed the epidemiology and prevention of oral disease and suggests that many opportunities exist for further prevention in clinical and public-health dental practice. One priority may be to improve the evidence-base for these purposes in parallel with those that have occurred in medical practice.

Further Reading

Levine, R. S. and Stillman-Lowe, C. R. (2004). *The Scientific Basis of Oral Health Education.* London: BDJ Books.

Nettleton, S. (1992). *Power, Pain and Dentistry.* Milton Keynes: Open University Press.

WHO (2003). *Diet, Nutrition and the Prevention of Chronic Diseases.* Geneva: World Health Organization.

References

References for this chapter can be found at www.oxfordtextbooks.co.uk/orc/yarnell. Where possible, these are presented as *active links* which direct you to an electronic version of the work. If you are a sub-scriber to that work (either individually or through an institution), and depending on your level of access, you may be able to peruse an abstract or the full article if available. 🖥

Model answers

Q1

● Fluoride levels below 0.3 ppm in existing water supply.

● Prevalence of caries in health district above national average.

● Socioeconomic distribution such that many children have limited access to dental care.

Q2

This may be associated with an increase in tobacco smoking among women.

Clinical and Public-Health Applications

CHAPTER 20

Clinical epidemiology and evidence-based practice

This chapter provides a brief introduction to clinical epidemiology and an overview of the principles that guide the use of evidence in clinical and public-health practice. The elements of critical appraisal of research findings are illustrated in a series of topical, health-related scenarios and relevant published studies. These use the techniques of: (1) cross-sectional design (evaluation of a diagnostic test for venous thrombosis), (2) a randomized controlled trial (two options for the delivery of antenatal care); and (3) systematic review (workplace smoking bans on employees' smoking habits). A practical guide including sources of evidence and critical appraisal is provided.

20.1 Clinical Epidemiology

One simple definition of clinical epidemiology is 'epidemiology in patient populations rather than in general populations'. Fletcher *et al.* (1996), ▯ authors of an excellent pioneering textbook in this area, stress that the discipline seeks to answer clinical questions, and to guide clinical decisions with the best available evidence. Clinical epidemiology thus utilizes most of the epidemiological tools and biostatistical methods described in our previous chapters, and is the cornerstone of evidence-based practice. Fletcher *et al.* (1996) ▯ have summarized the main clinical questions that fall within its remit (Box 20.1).

Scrutiny of the topics and questions shown in the box reveals all the key issues dealt with in earlier chapters of this book: philosophical question of disease definition, diagnosis, risk, prevention, etc. The validation of diagnostic tests is reviewed in detail in Chapter 5

BOX 20.1 CLINICAL QUESTIONS IN EPIDEMIOLOGY

Issue	Question
Abnormality	Is the patient sick or well?
Diagnosis	How accurate are tests used to diagnose disease?
Frequency	How often does a disease occur?
Risk	What factors are associated with an increased risk of disease?
Prognosis	What are the consequences of having a disease?
Treatment	How does treatment change the course of disease?
Prevention	Does an intervention on well people keep disease from arising? Does early detection and treatment improve the course of disease?
Cause	What conditions lead to disease? What are the pathogenic mechanisms of disease?
Cost	How much will care for an illness cost?

Source: Fletcher, R. H., Fletcher, S. E. and Wagner, E. H. (1996). *Clinical Epidemiology. The Essentials.* Baltimore, MD: Williams and Wilkins.

BOX 20.2 THE FIVE STEPS OF EVIDENCE-BASED PRACTICE

1 Formulate a structured question.
2 Undertake an effective and efficient search for information.
3 Appraise the information gathered for relevance, validity, and usefulness.
4 Apply the information in practice, taking account of individual or population characteristics, preferences, and values.
5 Evaluate the impact of the information and the process on the patient, clinical practice and the service through self appraisal and audit.

Adapted from: Sackett, D. L., Straus, S. E., Richardson, W. S., Rosenberg, W. and Haynes, R. B. (2000). *Evidence-Based Medicine. How to Practice and Teach EBM* (2nd edn). Edinburgh: Churchill Livingstone.

(section 5.3) because such tests have much in common with those for population screening. Issues of cost in clinical and preventive health care are briefly reviewed in Chapter 21 (section 21.4).

20.2 Evidence-Based Practice

In certain respects the use of evidence-based practice may seem self-evident to the modern practitioner; why would we not choose the most effective treatment for our patients? **Patients** are entitled to receive the best possible care or advice that is appropriate to their needs. **Practitioners** wish to deliver the best possible service, and those in public health or clinical practice who are responsible for allocating funding for services expect the best possible use of scarce health-care resources. Surprisingly, however, evidence-based practice is a comparatively recent development, fuelled by spiralling health costs and Cochrane's seminal work in the 1960s which showed that less than half of routine medical and surgical treatments were based on solid scientific evidence (Cochrane 1972).

Sackett *et al.* (2000) ▣ have identified the key steps of evidence-based practice which, in essence, provide a review of current practice, with a view to its improvement (Box 20.2).

The value of asking a **structured** (and answerable) **question** is twofold: firstly it defines the problem to be addressed; and secondly it provides terms that can be used in searching electronic databases for relevant information.

The elements of a structured question are determined by identifying the type of patient or problem for which information is being sought; defining the intervention and possible alternatives being considered; and considering which outcomes are of particular interest. Some examples are given in Table 20.1.

The first two questions relate to routine clinical problems in general practice, but both may require extra research and advice tailored to individual patient needs. The third example questions routine practice in an outpatient setting, and the remaining examples are from public-health practice.

20.3 Three Case Scenarios

To provide some worked examples of critical appraisal the following three case scenarios are derived from different branches of medicine. In the first example a simple, rapid screening test for deep-vein thrombosis is evaluated. In the second scenario you consider the

TABLE 20.1	Examples of structured clinical questions			
	Elements of the structured question			
	Patients or populations	**Problem**	**Intervention**	**Outcome**
A 58-year-old lady with a previous deep vein thrombosis requests hormone replacement therapy; you are aware of an increased risk of venous thrombo-embolism with this treatment and wish to discuss the issues with her to enable her to make an informed choice.	Post-menopausal women	History of deep vein thrombosis	Hormone replacement therapy	Risk of venous thrombo-embolism
A 75-year-old man presents with symptoms and signs of heart failure. You are considering digoxin therapy.	Elderly Patients	Heart failure	Digoxin therapy	Reduction in mortality
Patients in your OP clinic with anaemia routinely have serum ferritin levels measured. You want to know if this is helpful in distinguishing those with iron deficiency.	Patients	Anaemia	Ferritin measurement	Presence of iron deficiency
Your health board is implementing a breast screening programme and want to set a target against which to audit its effectiveness	Women	Death from breast cancer	Screening by mammography	Reduction in incidence
There has been a fall off in uptake of the MMR vaccine in your area and you have been tasked with preparing a case to present to the local media to increase awareness of the benefits of this programme.	Children under 5	Severe complications of measles	MMR vaccination	Reduction in incidence
You are preparing a teaching session on the benefits of seat-belt legislation for your local secondary school.	Car users	Death in road traffic accidents	Seat belt legislation	Reduction in traffic accident fatalities

evidence for restructuring the delivery of postnatal care in general practice. In the third case you are working as a public-health physician, and you are asked to advise on the effectiveness of workplace smoking bans.

Abstracts have been provided but readers may require the complete reports to fully work through these practical examples of the process of critical appraisal. Finally, the evidence-base is based on a continuous, dynamic process, and a current search of the research literature should always be made before recommending a change in medical practice.

Scenario 1: Evaluation of a study of a diagnostic test

You are a radiologist working in a UK hospital, with responsibility for providing duplex ultrasonography (DUS) for the investigation of patients suspected of having a deep-venous thrombosis (DVT). You have noticed that the demand for this test has increased to such an extent that you are no longer able to provide a timely service to referring clinicians. You have also noticed that less than 25 per cent of patients referred for DUS are shown to have a DVT. You recall a presentation at a conference you attended a couple of years ago where a unit, which seemed similar to yours, employed rapid fibrin D-dimer testing (a marker for clotting) before DUS. You find the paper relating to the conference presentation (Aschwanden et al. 1999) 💻 *and read it to assess whether the study is robust and relevant to your practice.*

ABSTRACT 1

Purpose Large studies have shown that most cases referred for duplex sonography for suspected deep-vein thrombosis (DVT) have normal scan results. For medical and economic reasons, a preselection procedure, which allows the detection of true-negative cases before duplex scanning, is required; this procedure should be characterized by a high sensitivity and a high negative predictive value.

Methods In 343 patients (398 lower extremities) with suspected DVT, the DVT probability was clinically assessed, and a whole blood D-dimer agglutination test and a duplex scan were performed. The diagnostic sensitivities of the D-dimer test alone, a high clinical DVT probability alone, and the combination of both were evaluated.

Results The sensitivity values for the D-dimer test to diagnose proximal and distal DVTs were 88.7 per cent and 80.9 per cent, the negative predictive values (NPV) were 96.3 per cent and 97.9 per cent, and the specificity and the positive predictive value (PPV) were 54.8 per cent and 49.6 per cent and 26.6 per cent and 8.2 per cent, respectively. The sensitivities of the clinical DVT probability assessment for the diagnosis of proximal and distal DVTs were 83.9 per cent and 66.7 per cent, respectively; the corresponding NPVs were 94.9 per cent and 96.5 per cent, respectively. The specificity was 56.1 per cent and 50.8 per cent, and the PPVs were 26.1 per cent and 7.0 per cent, respectively. The combined use of the results of the clinical probability assessment and the D-dimer test resulted in sensitivities for proximal and distal DVTs of 98.4 per cent and 90.5 per cent, NPVs of 99.3 per cent and 98.6 per cent, a specificity of 43.4 per cent and 38.4 per cent, and PPVs of 24.3 per cent and 7.6 per cent, respectively.

Conclusion The combined use of a clinical DVT probability assessment scheme and the D-dimer test largely avoids false negative results, has a high sensitivity and NPV, helps to reduce the costs of DVT diagnosis, and may, in the future, be useful as a preselection procedure before duplex sonography.

Reprinted from: Aschwanden, M. *et al.*, (1999) 'The Value of Rapid D-Dimer Testing Combined with Structured Clinical Evaluation for the Diagnosis of Deep Vein Thrombosis'. *Journal of Vascular Surgery*, **30** (5), 929–35. Copyright (1999), with permission from The Society of Vascular Surgery.

1. Are the results of the study valid?

(a) Was there an independent, blind comparison with a reference standard? *All patients in the study underwent structured clinical evaluation, a rapid D-dimer assay and the gold standard test, duplex ultrasonography. Operators applying each test were blind to the results of the other two tests.*

(b) Did the patient sample include an appropriate spectrum of patients to whom the diagnostic tests will be applied in clinical practice? *The study investigated consecutive patients referred to the Angiology Department of a university hospital in Switzerland in a 4 month period for investigation of suspected DVT. Seventeen out of*

360 patients were excluded because independent D-dimer testing was unavailable. No other exclusion criteria were applied. A wide range of ages, both sexes, and inpatients and outpatients were included.

(c) Did the results of the test being evaluated influence the decision to perform the reference standard? *All patients underwent all three tests.*

(d) Were the methods for performing the test described in sufficient detail to allow replication? *A commercial D-dimer assay was used, the manufacturer's details were provided, and a detailed description of how to use the test was referenced. The structured clinical evaluation used had been previously published and was referenced and its main components were listed.*

2. What are the results of the study?

(a) Are likelihood ratios for the test results presented or data necessary for their calculation provided? *Likelihood ratios were not presented but sensitivities, specificities, negative and positive predictive values (NPVs and PPVs) (for proximal and distal DVTs) were provided for the D-dimer assay alone and in combination with the result of the structured clinical evaluation (see Chapter 5 for NPVs and PPVs).*

(b) What are the main findings of the study? *The combination of a structured clinical evaluation and a rapid D-dimer assay has high sensitivity (98.4 per cent) and NPV (99.3 per cent) for identifying proximal DVTs. This means that, when applied together, the patients with a low clinical evaluation score and a negative D-dimer test were very unlikely to have a DVT. There was no difference in the performance of the combined tests (clinical evaluation and assay) between inpatients and outpatients.*

3. Will the results help me in providing a more timely investigative service for referring clinicians?

(a) Will the reproducibility of the test's results and their interpretation be satisfactory for my setting? *It would appear that all the tests applied in the study are reproducible within normal hospital practice.*

(b) Are the results applicable to my patients? *No specific exclusion criteria were applied so the findings should be applicable to patients from a similar setting. It may have been helpful for the authors to have included more information on their hospital (for example is it a tertiary referral centre) and the sources from which the patients were referred. This would enable you to judge how similar your setting and that of the study are.*

(c) Will the result of this study change your practice? *This is only one study and your literature review has identified a similar study published around the same time from a UK hospital. You need to obtain and assess this paper also. Perhaps a systematic review of all published studies has been done. To change your practice the agreement of referring clinicians is required. The more evidence you can muster, and the more robust it is, the more likely you are to receive their agreement. You could consider implementing the procedure within your department for a trial period and auditing the results.*

(d) Will patients benefit if your department employed a structured clinical evaluation and rapid D-dimer assay before DUS? *Any benefits to patients are likely to be indirect as DUS is a non-invasive procedure although access times for screening are likely to be faster. Cost savings and reduction of pressure on investigative services may enable resources to be invested in other important areas.*

Scenario 2

You are a UK general practitioner in a four-partner, semi-urban practice with a dynamic multidisciplinary primary health-care team and you have a particular interest in maternal and child health. At one of the team's monthly meetings the practice midwives draw your attention to the recently published results of a trial comparing redesigned midwife-led post-natal care to standard care (MacArthur et al. 2002). ⌨ The midwives would like your opinion on whether it would be appropriate to adopt this new approach to the delivery of post-natal care. You undertake to carefully assess the paper and discuss it, and its potential implications for the practice, at the next meeting of the primary health-care team.

Abstract 2

Background Much postpartum physical and psychological morbidity is not addressed by present care, which tends to focus on routine examinations. We undertook a cluster randomized controlled trial to assess community postnatal care that has been redesigned to identify and manage individual needs.

Methods We randomly allocated 36 general practice clusters from the West Midlands health region of the UK to intervention ($n = 17$) or control ($n = 19$) care. Midwives from the practices recruited women and provided care. 1087 (53 per cent) of 2064 women were in practices randomly assigned to the intervention group, with 977 (47 per cent) women in practices assigned to the control group. Care was led by midwives, with no routine contact with general practitioners, and was extended to 3 months. Midwives used symptom checklists and the Edinburgh postnatal depression scale (EPDS) to identify health needs and guidelines for the management of these needs. Primary outcomes at 4 months were obtained by postal questionnaire and included the women's short form 36 physical (PCS) and mental (MCS) component summary scores and the EPDS. Secondary outcomes were women's views about care. Multilevel analysis accounted for possible cluster effects.

Findings 801 (77 per cent) of 1087 women in the intervention group and 702 (76 per cent) of 977 controls responded at 4 months. Women's mental health measures were significantly better in the intervention group (MCS, 3.03 [95% CI 1.53–4.52]; EPDS, 1.92 [−2.55 to −1.29]; EPDS 13+, odds ratio 0.57 [0.43–0.76]) than in controls, but the physical health score did not differ.

Interpretation Redesign of care so that it is midwife-led, flexible, and tailored to needs, could help to improve women's mental health and reduce probable depression at 4 months' postpartum.

1. Are the results of the study valid?

(a) Was the assignment of patients to the intervention/non-intervention limb randomized? *Individual patients were not randomized within this trial, rather primary care practices were randomly allocated to intervention and non intervention limbs. 'Clustered' randomized controlled trials such as this are often the most appropriate method of assessing different methods of delivering care.*

(b) Were all patients who entered the trial properly accounted for and attributed at its conclusion? *All but one of the 37 practices that were randomized were accounted for at the end of the trial.*

(c) Was follow-up complete? *Women receiving postnatal care within these practices were recruited to provide information on their health and well-being and the quality of the care provided to them. Recruitment rates were similar in intervention and control practices. Response rates to the questionnaire at 4 months were 77 per cent and 76 per cent from intervention and control practices, respectively.*

(d) Were patients analysed in the groups to which they were randomized? *Yes, intention to treat analysis was* used and the clustered nature of the trial design was taken into consideration in the analysis.

(e) Were patients, health workers and study personnel blind to the intervention? *This was not possible, as is often the case in trials of the delivery of care.*

(f) Were the groups similar at the start of the trial? *There were some differences between intervention and control practices e.g. the proportion that were single handed practices, but the baseline characteristics of recruited women were very similar between the intervention and control limbs.*

(g) Aside from the experimental intervention were the groups treated equally? *Yes, and methods were used to try to minimize a possible Hawthorne effect (an additional positive bias) resulting from more enthusiastic care being delivered by midwives in the intervention limb.*

2. What were the results?

(a) What were the overall findings? *Physical health scores did not differ between the intervention and control groups but mental health scores were higher, (indicating better mental health), and post-natal depression scores lower, (indicating less depression) in the intervention group. Overall satisfaction with care did not differ between the groups. The mean total midwife visit duration time was 20 per cent higher in the intervention group. The mean number of home visits by GPs was the same in both groups.*

(b) How large was the treatment effect? *As the main outcome measures in this trial were physical and psychological well-being rather than the occurrence of an undesirable event, it is not possible to calculate absolute risk reductions as an event rate or numbers needed to treat to avoid such an event. The authors state that the three-point improvement in the mean mental health score seen in intervention group is similar to that associated with chronic lung disease, rheumatoid arthritis or vision impairment.*

(c) How precise was the estimate of the treatment effect? *The 95% confidence intervals around the difference in mean mental health score were 1.53 to 4.52.*

3. Will the results help you and the primary care team in delivering post-natal care to your patients?

(a) Are the results applicable to your primary care practice? *The trial was undertaken within primary care in the UK and practices were randomly selected to participate, although less than 50 per cent of eligible practices participated.*

The main reason for ineligibility was lack of agreement of midwife managers. The results should apply to your practice unless it differs substantially from other UK primary care practices.

(b) Were all clinically important outcomes considered? *The study concentrated on self-reported psychological well-being and patient satisfaction with the service, rather than on adverse events. This appears reasonable as childbirth is essentially a normal process.*

(c) Are the likely treatment benefits worth the potential harm and costs? *There was no evidence of harm occurring as a result of inclusion in the intervention group. The psychological well-being of women in the intervention group was improved but this was at some cost in terms of midwife time. A full cost-effectiveness analysis was not provided, but is planned. The resources required for midwife training appeared to be substantial.*

(d) Will you recommend that your primary care team adopt this approach to post-natal care? *The case for doing so is not yet clear as not all important outcomes were improved and a cost-effectiveness analysis has not been published. There are other important considerations that are likely to be beyond your control: agreement of midwife managers, training of midwives, changes to GP payment structures, indemnity issues, etc. It is unlikely that your practice can adopt this approach without the model being adopted on a regional or national basis. However, you may decide to accept an invitation to be the GP representative on your local Health Board's working group that is reviewing post-natal services.*

Scenario 3

You are working as a public-health physician within a Multidisciplinary Task Force whose remit is to provide policy advice to the UK Government on reducing smoking prevalence and population tobacco consumption. The Chairman has asked you report to the group on the effect of workplace smoking bans. You undertake a literature review and identify a recent **systematic review** *(Fitchenberg et al. 2002) 🖥 that has examined this issue. How will you assess whether the findings of this review are robust and report back to the group?*

Abstract 3

Objective To quantify the effects of smoke-free workplaces on smoking in employees and compare these effects to those achieved through tax increases.

Design Systematic review with a random effects meta-analysis.

Study selection 26 studies on the effects of smoke-free workplaces.

Setting Workplaces in the USA, Australia, Canada and Germany.

Participants Employees in unrestricted and totally smoke-free workplaces.

Main outcome measures Daily cigarette consumption (per smoker and per employee) and smoking prevalence.

Results Totally smoke-free workplaces are associated with reductions in prevalence of smoking of 3.8 per cent (95% confidence interval 2.8–4.7 per cent) and 3.1 (2.4–3.8) fewer cigarettes smoked per day per continuing smoker. Combination of the effects of reduced prevalence and lower consumption per continuing smoker yields a mean reduction of 1.3 cigarettes per day per employee, which corresponds to a relative reduction of 29 per cent. To achieve similar reductions the tax on a pack of cigarettes would have to increase from $0.76 to $3.05 ($0.78–3.14) in the USA and from £3.44 to £6.59 (£5.32–10.20) in the UK. If all workplaces became smoke-free, consumption per capita in the entire population would drop by 4.5 per cent in the USA and 7.6 per cent in the UK, costing the tobacco industry $1.7 billion and £310 million annually in lost sales. To achieve similar reductions tax per pack would have to increase to $1.11 and £4.26.

Conclusions Smoke-free workplaces not only protect non-smokers from the dangers of passive smoking, they also encourage smokers to quit or to reduce consumption.

Fichtenberg, C. M. and Glantz, S. A. (2002). *British Medical Journal*, **325**: 188, reproduced with permission from the BMJ Publishing Group.

1. Are the results of the study valid?

(a) Did the review address a focused question relevant to the task you have been charged with? *The review's objective was to quantify the effect of smoke-free workplaces (total workplace bans) on smoking by employees. The authors also aimed to compare the effects to those achieved by cigarette taxation increases.*

(b) Were the criteria used to select articles for inclusion appropriate? *Criteria for study selection were not clearly defined. Several types of study were included, all of which were observational in nature.*

(c) Is it unlikely that important relevant studies were missed? *All relevant databases were searched, as were other reviews and the references in identified studies. The authors do not mention that all relevant conference proceedings were examined or that experts in the field were contacted to identify suitable studies. However, a **funnel plot** (the effect estimate plotted against sample size) did not show evidence of publication bias.*

(d) Was the validity of the included studies appraised? *The studies were appraised but scant details on the process used were provided.*

(e) Were assessments of studies reproducible? *Details not provided.*

(f) Were the results similar from study to study? *There were no significant differences between study types for smoking prevalence, cigarette consumption per employee or relative change in consumption.*

2. What were the results?

(a) What are the main findings? *Implementation of totally smoke free workplace policies was associated with an absolute reduction (95% CI) in the prevalence of smoking of 3.8 (2.8, 4.7) and in daily cigarette consumption per continuing smoker of 3.1 (2.4, 3.8).*

(b) How precise were the results? *95% confidence intervals around the effect estimates were tight.*

(c) Were all relevant outcome measures assessed? *The effect on passive smoking was not assessed but this was not an objective of the review.*

(d) How do the results of the study relate to other work in the field? *The authors set the findings in context by comparing the effects of the workplace ban to those achieved by increasing taxation on cigarettes.*

3. Will the results assist you in reporting to the Task Force?

(a) Can the results be applied to 'your' population? *The studies included in the review were from Australia, Canada, Germany and the USA, but not the UK. However, the consistency of findings between countries indicates that they may be relevant to the UK population. Fewer workplaces in the UK than in the USA are smoke-free so country-wide legislation should be more effective in reducing cigarette consumption in the UK.*

(b) Are the benefits to the population worth the costs? *The costs of introducing workplace smoking bans were not assessed. However, large increases in cigarette taxation would be required to achieve the reduction in cigarette consumption possible from total workplace smoking bans.*

Estimates of the costs of implementing smoke-free work-place legislation in the UK are required.

(c) Are there alternative 'treatment' options? *Legislation for smoke-free work places is one of a range of options for reducing smoking prevalence and population tobacco consumption. Other possibilities include raising taxation, advertising bans, cessation assistance, etc. The Task Force needs to review and compare the evidence for and costs/benefits of each approach before reporting to the Government.*

4. General comment

Provision of more explicit detail on the methods used to appraise the studies reviewed would have enhanced confidence in the review's findings and enabled you to provide more definitive advice to the Task Force.

20.4 Working with Evidence-Based Practice

Figure 20.1 illustrates the major disciplines involved in the practice of health care and the multidisciplinary nature of the health service in a developed country.

In clinical practice, this has been defined as '**the conscientious, explicit and judicious use of current best evidence about the care of individual patients**' (Sackett *et al.* 1996). ▢ The need is for evidence about the accuracy of diagnostic tests, the power of prognostic markers, and the comparative **efficacy** and safety of interventions, all of which have been discussed in previous chapters. Clinical skills and clinical judgement are vital for determining whether the evidence (or guideline) applies to the individual patient at all and, if so, how. In addition, good practice in the care of patients requires consideration of the patient's wishes.

In public health practice, evidence used in this setting is to inform policy and public-health interventions rather than individual patient care. Nevertheless, the same principles may be applied and there is a similar need to integrate the findings from relevant research with the particular health needs and values of the population being served.

Between these two ends of the spectrum (the individual patient and the general population), lies the whole area of provision of health services, whose purpose is to benefit patient and population health. Here the perspective is the optimal pattern of care for groups of ill people; people with diabetes or breast cancer for example; or groups of people at risk of developing particular conditions, such as smokers or those with hypertension.

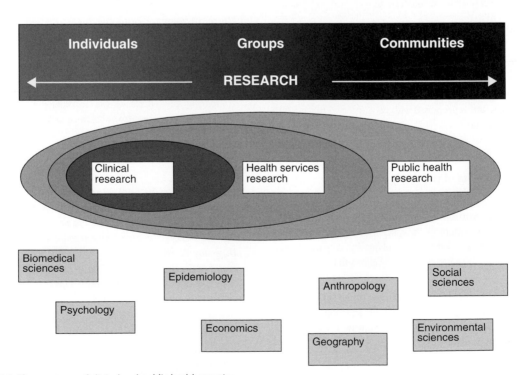

Fig. 20.1 The spectrum of clinical and public-health practice.

The evidence base for managed care is likely to include that used to inform both individual patient care and health-service organization. The former underpins the production of evidence-based guidelines (for example those produced by the National Institute for Clinical Excellence (NICE), and the Scottish Intercollegiate Group Network (SIGN)), whereas the latter could be expected to inform implementation strategies (for example the National Service Frameworks now available in the UK for coronary heart disease (CHD), for the Elderly, for Diabetes, and for Epilepsy, to name only a few topics).

Provision of health care is complex, and there are likely to be many more decisions, circumstances and questions than there is good quality evidence that will be able to inform all clinical decisions. Nevertheless, there is an obligation to be explicit about current practice and its evidence-base and what is uncertain, to make more balanced, cost-effective decisions about health care, and to inform the health-research agenda to address the gaps in knowledge.

A practical guide

In the examples quoted earlier in this chapter we have used the framework proposed by Sackett et al. (2000) ⌨ (Box 20.2) to guide the responses to the structured questions which were posed. Here we briefly review the remaining steps in achieving such outcomes in practice.

Effective and efficient searching

There is a bewildering range of information sources that may be considered in pursuit of evidence including textbooks, guidelines, consensus statements, original research, patients and colleagues, and electronic evidence databases. If the answer is not readily found in your textbook for your particular speciality then your search will probably turn to your computer.

The availability of electronic databases of published articles and original research such as PubMed, MEDLINE, and Embase can both aid and confound the search for relevant articles. A strategy is required before approaching these databases. The most efficient strategy is to look first among sources which have already been appraised, such as the Evidence-Based Reviews, the Cochrane Library which combines several databases, or evidence-based journals such as *Clinical Evidence* (BMJ Group), and *Best Evidence* (American College of Physicians) (see web addresses). If this draws a blank, then the original research literature must be searched and then appraised. While each electronic database will have its own instructions for use, the technique for efficient electronic searching has some common principles: consider the terminology used to define your patient population, intervention and outcome, and consider potential alternatives, particularly spelling; use Boolean operators ('and', 'or', 'not'); use limits such as language, subject, type of article; use 'clinical query' options where available. The resources of the local health library and its librarians should not be underestimated: they can provide helpful advice and training.

The type of evidence sought should be appropriate to the question being addressed: to address a question on therapy, the best evidence will be derived from a randomized controlled trial (RCT), or preferably a systematic review of several RCTs. To address a question on prognosis, a cohort study will produce the best information, while diagnosis would be best answered by information from a cross-sectional study (Chapter 3). The development of search filters designed to increase the relevant yield of articles in these categories has been helpful and is reviewed elsewhere (Haynes *et al.* 1994). ⌨

Critical appraisal of the literature

The evidence you have obtained from your search should be 'critically appraised' to discover whether it fully answers your question, for example 'How good is this treatment or intervention?' or 'How good is this test?' In evaluating the evidence presented, an assessment needs to be made of its **relevance** (generalizability) in relation to the setting in which it is to be used, whether or not it is **important** enough to implement, and whether or not it has **validity**.

Relevance

A study will be relevant if the results would help in caring for your patient or planning for your population. The assessment of relevance requires a comparison of the study subjects with your patient(s) or population; of the study setting and intervention with yours; and of the study outcome with the desired outcome for your patient(s) or population. In general, if your patient or population could have been included in the study, often the results are likely to be applicable to your situation. If there are differences in these elements, then the findings may need to be modified; if the differences are large, the study is unlikely to be able to address your question.

Importance

Any assessment of importance considers the measured outcome(s) of the study, the size of the effect and the level of statistical significance. Is the size of the effect likely to be important to your patient(s), to public health or to clinical diagnosis? For a study addressing an intervention the effect size may be presented as a difference, a ratio or as a 'number needed to treat' (NNT), along with the appropriate **confidence interval** (see Glossary). The importance of a study of the performance of a diagnostic test is assessed by asking how well the test distinguishes patients who have a specific disorder. This is summarized in measures of test performance (see Chapter 5) such as sensitivity, specificity, positive and negative predictive values, and likelihood ratios.

The study report should contain these estimates or at least present the data required for their calculation.

Validity

The validity of a study is assessed by determining to what extent study findings can be supported. **Internal validity** reflects the assessment of the adequacy of the study design and **external validity** places the study finding against those of other studies.

The specific criteria by which the validity of a study can be assessed will vary according to the type of question being addressed and the type of study design used. The validity of a study of therapy or prevention can be assessed by using the questions set out in Box 20.3 (Guyatt *et al.* 1993, 1994). 🖳

BOX 20.3 **VALIDITY OF A STUDY OF THERAPY/PREVENTION**

- Was the assignment of treatments randomized?
- Was follow-up complete and for long enough?
- Were all the patients analysed in the groups to which they were randomized (an intention to treat analysis)
- Were patients and clinicians kept 'blinded' to the treatment?
- Were groups treated equally?
- Were groups similar at the start of the trial?

Sources: Guyatt, G. H., Sackett, D. L. and Cook, D. J. (1993) 'Users' Guides to the Medical Literature. II. How to Use an Article about Therapy or Prevention. A. Are the Results Valid?' *Journal of the American Medical Association,* **270**: 2598–601.
Guyatt, G. H., Sackett, D. L. and Cook, D. J. (1994). 'Users' Guides to the Medical Literature. II. How to use an Article about Therapy or Prevention. B. What Were the Results and Will They Help Me in Caring for My Patients?' *Journal of the American Medical Association,* **271**: 59–63.

BOX 20.4 **VALIDITY OF A STUDY OF A DIAGNOSTIC TEST**

- Was there an independent, blind comparison with a reference 'gold standard'?
- Was the test evaluated in an appropriate spectrum of patients?
- Was the reference standard applied regardless of the diagnostic test result?
- Was the test validated in a second, independent group of patients?
- Were the methods for performance of the test described in sufficient detail to allow their replication?

Sources: Jaeschke, R., Guyatt, G. H. and Sackett, D. L. (1994a). 'DL Users' Guides to the Medical Literature. III. How to Use an Article about a Diagnostic Test. A. Are the Results of the Study Valid?' *Journal of the American Medical Association,* **271**: 389–91.
Jaeschke, R., Guyatt, G. H. and Sackett, D. L. (1994b). 'Users' Guides to the Medical Literature. III. How to Use an Article about a Diagnostic Test. B. What Were the Results and Will They Help Me in Caring for My Patients?' *Journal of the American Medical Association,* **271**: 703–7.

For diagnosis, the best evidence is derived from a cross-sectional study in which a comparison of the results of the test undergoing evaluation against a gold standard which is used to define the presence of disease. Both are applied to the same group of patients and an assessment made of the number of times the two tests agree or differ. Box 20.4 shows questions that can be used to assess such studies (Jaeschke *et al.* 1994a, b). 🖳

Reviews of evidence

In general, questions about health and health care are inadequately addressed by single studies. The most robust conclusions are derived from an examination of the totality of available evidence relevant to the question being addressed. Such literature reviews may include only one type of evidence, for example, several RCTs of a particular intervention. Alternatively, they may derive information from a range of study designs; for example, a review examining water fluoridation contained studies with a range of designs, from ecological to cohort studies (see Chapter 19, section 19.1).

As well as summarizing large amounts of information, reviews have the following merits: they increase statistical power; improve the accuracy and precision of the estimated effect, assess the consistency and generalizability of findings; and can help to explain heterogeneity among studies. All of these attributes provide better building blocks for decision making. Furthermore, they may prevent the unnecessary duplication of research effort.

The key element in producing a good quality review is that it is **systematic**: that is, it is prepared using an explicit, systematic approach to minimize biases and random errors. This means that its scope, evidence-base, criteria for inclusion and exclusion of primary studies, studies which use original data, and data extraction and analysis techniques, are clearly stated. In contrast to the conventional review which usually summarizes the information available from only the author's perspective a systematic approach minimizes bias arising from an incomplete selection of studies, inappropriate synthesis of data, and subjective interpretation of primary evidence (Cook *et al.* 1995). 🖳

A further requirement for a good quality review is that the primary studies selected are themselves of good quality. Therefore the inclusion criteria for the review should include those based on an assessment of the methodological quality of the primary studies, i.e. the internal validity of the individual primary studies.

The term **meta-analysis** is used to describe a quantitative synthesis of primary data which yields an overall summary statistic. The synthesis may involve the reanalysis of individual level data collected in the primary studies, or combining the published summary statistics from individual primary studies. It is generally only reasonable to do this if the results from primary studies are consistent. If individual study results show significant **heterogeneity**, an explanation for this should be sought and tested using a **sensitivity analysis** or meta-regression technique (Chapter 4). Figure 20.2 shows an example of a **meta-analysis** of the effectiveness of intensive advice for smoking cessation. In this example, three of the controlled trials eligible for inclusion showed inconclusive results, while two showed positive, statistically significant, results. The combined odds ratio was 1.32 (95% CI 1.18, 1.48) that the intensive advice was superior to routine practice.

In critically appraising a systematic review, relevance and importance are assessed as for primary studies. Relevance will be determined by the similarity of your population/patient/setting to the study populations, interventions and outcomes, which are the focus of the review. Significant heterogeneity (systematic differences in study populations, etc.) indicates that the relevance to general populations may be limited. Importance is assessed by considering

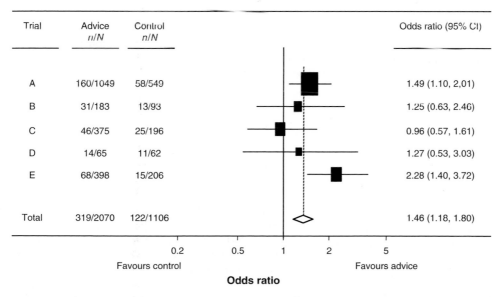

Trial	Advice n/N	Control n/N		Odds ratio (95% CI)
A	160/1049	58/549		1.49 (1.10, 2.01)
B	31/183	13/93		1.25 (0.63, 2.46)
C	46/375	25/196		0.96 (0.57, 1.61)
D	14/65	11/62		1.27 (0.53, 3.03)
E	68/398	15/206		2.28 (1.40, 3.72)
Total	319/2070	122/1106		1.46 (1.18, 1.80)

Odds ratio

Favours control   Favours advice

Test for difference between advice and control: $\chi^2 = 12.4$, d.f. = 1; $P < 0.001$.
Test for heterogeneity between trials: $\chi^2 = 6.02$, d.f. = 4; $P = 0.20$.

Fig. 20.2 Meta-analysis of quitting rates in controlled trials of intensive advice for smoking cessation. Data derived from: Ashenden, R., Silagy, C. and Weller, D. (1997). 'A Systematic Review of the Effectiveness of Promoting Lifestyle Change in General Practice'. *Family Practice*, **14**: 160–76.

BOX 20.5 APPRAISAL OF A SYSTEMATIC REVIEW

- Did the review address a clearly focused question in terms of the population studied, intervention applied and outcomes considered?
- Did the studies that were sought have the appropriate design to address the issue?
- Was the search strategy used to find primary studies described and was it appropriate and comprehensive? Could important studies have been missed?
- What were the criteria for inclusion and exclusion of primary studies? Did this include an appraisal of the primary studies for methodological quality?
- Were the results similar from study to study or was there heterogeneity among primary study results? If the results of primary studies were combined in a meta-analysis, was it appropriate to do so?
- Was a sensitivity analysis presented?
- Are the author's conclusions supported by the evidence presented?
- Are recommendations linked to the strength of the evidence presented?

Source: Oxman, A. D., Cook, D. J. and Guyatt, G. H. (1994). 'Users' Guides to the Medical Literature. VI. How to Use an Overview'. *Journal of the American Medical Association*, **272**: 1367–71.

BOX 20.6 ASSESSING THE USEFULNESS OF EVIDENCE

- Do the results apply to your patient/population?
- Is the treatment feasible in your setting?
- What are your patient's/population's potential benefits and harms from the treatment?
- What are your patient's/population's values and expectations for both the outcome you are trying to prevent and for the treatment you are offering?

Source: Sackett, D. L., Straus, S. E., Richardson, W. S., Rosenberg, W. and Haynes, R. B. (2000). *Evidence-Based Medicine. How to Practice and Teach EBM* (2nd edn). Edinburgh: Churchill Livingstone.

---

how big an effect is evident, how precise is the estimate of effect, and whether the effect is clinically significant.

The assessment of validity is an evaluation of the methodology used in the review. Some of the validity criteria for the review will be the same as those presented for primary studies, and will depend on the focus of the review: therapy, diagnosis, etc. Additional questions that need to be addressed for appraisal of reviews are listed in Box 20.5.

Systematic reviews and meta-analyses, which will be increasingly available to guide medical practice and public-health policies, are discussed in further detail elsewhere (Eggar *et al.* 1997, 2002). ▢

Applying the evidence

Once relevant, valid, and important information is identified, it needs to be applied to the care of a particular patient or to the provision of a service or information for a particular population. This requires integrating the evidence with the particular

circumstances and values of the patient or population concerned. An assessment of usefulness would include the questions in Box 20.6 (Sackett *et al.* 2000). ▢

The evidence may point to a particular action but the individual benefit to a patient may be small enough to warrant doing nothing. Other obstacles to implementing the evidence include patients' values and preferences, geography, economics, administrative or organizational characteristics, traditions and 'expert' opinion. Ultimately, only the first of these is an acceptable reason for not applying evidence in practice. Implementing evidence may also require a change in behaviour from service providers and/or patients. This may not be achievable: all that evidence can do is to specify the recommended behaviour.

There will often be evidence to suggest change in several areas. In balancing the cost of applying one guideline rather than another cost-effectiveness criteria may be useful (see Chapter 21).

Evaluating the impact of evidence on your routine practice

Just as evidence is sought for the effectiveness of health-care practices, so should we assess whether this has become incorporated into our routine practice. This can be approached through the process of **health-care audit**, looking at both processes and outcomes of care, and through an assessment of personal practice. The questions in Box 20.7 are useful in assessing your personal practice (Sackett *et al.* 2000). ▢

The scheme illustrated in Figure 20.3 sets out the three dimensions of personal practice of evidence-based medicine; the clinical problem; sources of evidence used; and level of critical appraisal skills.

Traditionally, during professional training students tend to start at the origin of these three scales using supplied information that is not necessarily linked to specific clinical or public-health problems, and followed intuitively. Increasingly, however, curricula are moving towards **problem-based learning** incorporating many of the principles discussed in this chapter. On graduating to clinical practice, clinicians move on to the clinical problem scale with information needs firmly grounded in patient and service issues. Attainment of fully established evidence-based practice requires continuous development of personal skills in searching research databases and in critical appraisal. New studies are continuously added to research databases, and periodic updating of your routine practice should become an integral part of any programme of continuous professional development.

In this chapter we have briefly described the discipline of clinical epidemiology and shown how epidemiological tools can be used in routine clinical or public-health practice. The development of critical appraisal skills is likely to develop during undergraduate training, and in clinical practice should be incorporated into a programme of continuous professional development.

Further Reading

Brownson, R. C., Baker, E. A., Leet, T. and Gillespie, K. N. (2003). *Evidence-Based Public Health*. New York, NY: Oxford University Press.

Cochrane, A. L. (1972). *Effectiveness and Efficiency*. Nuffield Provincial Hospitals Trust.

Eggar, M., Davey Smith, G. and Sterne, J. A. C. (2002). 'Systematic Reviews and Meta-analysis', in R. Detels, J. McEwen, R. Beaglehole and H. Taneka (eds.), *Oxford Textbook of Public Health*, vol. 2 (4th edn). Oxford: Oxford University Press, 655–75.

Fletcher, R. H., Fletcher, S. E. and Wagner, E. H. (1996). *Clinical Epidemiology. The Essentials*. Baltimore, MD: Williams and Wilkins.

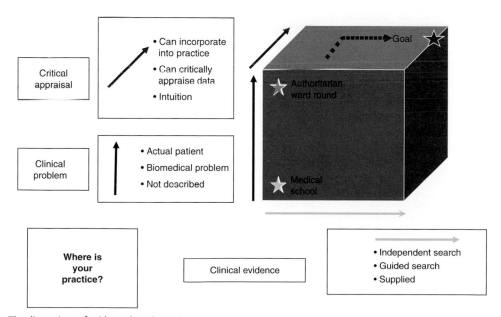

Fig. 20.3 The dimensions of evidence-based practice.

Muir Gray, J. A. (2001). *Evidence-Based Healthcare. How to Make Health Policy and Management Decisions* (2nd edn). Edinburgh: Churchill Livingstone.

Sackett, D. L., Haynes, R. B., Guyatt, G. H. and Tugwell, P. (1991). *Clinical Epidemiology. A Basic Science for Clinical Medicine* (2nd edn). Boston, MA: Little, Brown and Company.

Sackett, D. L., Straus, S. E., Richardson, W. S., Rosenberg, W. and Haynes, R. B. (2000). *Evidence-Based Medicine. How to Practice and Teach EBM* (2nd edn). Edinburgh: Churchill Livingstone.

Web Addresses

Annals of Internal Medicine (American College of Physicians) (Best Evidence Series), www.annals.org.

Cochrane Library, www.cochrane.org, www.update-software.com.

National Electronic Library, www.nelh.nhs.uk.

National Institute of Clinical Excellence, www.nice.org.uk.

NHS PRODIGY, www.prodigy.nhs.uk.

BMJ Clinical Evidence Series, www.clinicalevidence.com.

Effective Health Care Reviews, www.york.ac.uk/inst/crd.

Scottish Intercollegiate Guidelines Network, www.sign.ac.uk.

Centre for Evidence-Based Medicine, www.cebm.org. The ScHARR Introduction to Evidence-Based Practice on the Internet, www.nettingtheevidence.org.uk.

References

References for this chapter can be found at www.oxfordtextbooks.co.uk/orc/yarnell. Where possible, these are presented as *active links* which direct you to an electronic version of the work. If you are a subscriber to that work (either individually or through an institution), and depending on your level of access, you may be able to peruse an abstract or the full article if available. 🖳

Epidemiology in public-health practice

This chapter introduces the topic of public-health practice, of which epidemiology is a core science. International, national, and local public-health practice are reviewed under five broad headings: health protection and disease prevention (see also Chapter 16); health improvement (see Chapter 17); the evaluation of public and personal health-care services; economics of health care; and prevention in public-health and clinical practice. Key themes in this chapter are the importance of adopting a systematic approach to population health assessment, and generation of pragmatic and workable public-health strategies. Several important sources of information, mostly electronic, are given at the end of this chapter and are intended for additional self-directed learning.

Introduction

The public-health function has been defined as '**the science and art of preventing disease, prolonging life and promoting health through organized efforts of society**' (Acheson 1988). 🖳 The 'science of public health' requires a robust, systematic, and evidence-based approach to describe and understand population health issues, and to identify optimal solutions for health improvement from available resources. The 'art of public health' refers to the interpersonal and organizational skills needed to work in partnership with others, influence decisions, support implementation of policy, programmes or projects, and to produce significant improvements in health indicators.

Core activities in public health are summarized in Box 21.1.

BOX 21.1 CORE ACTIVITIES IN PUBLIC HEALTH

1 Preventing epidemics.
2 Protecting the environment, workplaces, food and water.
3 Promoting healthy behaviour.
4 Monitoring the health status of the population.
5 Mobilizing community action.
6 Responding to disasters.
7 Assuring the quality, accessibility, and accountability of medical care.
8 Reaching out to link high-risk and hard-to-reach people to needed services.
9 Research to develop new insights and innovative solutions.
10 Leading the development of sound health policy and planning.

Source: Pencheon, D., Guest, C., Melzer, D. and Muir Gray, J. A. (eds.) (2001). *Oxford Handbook of Public Health Practice.* Oxford: Oxford University Press.

21.1 Health Protection and Disease Prevention

The prevention of disease and maintenance of health in the population have long been core functions of public health requiring key epidemiological skills. These skills include *surveillance* and *monitoring* skills, both for disease, risk factors, and for health status, and *organizational* and *implemental* skills in dealing with outbreaks of infectious diseases or influencing health-related behaviours. Increasingly, public-health practitioners will be required also to have basic skills in *health economics*, both for the role of managing health-care resources and in the development of cost-effective models for disease prevention. In summary, public-health practitioners work to improve and protect population health by public-health actions (at any organizational level), and to develop or modify health systems.

The **World Health Organization** (WHO) has two major key roles in global public health; surveillance and monitoring of disease and health status; the development of strategies to control infections, both epidemic and endemic, and chronic, non-infectious disease, in adults and children. The WHO was established

under the auspices of the United Nations in 1948 as a response to the dire state of European and world health after World War II, which was caused by five years of intense conflict, destruction of cities, towns, and villages, and inadequate food supplies. The work of the WHO in developing **health information systems** such as the International Classification of Diseases was summarized in Chapter 2, while its role in combating epidemics of cardiovascular disease (Chapter 6), obesity and diabetes (Chapter 8), emerging infectious diseases (Chapter 16), and tobacco control (Chapter 17), have been noted. Several special programmes to eliminate diseases such as smallpox (the first successfully eradicated major infectious disease), polio and leprosy, to reduce the global burdens of tuberculosis, malaria and acquired immune deficiency syndrome (AIDS), and international public-health programmes to attempt to control tobacco use, are among the many activities coordinated by WHO. The major work programmes of WHO in 2004 are summarized in Box 21.2.

At national levels, different organizational structures are found which promote public-health practice. In the USA the Centers for Disease Control (CDC) have been established for many years and provide the main focus for the policy support for the public-health service, whereas in the UK this is provided by the Faculty of Public Health (London). In the UK the Health Protection and the Food Standards Agencies were recently formed to oversee standards and control policies in environmental and food hazards with a view to future developments at a European level.

The CDC has a mission statement which reads '... working with partners throughout the nation and world to monitor health, detect and investigate health problems, conduct research to enhance prevention, develop and advocate sound public health policies, implement prevention strategies, promote healthy behaviors, foster safe and healthful environments, and provide leadership and training'. Twelve centres with different functions form the basis of CDC programmes and activities; these are listed in Box 21.3. Further information for each of the programmes is available at the CDC website (CDC 2004). 💻

In contrast, the UK Health Protection Agency, which combines several existing organizations, is in its infancy and recently published its strategic goals (Ayres and Agius 2004) 💻 (Box 21.4). Its work in the control of communicable disease is discussed in Chapter 16. A broader, long term, view of health and its determinants was highlighted by recently proposed indicators of

BOX 21.2 MAJOR WORK PROGRAMMES OF THE WORLD HEALTH ORGANIZATION 2004

Sustainable Development and Healthy Environments

- Protection of the Human Environment
- Food Safety
- Health Millennium Development Goals
- Health and Development Policy
- Ethics, Trade, Human Rights and Law

Evidence and Information for Policy

- Health System Financing, Expenditure and Resource Allocation
- Health System Policy and Operations
- Human Resources for Health
- Knowledge Management and Sharing
- Measurement and Health Information Systems
- Research Policy and Cooperation

HIV/AIDS, TB and Malaria

- HIV/AIDS
- Stop TB Partnership
- Roll Back Malaria Partnership
- Strategic Planning and Innovation

Health Technology and Pharmaceuticals

- Essential Drugs and Medicines Policy
- Essential Health Technologies

Family and Community Health

- Child and Adolescent Health and Development
- Reproductive Health and Research
- Making Pregnancy Safer and Women's Health
- Immunization, Vaccines and Biologicals

Non-Communicable Diseases and Mental Health

- Health Promotion, Surveillance Prevention and Management of Non-communicable Diseases
- Injuries and Violence Prevention
- Nutrition for Health and Development
- Mental Health and Substance Abuse
- Tobacco Free Initiative

Communicable Diseases

- Communicable Diseases Surveillance and Response
- Communicable Diseases Control, Prevention and Eradication
- Special Programme for Research and Training in Tropical Diseases

Source: WHO (2004).

sustainable development from the UK Department of Environment, Food and Rural Affairs (DEFRA), also shown in Box 21.4. The need to co-ordinate strategic goals between different government agencies has been stressed by Ayres and Agius (2004), ▢ and the recognition that these goals fall under the general remit of national, local, and international public health should assist this process. Further information on the organization and function of the Health Protection and Food Standards Agencies is provided on their respective websites (Health Protection Agency 2005; Food Standards Agency 2005). ▢

21.2 Health Improvement

A key skill for public-health practice, and a prerequisite for health improvement, is 'health (care) needs assessment'. This has been defined specifically as 'the assessment of the population's ability to benefit from health care' (Stevens *et al.* 2004). ▢ In public-health terms, 'needs' should incorporate both a description of the difference between the current situation and the optimal population health status, and the capacity to reduce any 'gap' by a specified health action. The perspective of the public-health practitioner is related to populations

BOX 21.3 ORGANIZATIONAL GROUPINGS OF THE CENTERS FOR DISEASE CONTROL (USA)

National Center on Birth Defects and Developmental Disabilities (NCBDDD) provides national leadership for preventing birth defects and developmental disabilities and for improving the health and wellness of people with disabilities.

National Center for Chronic Disease Prevention and Health Promotion (NCCDPHP) prevents premature death and disability from chronic diseases and promotes healthy personal behaviours.

National Center for Environmental Health (NCEH) provides national leadership in preventing and controlling disease and death resulting from the interactions between people and their environment.

National Center for Health Statistics (NCHS) provides statistical information that will guide actions and policies to improve the health of the American people.

National Center for HIV, STD, and TB Prevention (NCHSTP) provides national leadership in preventing and controlling human immunodeficiency virus infection, sexually transmitted diseases, and tuberculosis.

National Center for Infectious Diseases (NCID) prevents illness, disability, and death caused by infectious diseases in the United States and around the world.

National Center for Injury Prevention and Control (NCIPC) prevents death and disability from non-occupational injuries, including those that are unintentional and those that result from violence.

National Immunization Program (NIP) prevents disease, disability and death from vaccine-preventable diseases in children and adults.

National Institute for Occupational Safety and Health (NIOSH) ensures safety and health for all people in the workplace through research and prevention.

Epidemiology Program Office (EPO) strengthens the public health system by co-ordinating public health surveillance; providing support in scientific communications, statistics, and epidemiology; and training in surveillance, epidemiology, and prevention effectiveness.

Public Health Practice Program Office (PHPPO) strengthens community practice of public health by creating an effective workforce, building information networks, conducting practice research, and ensuring laboratory quality.

Office of the Director (CDC/OD) manages and directs the activities of the Centers for Disease Control and Prevention; provides overall direction to, and co-ordination of, the scientific/medical programs of CDC; and provides leadership, coordination, and assessment of administrative management activities.

CDC performs many of the administrative functions for the Agency for Toxic Substances and Disease Registry (ATSDR), a sister agency of CDC, and one of eight federal public health agencies within the Department of Health and Human Services. The Director of CDC also serves as the Administrator of ATSDR

Future challenges

Challenges that CDC faces in the future are highlighted below. CDC's mission and programs clearly focus upon these challenges. Specific action steps for each challenge are described briefly.

Improving People's Health by Putting Science into Action

Preventing Violence and Unintentional Injury

Meeting the Health and Safety Needs of a Changing Workforce

Utilizing New Technologies to Provide Credible Health Information

Protecting Individuals against Emerging Infection Diseases including Bioterrorism

Eliminating Racial/Ethnic Health Disparities

Fostering Safe and Healthy Environments

Working with Partners to Improve Global Health

Futures Initiative

Source: Centers for Disease Control (2004), http://www.cdc.gov/.

BOX 21.4 1. HEALTH PROTECTION AGENCY: STRATEGIC GOALS

To prevent and reduce impact and consequences of infectious diseases.

To anticipate and prevent the adverse health effects of acute and chronic exposure to hazardous chemicals and other poisons.

To reduce the adverse effects of exposure to ionizing and non-ionizing radiation.

To identify, prepare, and respond to new and emerging diseases and health threats.

To identify and develop appropriate responses to childhood diseases associated with infections, chemical or radiation hazards.

To improve preparedness of responses to health protection emergencies, including those caused by deliberate release.

To strengthen information and communication systems for identifying and tracking diseases and exposures to infectious, chemical, and radiological hazards.

To build and improve the evidence base through a comprehensive programme of research.

To develop a skilled and motivated workforce.

To manage knowledge and share expertise and strengthen international working.

To build on and develop the intellectual assets of the organization in partnership with industry and other customers.

To raise the understanding of health protection and the involvement of the public so that there is access to authoritative, impartial, and timely information and advice.

2. Headline Indicators of Sustainable Development

Economic
Economic output
Investment
Employment
Social
Poverty and social exclusion
Education
Health
Housing
Crime
Environmental
Climate change
Air quality
Road traffic
River water quality
Wildlife
Land use
Waste

Source: Ayres, J. G. and Agius, R. (2004). 'Health Protection and Sustainable Development: Time for Joined Up Thinking'. *British Medical Journal*, 328: 1450–1, reproduced with permission from the BMJ Publishing Group.

---

rather than to individuals, and **population health gain** does not necessarily mean that the health of *every* individual in a population will be positively affected. In recognition of the scarcity of resources, the discipline of economics differentiates between *wants*, *demands*, and *supply*, whereas sociologists refer to *felt*, *expressed*, and *normative* needs (Figure 21.1). It is unreasonable to generalize needs assessment findings from one population to another without local consultation, as the definition and interpretation of 'need' may be subject to many external influences (Figure 21.2).

The epidemiological approach to health assessment

The epidemiological approach (Box 21.5A) provides a generic framework to quantify and describe the health of a given population. A cautionary note is provided by a former Nobel prizewinner (Box 21.5B).

It is not possible to assess every health issue so activities are often focused on 'fire-fighting' and on 'apparent' problems. However, specific assessments (Box 21.6) may be indicated following: the results of previous assessment; political or public input; allocation of 'ring-fenced' funding for service development; the occurrence of a critical or major incident; or the publication of new research, guidelines or standards.

Although the epidemiological approach can provide an estimate of the size of a particular health issue, this may not be sufficient to capture all potentially relevant factors (for example political and bureaucratic). Identifying feasible solutions often requires the use of methodology from other disciplines such as the social

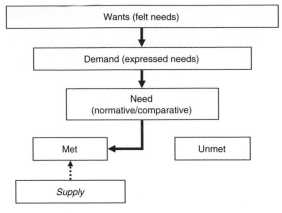

Fig. 21.1 Economic and sociological constructs of need.
Adapted from: Wright, J., Williams, D. R. R and Wilkinson, J. (1998).
'The Development of Health Needs Assessment', in *Health Needs Assessment in Practice* (ed. J. Wright), London: BMJ Books, 1–11.

BOX 21.5 **EPIDEMIOLOGICAL APPROACH TO HEALTH ASSESSMENT**

A.   I. Scope and define the health issue(s).

    II. Agree population health assessment aims and objectives.

    III. Define and profile the 'population base' and subgroups: denominator(s).

    IV. Define health events or health related factors: numerator(s).

    V. Collect, collate, and analyse data.

    VI. Interpret results appropriately.

    VII. Disseminate findings to support informed decisions and choices.

B.   'Not everything that counts can be counted and not everything that can be counted, counts.'

           Albert Einstein (letter to President Roosevelt)

Source: Stevens, A., Raftery, J., Mant, J. and Simpson, S. (eds.) (2004). *Health Care Needs Assessment: The Epidemiologically Based Needs Assessment Reviews*. Oxford: Radcliffe Publishing, http://hcna.radcliffe-oxford.com/ (accessed 2004).

---

sciences, psychology, economics, management, and politics.

Public-health observatories

In recognition of the wider socioeconomic determinants of health status, the Chief Medical Officer for England launched the Public Health Observatories in English NHS regions in the year 2000 to provide health information to examine and reduce health inequalities between local authority districts and to monitor

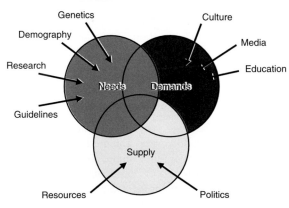

Fig. 21.2 External influences and relationship between needs, demands, and supply.
Adapted from: Stevens, A., Raftery, J., Mant, J. and Simpson, S. (eds.) (2004). *Health Care Needs Assessment: The Epidemiologically Based Needs Assessment Reviews*. Oxford: Radcliffe Publishing. Available from: http//hcna.radcliffe-oxford.com/(accessed 2004).

improvements over time (Association of Public Health Observatories 2004). ⌨ Currently, data are taken from the annual Health Surveys for England, and re-analysed at Health Authority level; comparable data are not available for other UK regions. However, across the UK *Health Improvement Areas* have been designated at local level to undergo pilot projects which seek to improve the health of people living in materially deprived local districts. It is hoped that future public-health initiatives to reduce health inequalities will use the results of these pilot studies to develop wider policies. The issues have been recently well summarized in a government-sponsored report 'Public health policy in England: lessons to be learnt' (Wanless *et al.* 2004). ⌨

21.3 **Evaluation of Public Health and Personal Health Care**

Just as epidemiological skills are required in the evaluation of public-health strategies, policies, and programmes, such skills are also required for the evaluation of the personal (clinical) health-care services. In most countries such services can be broadly divided into primary care and the specialist hospital services, either as

---

BOX 21.6 EXAMPLES OF POPULATION-LEVEL HEALTH ASSESSMENTS

Health status assessment: to identify, scope, characterize and quantify health issues or problems experienced by a specified population.

Health needs assessment: to determine and implement the optimal local solution to a specified population health issue or problem, on the basis of robust evidence, feasibility, stakeholder input, and available resources.

Health impact assessment (HIA): to estimate potential health effects resulting from a specified action, not primarily undertaken to impact on health. The actions may range in scope and scale from a local project (for example new industrial installation – Integrated Pollution Prevention and Control regulatory system) to national policy (for example integrated transport strategy).

Health risk assessment: to estimate the potential impact of a chemical, biological, physical, or social agent on a specified human population system under a specific set of conditions and for a certain timeframe.

Health care assessment: to evaluate existing services, and identify potential quality improvement through redesign, modification, or development.

---

mortality (McKeown 1976) 💻 (Figure 1.1). At the beginning of the twenty-first century child and adult mortality have been further reduced but now personal health care may also play an important role in national health status. How can health service **inputs** and **outcomes** be best measured and compared? Clearly standard indicators available for most countries are required. In early studies (for example Cochrane *et al.* 1978) 💻 input was measured by health-service expenditure (adjusted to a standard cost of living index) and health-service staffing; and output measured by infant, maternal, and premature adult mortality, and life expectancy. More recently, coverage of primary care has been added to input together with several additional outputs, which include life expectancy adjusted for quality (QALY) or disability (DALY) (see Chapters 12, 13, and 17). A recent WHO Annual Report (WHO 2000) 💻 addressed the question 'How well do health systems perform?' and produced a combined output index based on three indicators: disability-adjusted life expectancy (DALE), responsiveness (a measure of patient satisfaction based on the perceived responsiveness of health service personnel to personal need) and financial fairness (a measure of equality of access) (WHO 2000). 💻 The rank order for a sample of countries according to this index of 'health output' was: France 1, Italy 2, Norway 11, UK 18, Ireland 19, Switzerland 20 and US 37. Rank order based on DALE alone was: Japan 1, Australia 2, France 3, Sweden 4, Italy 6, Switzerland 8, UK 14, US 24, Ireland 27, but the range of DALEs in these developed countries was only five years: from 74.5 years (Japan) to 69.6 years (Ireland).

In the 50 countries with the lowest life expectancies it is unsurprising that most are in Africa; Bangladesh is among the handful of countries outside that continent (49.9 years) while South Africa, Ethiopia, Zimbabwe, Uganda, and Sierra Leone record DALEs of 39.8, 33.5, 32.9, 32.7, and 25.9 years, respectively. AIDS, malnutrition, and civil war largely account for this premature mortality. Models of health service inputs and outputs are still in their infancy and require further development.

Individual health care

Individual health care operates at three points in the development of disease: at the primary, secondary, and tertiary stages. Although public-health prevention mainly operates at the primary and secondary stages, increasingly primary care, in the UK at least, is taking a greater role in primary prevention. Evaluation of treatments and other medical interventions are fully

in- or out-patients. Primary care (general) practitioners are the 'gatekeepers' for access to specialist services in many countries, and health systems which allow direct access may be more wasteful of resources, and costly to maintain. Clearly the diversity of health-care systems and the absence of any experimental data make comparisons of the **effectiveness** and **efficiency** of different health-care systems very difficult. Nevertheless, such international comparisons have been made, and may be essential to future developments of health-care systems, both in the poorest countries with underdeveloped health sectors, and in wealthy countries where costs and public expectations have spiralled ever upwards.

International comparisons

In Chapter 1 we noted that improved living conditions and nutrition had a major impact in reducing childhood

discussed in Chapter 20 and in the evaluation of screening programmes in Chapter 5. The 'gold standard' in such evaluations is the randomized controlled trial, which is used in all branches of medicine, including public health. The process of continuously updating the evidence of benefit for patients may cause upheavals in medical practice, particularly for treatments that are popular with patients and well-established in practice. One example is provided by hormone-replacement therapy, which appeared beneficial and justified from observational studies, but an expensive, long-term trial was prematurely stopped in the USA when a significant excess of cardiovascular and cancer (breast and endometrial) events was reported (Grodstein *et al.* 2003). 🖳 Full discussion of the evaluation of clinical preventive services and public-health initiatives is beyond the scope of this textbook, but useful summaries are available elsewhere (Haddix *et al.* 2003). 🖳

Clinical governance

Epidemiological, organizational, other multidisciplinary and clinical skills are required in the setting of standards of quality in clinical care (clinical governance), which is required in all specialities. These standards encompass both the optimal cost-effective delivery of health care under differing systems, and clinical standards that may be expected by patients. The UK government established a Patients' Charter to provide baseline standards for the NHS for waiting times, bed-availability, and complaints procedures (Press for Change 1999). 🖳 More recently, the Patients' Charter has been incorporated into The NHS Plan (Department of Health 2005). 🖳 The NHS Plan for England includes the reintroduction of school nurses to help combat obesity and sexually transmitted diseases, and health trainers, who have a broader role. It is planned that over 80 per cent of the NHS budget in England will be controlled by Primary Care Trusts (Department of Health 2005). 🖳 Mechanisms and frameworks that can evaluate quality in medical care are still evolving but some examples of proposed frameworks are shown in Box 21.7. Routine methods of assessing quality of medical care should be simple, unbureaucratic, and equally fair to patients and to their doctors and other health professionals.

BOX 21.7 HEALTH CARE EVALUATION FRAMEWORKS AND DIMENSIONS OF QUALITY

[1]Effectiveness Efficiency Accessibility Equity Social acceptability Relevance to population needs	[2]Professional performance (technical quality); Resource use (efficiency); Risk management (the risk of injury or illness associated with the service provided); and Patients' satisfaction with the service provided.	[3]Health improvement Fair access Effective delivery of appropriate health care Efficiency Patient / carer experience Health outcomes of NHS care	[4]Effectiveness Safety Timeliness Patient centredness Equity

Sources: 1, Maxwell (1984); 2, World Health Organization; 3, Department of Health (1999); 4, Agency for Healthcare Research and Quality (2002).

Maxwell, R. (1984). 'Quality Assessment in Health'. *British Medical Journal*, **288**: 1470–2.

WHO (2000). The World Health Report 2000. Health Systems: Improving Performance, http://www.who.int/whr/en/ (accessed 2004).

WHO (2002). The World Health Report 2002. Reducing Risks, Promoting Healthy Life, http://www.who.int/whr/en/ (accessed 2004).

Department of Health (1999). The NHS performance assessment framework, http://www.dh.gov.uk/Publications AndStatistics/Publications/PublicationsPolicyAndGuidance/PublicationsPolicyAndGuidanceArticle/fs/en?CONTENT_ID=40091 90andchk=riXW/M (accessed 2004).

Agency for Healthcare Research and Quality (AHRQ) (2002). NHQR Preliminary Measure Set. Background, http://www.ahrq.gov/qual/nhqr02/nhqrprelim.htm (accessed 2004).

21.4 **Economics of Health Care**

Increasingly, clinicians, policy makers, planners, and politicians are faced with stark choices about how to allocate scarce NHS resources. Such decisions are no longer left to the discretion of managers, several steps removed from the bedside. Doctors may reasonably ponder whether their only duty is to be an advocate for their patient or whether they have a duty to distribute (some would say 'ration') services. However, the General Medical Council makes it clear that doctors have duties both to serve their individual patients and to ensure that their service is planned and delivered as effectively and efficiently as possible (General Medical Council 2004). ⌨ Perhaps renal specialists appreciate these realities better than most; routinely they are involved in decisions about which patient should get the next available donor kidney, or what facilities can be freed up to accommodate another patient in the schedule for dialysis (see Chapter 10).

In an equitable health service if a service exists or a new treatment has been devised, then theoretically it should be available to all who may benefit. In fact, the NHS has never been capable of operating such a principle and clinicians have to recognize that, irrespective of the actual level of resources that the Government makes available, these resources will always be finite. Choices between competing groups of patients or between treatments will always have to be made. What are required are some guiding principles that can help make the choices better informed. A variety of health economic tools exists to aid the decision making process, but, in debates about how resources should be allocated, there is ultimately no formula or algorithm that will give us the 'right answer'. There is rarely a single 'right answer'; value judgements will always have to be made, whether about which principles should guide us, or how they are weighed and applied. Consideration of the following issues, nevertheless, helps provide a framework for the decision-making process and a path towards resolution.

Some fundamental questions

Box 21.8 lists a few key issues that need to be clarified at an early stage for the resolution of any problems of resource allocation.

It is always useful to start by first considering whose voice needs to be heard. Whereas in the past health professionals may have been useful advocates or proxies for their patients, finding someone who can be completely dispassionate is difficult. In the past, the

---

> **BOX 21.8 KEY ISSUES IN RESOURCE ALLOCATION**
>
> Whose values are important to the debate?
>
> What are the overall objectives of the NHS?
>
> How explicit need the decision-making processes be and what accountability mechanisms are required?
>
> What are the ethically defensible criteria for discriminating between competing claims?

public's voice might have been heard through the representation on the Health Authority (HA) committees of locally elected officials (local councillors, for example) but more recently several HAs have employed 'citizen's juries' to help them wrestle with difficult choices (Lenaghan *et al.* 1996). ⌨ Perhaps the most famous of these types of initiative was that in the state of Oregon in the USA (Walsh and Hendrickson 2003). ⌨ Though many may take differing views of the success of these ventures, no one disputes the necessity of having more than the health professional and managers' viewpoints heard. For example, in planning renal dialysis services for Northern Ireland and deciding upon the optimal location of new facilities, the work of the strategy group was greatly assisted by the input of the representatives of patients (DHSSPSNI 2003). ⌨

Deciding upon any problem of resource allocation in the NHS also requires clarity about what the core objective of the NHS should be. Maximizing health or health gain is an obvious priority but reducing health inequalities across socioeconomic groups, or between areas and their populations, is also of major importance. In deciding where to locate new renal dialysis facilities in Northern Ireland, note was taken of the likely travelling times which patients would face to reach the nearest facility.

There is also unresolved debate on what constitutes equitable or fair treatment. If a treatment like renal dialysis can equally effectively prolong the life of a 35-year-old or a 75-year-old, who should get priority when there is only one dialysis station available? There is no easy solution to this issue; perhaps the most that we, as consumers, can hope for is that those charged with making the decisions can make the basis for their judgements as explicit as possible. Part of the difficulty is that the success of any health intervention can be measured in different ways across several dimensions.

At a population level we may count: (i) lives saved; (ii) life-years gained; (iii) symptom-free survival; (iv) complications avoided; (v) cases successfully diagnosed; or (vi) prevented; and the currency chosen may influence our judgements about our effectiveness, efficiency, or our attempts at equity. Health economists have developed indices to help with such judgements, such as the **quality-adjusted life-year** (QALY) whereby each life-year (for example saved by a treatment intervention) is allocated a quality 'weighting' (1 for the best possible quality and 0 for the worst possible quality of life) (see also Chapters 2, 12, 13, and 17). The aim is to produce a common currency with which to measure the outcome of different health interventions. Using a measure such as this certainly has potential advantages if one is trying to maximize the overall benefit to a community, as Box 21.9 illustrates. When compared with a scheme that would allocate our resources on the basis of treatment effectiveness (option 1), or on the basis of the number of subjects affected, namely the burden of disease (option 2), allocating resources to those interventions with greatest cost-effectiveness, for example in ascending order of cost per QALY (option 3), would result in more aggregate benefit to the population.

On one level a tool like this may be very helpful in ensuring the maximum dividend to the NHS but there remain many difficult and unresolved questions about how QALYs are devised, not only in the minds of some clinicians but also among many health economists. For example, one of the ways of 'measuring' a QALY (the 'time trade-off' approach) involves looking at the way we are prepared to trade the quality of life against its duration. But when you are 40 years old, are you

---

BOX 21.9 ILLUSTRATION OF TOTAL NUMBER OF PATIENTS TREATED WITHIN PURCHASING UNIT WITH TEN DIFFERENT DISEASES USING DIFFERENT PURCHASING OPTIONS

Number of patients with each treatable disease	Units of health benefit (UHB)	Total UHBs	Cost per patient (£)	Total Cost (£)	CE ratio	Option 1 Based on	Option 2 Based on	Option 3 Based on
(a)	(b)	$(a \times b)$	(c)	$(a \times c)$	$(a \times c)/(a \times b)$	(b)	(a)	$\left(\dfrac{CE}{ratio}\right)$
A. 20	9.5	190	3000	60 000	316	1		6
B. 15	9.0	135	3800	57 000	422	2		7
C. 30	8.6	258	2300	69 000	267	3		5
D. 5	8.3	42	1000	5 000	119	4		2
E. 70	7.5	525	5200	364 000	693	5	2	
F. 40	6.8	272	950	38 000	140	6		3
G. 84	5.4	454	3000	252 000	555		1	9
H. 18	4.3	77	2200	39 600	512			8
I. 65	4.0	260	875	56 875	219			4
J. 50	3.8	190	300	15 000	80			1
397		2403		956 475				

Notes: This illustration shows the effect of different purchasing options on the total number of patients treated within a purchasing unit (for example hospital or trust). The available budget is £600 000 but the cost of treating **all** patients is £956 475 (total cost). Three options are available:

Option 1: Select most effective treatments until budget exhausted.

Option 2: Select treatments benefiting the greatest burdens until budget exhausted.

Option 3: Select most cost-effective treatments until budget exhausted.

Option 1: Most effective treatment: Cost: £593 000; Patients treated: 180; Health benefit: 1422

Option 2: Burden of disease: Cost: £616 000; Patients treated: 154; Health benefit: 979

Option 3: Cost effectiveness: Cost: £592 475; Patients treated: 327; Health benefit: 1878

prepared to trade quality of life for duration in exactly the same way as when you have reached 80 years? Even if such measurement issues can be resolved, is one man's (or woman's) QALY the same as any other man's QALY? To maximize public welfare overall, should the needs of economically active people be valued more highly because their taxes help fund health and social services? Should the QALYs (and needs) of smokers, alcoholics, or drug addicts be regarded any less highly?

Clearly a health economist may help answer these questions only up to a point, for they are as much about ethics as economics. In practice, nephrologists' judgements about who should receive priority for renal dialysis are little influenced by 'non-clinical factors' (Kee *et al.* 2002) 💻 and, indeed, guidelines devised by professional bodies will seldom, if ever, refer to the socioeconomic attributes of patients. On the other hand, the health professions are now served at a national level by the National Institute for Clinical Excellence (NICE), which produces evidence-based appraisals of new treatments and services, and on their cost effectiveness. It would seem that many of their statements of support for the introduction of a new treatment or service are below a threshold of approximately £30 000 per QALY (Raftery 2001). 💻 Interventions above this threshold, the more expensive interventions, seldom get support from NICE. NICE recommendations are meant to be implemented by local health authorities, but the problem with this requirement is that it gives no consideration to other local priorities and *opportunity cost*. **Opportunity cost** merely expresses the idea that we must not think only of the economic cost of an intervention, but also in terms of what other beneficial intervention may be forgone if we choose the new intervention. The rising costs of health care will necessitate careful economic evaluation of new therapies and procedures in future years, and a wider knowledge of the basic tools of health economics among health professionals. Further discussion of these issues is available elsewhere (Haddix *et al.* 2003). 💻

21.5 **Prevention in Public Health and Clinical Practice**

A core aim of this textbook is to show the role of epidemiology in examining the scope for prevention of disease in a limited text. A secondary aim is to encourage students in their future careers to question medical dogma and myth and to ask the question 'why?' more often than their predecessors. We examined in Chapters 1–3 the role of epidemiology in unravelling the natural history of disease, in establishing risk factors, and in estimating the proportion of disease that could be attributed to individual risk factors. There have been some epidemiological success stories in the past few decades; for example, linking the natural history of human immunodeficiency virus and bovine spongiform encephalopathy with 'infectious' agents (necessary causes), and cardiovascular disease with multiple causes. To explain a 62 per cent reduction in coronary heart disease (CHD) mortality in men, and a fall of 45 per cent in women, in England and Wales in the last two decades of the twentieth century, Unal *et al.* (2004) 💻 examined the influence of changes in population levels of risk factors such as smoking, hypertension, and cholesterol, and of improvements in medical care. Fifty-eight per cent of the reduction could be attributed to changes in risk factors. In contrast, medical and surgical treatments in hospital accounted for 42 per cent of the reduction, and only 4 per cent was due to coronary artery bypass surgery, although this was responsible for a substantial proportion of hospital costs. Unal *et al.* (2004) 💻 noted adverse risk factor trends for physical activity, obesity, and type 2 diabetes mellitus (discussed in Chapter 8); to counter the medical implications of these changes a concerted effort by public health and clinical practitioners, in collaboration with policy makers and others, will be required in the UK and elsewhere in the next few decades. The case for an increased emphasis on the primary prevention of diabetes by public health and policy interventions is strongly argued by McKinley and Marceau (2000). 💻

Although understanding and control of risk factors can be effective in reducing disease incidence (primary prevention), interruption of the natural history of diseases by early effective interventions can also have an effect on the burden of disease (secondary prevention). Chapter 5 discussed screening methods, including those for the early detection of cancers, which are now an increasing public health and clinical problem as life expectancy increases and overall mortality from cardiovascular disease declines. Early detection of cancers and improved treatments are the best hope for patients, unless the natural history is strongly linked with risk factors such as smoking or occupational carcinogens. Epidemiological methods are required to evaluate screening and treatment trials, which often have to be conducted on large numbers of patients in multi-centre studies. The latest databases of evidence for these interventions (discussed in Chapter 20) will be increasingly required by practitioners to ensure optimal treatment of their patients. Monitoring and audit by special surveys of the treatment of CHD in Europe showed considerable variation in the quality of medical care in European countries (EUROASPIRE Study Group 1997). 🖳 To address such concerns in the UK, National Service Frameworks and guidelines for investigation and treatment are issued at intervals, either directly through the Department of Health (for example National Clinical Frameworks for CHD, for the Elderly, and for Diabetes), or, indirectly, through agencies such as NICE. Guidelines and frameworks such as these provide summaries of the evidence-base and opportunities for self-audit, but probably best improve the quality of care for patients by raising awareness of innovations in treatments and care.

As noted earlier in this chapter, costs of health care have increased disproportionately in most developed countries, particularly for specialist care in hospitals (section 21.4 and Box 21.9). Preventive efforts, particularly those that require mass screening can be costly also; but costs of population prevention programmes are generally small compared with those required in the hospital sector and for the institutionalized elderly. Recent data have indicated a tenfold increase in health-care costs in the last year of life compared with that five years before death, although costs begin to increase 15 years before death (Seshamari and Gray 2004). 🖳 League tables based on cost-effectiveness have been developed for the preventive services in the USA (Messonnier *et al.* 1999; Coffield *et al.* 2001), 🖳 and epidemiological principles and methods in addition to economic skills will be required to develop these approaches further in the future. In the meantime, however, public-health policies should be based on pragmatic solutions that are both acceptable to the public, and can produce cost–benefit in terms of validated indicators.

This chapter has reviewed the use of epidemiological tools in public-health practice, particularly from a UK perspective, although practice in most developed countries would share most of the elements discussed. What appears evident is that public health is a highly diverse and challenging discipline requiring a sound knowledge of epidemiological theory and continuous updating of practice to maintain and improve the health of the population that we serve.

Further Reading

Brown, R. C., Baker, E. A., Leet, T. L. and Gillespie, K. N. (2003). *Evidence-Based Public Health*. New York, NY: Oxford University Press.

Donaldson, L. J. and Donaldson, R. J. (2003). *Essential Public Health* (3rd edn). Libra Pharm Ltd, Petroc Press.

Haddix, A. C., Teutsch, S. M. and Corso, P. A. (eds.) (2003). *Prevention Effectiveness. A Guide to Decision Analysis and Economic Evaluation* (2nd edn). New York, NY: Oxford University Press.

Pencheon, D., Guest, C., Melzer, D. and Muir Gray, J. A. (eds.) (2001). *Oxford Handbook of Public Health Practice*. Oxford: Oxford University Press.

Web Addresses

Agency for Healthcare Research and Quality (AHRQ) (2002). NHQR Preliminary Measure Set. Background, http://www.ahrq.gov/qual/nhqr02/nhqrprelim.htm (accessed 2004).

Association of Public Health Observatories (2004). http://www.apho.org.uk.

Centers for Disease Control (2004). http://www.cdc.gov/.

Department of Health (1997). Communicating about risk to public health. HMSO, London, http://www.dh.gov.uk/PublicationsAndStatistics/Publications/PublicationsPolicyAndGuidance/PublicationsPolicyAndGuidanceArticle/fs/en?CONTENT_ID=4006604&chk=f3sSqN (accessed 2004).

Department of Health (1999). The NHS performance assessment framework, http://www.dh.gov.uk/PublicationsAndStatistics/Publications/PublicationsPolicyAndGuidance/PublicationsPolicyAndGuidanceArticle/fs/en?CONTENT_ID=4009190andchk=riXW/M (accessed 2004).

Department of Health (2005). NHS Improvement Plan, http://www.dh.gov.uk/Home/fs/en.

Department of Health, Social Services and Public Safety (2002). Investing for Health strategy, http://www.investingforhealthni.gov.uk/default.asp (accessed 2004).

DHSSPSNI (2003). Regional Review of Renal Services, http://www.dhsspsni.gov.uk/show_publications?txtid=7536.

General Medical Council (2004). Maintaining Good Medical Practice, http://www.gmc-uk.org/global_sections/sitemap_frameset.htm.

Donaldson, L (2001). The Report of the Chief Medical Officer's Project to Strengthen the Public Health Function. London: Department of Health, http://www.doh.gov.uk/cmo/phfunction.htm (accessed 2004).

Faculty of Public Health (2003). Public Health and the Role of the Faculty, http://www.fphm.org.uk/ (accessed 2004).

Food Standards Agency (2005). http://www.food.gov.uk.

Health Protection Agency (2005). http://www.org.uk.

Institute of Medicine (2000). Promoting Health: Intervention Strategies from Social and Behavioral Research, http://books.nap.edu/books/0309071755/html/37.html (accessed 2004).

Institute of Medicine (2002). Board on Health Promotion and Disease Prevention (HPDP). *The Future of the Public's Health in the 21st Century*, http://www.nap.edu/books/030908704X/html/ (accessed 2004).

NHS Modernisation Agency (2004). Improvement Leaders' (series 3) Guide to Working in Systems, http://www.modern.nhs.uk/home/key/docs/workingwithsystems_final.pdf (accessed 2004).

Press for Change (1999). The Patients Charter for England. Putting the Citizen's Charter into Practice in the National Health Service, http://www.pfc.org.uk/Service.medical/pchit-e1.htm.

Stevens, A., Raftery, J., Mant, J. and Simpson, S. (eds.) (2004). *Health Care Needs Assessment: The Epidemiologically Based Needs Assessment Reviews*. Oxford: Radcliffe Publishing, http://hcna.radcliffe-oxford.com/ (accessed 2004).

Wanless, D. (2004). Securing Good Health for the Whole Population, http://www.hm-treasury.gov.uk.

WHO (2000). The World Health Report 2000. Health Systems: Improving Performance, http://www.who.int/whr/en/ (accessed 2004).

WHO (2002). The World Health Report 2002. Reducing Risks, Promoting Healthy Life, http://www.who.int/whr/en/ (accessed 2004).

References

References for this chapter can be found at www.oxfordtextbooks.co.uk/orc/yarnell. Where possible, these are presented as *active links* which direct you to an electronic version of the work. If you are a subscriber to that work (either individually or through an institution), and depending on your level of access, you may be able to peruse an abstract or the full article if available. ⌨

Glossary

absolute risk The probability of the occurrence of a future adverse event such as death, a disease, condition, trait or a complication of disease (cf. relative risk).

alternative hypothesis Usually the hypothesis of interest rather than the null hypothesis, which is the hypothesis actually tested by a particular statistical test. Often the opposite of the null hypothesis.

analytical study (cf. descriptive) A study that tests a particular hypothesis or several hypotheses.

ascertainment The methods, definitions and protocols used to define a particular disease or condition.

ascertainment bias Systematic errors in the methods used to define a disease or condition.

association A statistical relationship between two variables. This may arise due to chance, confounding or as part of a causal relationship.

attack rate In infectious disease epidemiology the term is used to describe the cumulative incidence during the period of an epidemic. In chronic disease epidemiology attack rate indicates the combined occurrence of new and recurrent cases of disease in a defined population in a given time period.

attributable fraction The proportion of disease that could be prevented by eliminating a particular exposure (see also population attributable fraction).

attributable risk The proportion of disease that can be attributed to a particular factor.

avoidable mortality Mortality that could be avoided by control of risk factors (primary prevention) or routine treatment (secondary prevention)

backward elimination See stepwise selection.

bar chart Graphical display of the frequencies or relative frequencies of the classes of a categorical variable in the form of bars or columns. The bars are usually separated along the descriptive axis (see Figures 6.2 and 13.4). (In contrast, a histogram shows a continuous distribution in which bars are contiguous.)

Bayes's theorem A procedure for updating the probability of a state or an event given new evidence. For example, the probability that an individual has a disease will increase with the knowledge that the individual has a positive result on a screening test.

bias The presence of a systematic error or systematic deviation from the true value in a measurement or estimate.

binary logistic regression See regression analysis.

body mass index Any index which estimates the proportion of body fat using standard anthropometric indices such as height and weight. Quetelet's index is the most commonly used and is calculated from the weight (in kilograms) divided by height (in metres) squared.

case definition The definition used to distinguish a person affected, or having a disease, from a person unaffected or without the disease. A case is defined from the information available and may differ, for example, in hospitalized and non-hospitalized cases or in countries with different levels of health care.

case finding The process of defining and locating cases for study.

case series or reports Usually a consecutive series of clinical cases of a particular disease which have attended a particular hospital or out-patient department.

case–control A study design in which potential exposures for a disease are measured in a group of controls selected for comparison with a group of cases. Controls are often matched for factors that could interfere or confound a hypothesis under test. Case–control studies are usually retrospective in nature when past exposures are measured, but nested or prospective case–control studies represent a special type of prospective study in which controls have been selected from the population being followed.

case-fatality The proportion of patients acquiring a disease who die within a given time period. Often this period is 28 days or one month, but shorter or longer periods are also used.

categorical variable A variable which represents different classes of some characteristic. Examples are gender and marital status, the latter being a non-ordered or **nominal categorical** variable. A categorical variable where the classes have a natural ordering is described as **ordered** or **ordinal**, for example highest level of educational attainment or smoking habit.

cause – external Any cause that does not arise within the human organism itself.

cause – multiple Of a disease or condition in which several causes usually operate together to produce the disease (synonym multifactorial condition).

cause – necessary A cause which always has to be present if a disease is to be produced. Micro-organisms which cause specific infectious disease are examples of necessary causes.

cause – sufficient A cause which is alone sufficient to produce a disease. In practice only genetic and highly infectious agents can be classed as single sufficient causes.
Multiple causes, acting together, are sometimes referred to as a **combined sufficient cause**.

clinical decision making A branch of evidence-based medicine which examines by different methods, the process of clinical diagnosis and treatment. Clinical pathways may be traced by algorithmns known as 'decision trees'.

cluster randomized trials A trial in which the unit of allocation of treatment is a cluster of individuals such as a school or a workplace.

cluster sampling In which the sampling unit is not the individual but is a group or cluster of individuals, for example a school or workplace. Because of possible similarities between individuals within a cluster, it may be necessary to make some statistical adjustment when analysing data from such a design. There may be several clustering steps, for example schools,

classes within schools and this is termed **multi-stage, cluster sampling**.

coefficient of variation The ratio of the standard deviation to the mean, often expressed as a percentage. It is used to compare the variation of measurements made in different units, and is often used to quantify measurement error in laboratories.

cohort A group of individuals who are examined together over a period of time, for example workplace (occupational cohort) or a year of birth (birth cohort).

cohort study A study in which a group of individuals, (usually a large group) is studied over a period of time, and particular endpoints are examined in relation to exposure data collected at the beginning of the study.

community intervention An intervention which is applied to groups of individuals based on their geographical distribution or social characteristics, for example fluoridation of water supplies or health promotion programmes directed at particular communities.

concordance A term used in family and twin studies to measure the similarity or concordance of individual traits in family members.

condition A term used in a medical context to indicate a disorder of a particular bodily system.

confidence interval A method of estimation in which an interval is calculated from sample data so that it includes an unknown population parameter with a chosen level of confidence, usually the 95% level, that is 95% of such intervals will contain the parameter.

confidence limits These are the upper and lower limits of the confidence interval.

confounding variable A confounding variable is one which is associated with the exposure variable and also

influences the disease or outcome. Age is often a confounder.

contagious Spread by touch or close bodily contact.

contingency table A two-way table of counts or frequencies, obtained by classifying samples of individuals by two categorical variables.

continuous variable A variable which theoretically has an infinite number of possible values along a continuum, for example height, weight, total cholesterol.

controls Any comparison group in epidemiological studies. Controls may be matched for certain characteristics which may affect the outcome of interest. In experimental studies when the exposures for treatments are allocated by the investigators, this may be done at random to ensure comparability between cases and controls in all relevant characteristics other than the intervention under investigation.

correlation analysis A method for measuring the degree of association between two variables. Perfect agreement, when the variables are essentially measuring the same phenomenon, as represented by a value of $r = 1$; and a value of $r = 0$ indicates no association between the variables. Correlations between continuous measurements are estimated using the **Pearson's coefficient**, while correlations of ordered or ranked categorical variables are estimated using **Spearman's coefficient**.

cross-sectional A study or analysis in which all exposure and disease variables are measured at the same time point.

demographic Relating to the structure or formation of a population.

descriptive epidemiology A type of epidemiology which is characterized by describing characteristics of individuals within a population with a particular disease or condition. Characteristics can be broadly classified under the headings of **person, place** and **time**. Such **studies**

are generally a prerequisite of analytical epidemiological studies in which specific hypotheses relating to particular causes (exposures) for the disease in question can be tested.

dichotomous A variable or distribution that can be divided conveniently into two divisions, for example sex, mortality status.

disability A bodily state that may indicate sub-optimal physical or mental health.

disability-adjusted life-years (DALYs) The anticipated length of life (in years) discounted by a factor, for example life expectancy (years) × 0.8 (to indicate disability status).

discrete variable A variable which takes only integer values, for example the number of children in a family or the number of disease episodes per year.

disease Any disorder of physical or mental function in an individual and perceived as such by others.

disease heterogeneity A situation in which one disease with similar clinical manifestations may in reality represent several diseases with potentially different causes.

disorder Any permanent or recurring malfunction of an individual bodily system.

dose–response An association or relationship characterized by a graded or incremental relation between disease risk and the level of exposure.

ecological fallacy The erroneous assumption that an association detected at an ecological (or aggregate) level is true at the individual level.

ecological studies Studies of disease associations with particular exposures in different geographical areas in which the outcome variables (disease) are measured in different individuals to the exposure variables. The term should probably be confined to the situation where the variables measured are a feature of the place rather than necessarily of the individual.

effect modification When the effect of an exposure on a disease is modified by another variable. For example age and smoking habit modify risk from exposures such as asbestos or infectious agents. A statistical test of interaction is often used to detect effect modification.

efficacy The impact of an intervention or treatment measured under ideal circumstances, ideally under the conditions of an adequately sized randomized controlled trial. In contrast the **effectiveness** of an intervention implies the same measure made under conditions of everyday clinical practice.

end points Any outcome measurement in a trial or cohort study used to determine the results. Examples include mortality, new episodes of disease, biochemical or physiological measurements and quality of life measures made by questionnaire.

endemic Describes a disease or disorder which is constantly present without fluctuating greatly in incidence in the population.

epidemic Describes a disease which fluctuates greatly in the population over a period of weeks, months, and years in the case of infectious diseases and, for chronic diseases, over decades.

epidemic curve A graphical representation of the distribution of cases according to the time of symptom onset which is used to plot the development of outbreaks of infectious disease.

estimate In statistical terms a measurement which is likely to incorporate a degree of error. Confidence intervals give an indication of the likely error for a particular sample or study.

estimation A form of statistical inference in which an estimate (with associated confidence interval) of an unknown population parameter is calculated from a sample of data.

excess or attributable risk In a particular study the difference between the risks in those exposed to a particular cause compared with that in those not exposed to the cause.

experimental or intervention studies Any study in which the exposure is assigned to participants by the investigator. In clinical medicine the randomized trial is the study design of choice.

exposure Any postulated cause which can be measured.

false negative A negative result in a screening test when the disease is present (in contrast to true negative).

false positive A positive result in a screening test when the disease is absent (in contrast to true positive).

familial trait A characteristic or trait that occurs within families more often than expected by chance and which may be genetic in nature.

forward selection See stepwise selection.

frequency table A table showing the number of occurrences of each particular value in the entire distribution of a variable in a study.

funnel plot A figure constructed in meta-analyses to detect publication bias. Conformity to a funnel shape indicates that publication bias is unlikely, whereas when small negative studies have not been published the funnel shape will be incomplete.

gestational age The age of a foetus *in utero* according to the exact chronological age measured from conception.

gold standard This usually refers to a protocol or method of measurement which is known to evaluate a particular disease, physiological measurement or a scientific experiment to the highest achievable standard of accuracy.

growth standards Frequency distribution for attained height and weight in childhood derived from large reference populations. Growth standards maybe set at particular cut points, for example 5th centile for either underweight or overweight, in order to compare the prevalence of under- or over-nourished children in the study population with those in the reference population.

health-care audit A general description of evaluating the structures, processes or outcomes of health care, usually by measuring simple indicators, but can be applied to more significant outcomes such as mortality.

health impact assessment A term used in public health to indicate an overall evaluation of the effect of introducing a new clinical or public-health intervention on the population health, usually for a given geographical area.

health technology assessment The process of evaluating any new clinical diagnostic or investigative technique by appropriate epidemiological and biostatistical methods.

herd immunity The proportion of the human or animal population having immunity to a particular micro-organism either naturally or by immunization procedures. Typically levels of herd immunity need to approach 80–95 per cent of the population to prevent epidemics of common significant human infectious diseases.

heritability The proportion of a disease or trait which can be attributed to genetic causes estimated from regression/correlation analyses among twins or other close family members.

histogram Graphical display in the form of bars or columns of the frequencies or relative frequencies in defined classes of quantitative variable data. The bars are arranged contiguously, for example Figure 4.1.

hospital episode statistics Data derived from hospital-inpatient episodes. Typically the discharge diagnosis is International Classification of Diseases (ICD) coded but usually re-admissions for existing disease cannot be easily distinguished from first admissions.

host A person or animal harbouring a particular micro-organism.

host susceptibility/resistance The level at which the hosts immunological system responds to the invading micro-organism.

hygiene Public health and clinical principle restricting the spread of infectious diseases and, in the case of chronic disease, of promoting and preserving health.

hypothesis testing A form of statistical inference in which sample data are assessed for consistency with hypotheses about the populations from which the samples were selected.

illness The experience of an individual having a disease.

incidence The number of **new cases** of disease occurring in a given time period (usually per annum).

incidence rate The number of new cases in a given time period per unit of the specified population. Clearly the denominator needs to be specified to permit comparisons of incidence rates between different populations, but commonly incidence rates are referred to as incidence.

independence (of events, e.g. exposure and outcome) when the occurrence of an event cannot be predicted from the occurrence of another (i.e. the two events are not associated).

independent variable Any variable which is included in a regression analysis to predict or explain a particular outcome or dependent variable.

infant mortality Usually used in a sense of infant mortality rate: the number of deaths in the first year of life per 1000 live births in the population.

interaction This may be used in the biological sense to indicate the mutually dependent actions of two or more causes to produce a disease or a biological effect. Also in the statistical sense to indicate that relationship between two variables is not constant across levels of a third of the variables,

which may be detected by the inclusion of an interaction term in the regression.

inter-ictal Period between epileptic seizures.

inter-quartile range Range of values between the 25th centile and the 75th centile of a given distribution or sample.

intervention Any clinical treatment or public health measure designed to reduce the incidence or modify the effects of particular diseases.

lead time bias A systematic error due to comparisons of time gained (survival time) in two or more populations in which the disease is detected at different stages of its natural history, for example malignancy detected by screening compared with clinically detected cases.

length bias A systematic error due to the inclusion of a larger proportion of cases surviving for a longer period in one group but not in another, for example longer duration cases are more likely to be captured in a screening programme than acute, fatal cases.

life tables Tables based on current mortality and census-based population structure indicating current life expectancy at given ages. In practice life expectancies at birth, at one year, and at 65 years, are commonly quoted to provide comparative indicators between countries at different levels of development.

life-years lost A summary statistic of years of life lost due to specific causes of premature mortality (formerly premature was defined as less than 65 years but for developed countries is usually less than 75 years).

logarithmic transformation Conversion of the numerical values for a particular variable into logarithms. For a positively skewed distribution this usually has the effect of making the distribution more like that of a normal distribution, which is a prerequisite for many statistical tests.

longitudinal (or prospective study) A study conducted over a period of time in which (baseline) measurements are taken at the beginning of the study, and outcome measures are made during a period of follow-up of the study members.

mean The average value of a group of observations or results in a given distribution.

median The value at the mid point (**fiftieth percentile**) of a given distribution. In distributions which are normally (symmetrically) distributed the median and the mean are identical, but in skewed distributions the mean value will be above or below that of the median.

meta-analysis A systematic review of published studies (and when possible also unpublished studies) using strict inclusion and exclusion criteria and appropriate statistical techniques to provide an overall estimate of the size of an effect in experimental or observational studies.

misclassification The incorrect placement of an individual in the wrong exposure or disease category. This may cause particular problems if misclassification has been selective or differential between different exposure/disease groups (**misclassification bias**).

mode (modal value) The most commonly occurring value of a frequency distribution.

multifactorial Diseases or disorders which arise from two or more causes which may also possibly interact with each other.

multiple linear regression See regression analysis.

multi-stage cluster sampling See cluster sampling.

natural experiment A situation occurring naturally or in an uncontrolled manner which mimics an experiment in which exposures are assigned by investigators. Natural experiments can occur in isolated communities or if a differential exposure is unintentionally made.

Fluoridation provides the most obvious example of a natural experiment as, firstly, the prevalence of dental decay was initially studied in areas with high naturally occurring fluoride levels and, secondly, the change in prevalence in dental decay was observed in areas in which fluoridation was introduced.

natural history A description of the full, naturally-occurring, course of disease progression from its causes, inception and clinical and pathological consequences, without interruption from treatment.

need – population Usually used in the sense of the need for health care in a given population with a particular set of epidemiological and demographic characteristics. Mainly used in the sense of **normative need**, i.e. health care needs from which there are known, recognized benefits.

need – unmet Health care needs not currently being met in the population under consideration.

needs-assessment studies Studies which evaluate a need for health care in given populations.

negative predictive value The probability that a negative screening test result is truly negative (the subject does not have the condition)

neonatal mortality (rate) The number of deaths in the first 28 days of life usually expressed as a rate per 1000 live births in the population.

nested or prospective case–control studies A longitudinal study in which exposure measures are measured at the time of the base line examination (sometimes using stored biological samples), but outcomes are measured in cases occurring during the follow-up period. A sample of controls is selected from those who do not develop the outcome.

non-parametric test Used if a distribution does not conform to a normal distribution and cannot be converted to such a distribution.

non-response bias Error due to differences in characteristics between those who respond and participate in a particular study and those who do not.

normal distribution A symmetrical distribution (also termed the Gaussian distribution) which is the basis for many statistical techniques.

normal (or reference) range Often used by laboratories to indicate the range of measurements of some factor in healthy subjects. If the factor is normally distributed, the 95% range is given by the mean $\pm 2 \times$ standard deviations.

notification – infectious disease A system of routine reporting of significant infectious diseases from clinical and biological sources which may vary from country to country.

null hypothesis The statistical proposition that the result or estimate occurred by chance and that there is, in reality, no difference or no association.

number needed to treat A measure of the overall effect of a treatment used for comparative purposes. It estimates the number of patients treated in order to prevent a single event (a disease outcome or death). It is calculated as the inverse of the absolute risk reduction (see also Chapter 20).

observational studies Epidemiological studies in which a subject's exposures are observed, rather than being assigned or modified by investigators, as in experimental studies.

observer bias Systematic difference between a true value and the observed value caused (usually unintentionally) by the interpretation of the observer. Any clinical measurement which depends in part on the interpretation of the observer may be subject to observer bias.

odds The ratio of the probability of an event occurring to that of an event not occurring.

odds ratio The ratio of the odds of an event in two groups, also termed the cross product ratio, or the relative odds.

opportunistic screening A type of medical screening in which the opportunity to conduct a particular screening test is taken, usually by a general practitioner, when the patient has attended for an unrelated reason.

organogenesis The process of formation of organs in the developing foetus.

outbreaks Clusters of cases of infectious disease against a continuous background of sporadic cases of endemic disease.

outcome A measure by which the result of a study is judged. Also the end result of a natural or clinical process.

outcome event A clinical or non-clinical event by which the results of a study are judged.

parameter In statistics and epidemiology the term is used to denote a characteristic of some variable in a population, for example the mean, standard deviation. A population parameter is often estimated by the corresponding quantity calculated in a sample, for example the mean, standard deviation with appropriate confidence limits. The term tends also to be used much more loosely ranging from **boundary** and **limit** to **factor**, **criterion**, and **scope**.

parametric test In which assumptions can be made about the distribution of the variables, for example a normal distribution can be assumed.

pedigree A family tree which enables inherited traits to be detected and the mode of inheritance ascertained.

perinatal mortality This is a measure of late foetal deaths (after 28 weeks), often termed stillbirths, and deaths within the first week of life per 1000 total births per annum. In developing countries late foetal deaths may not be accurately recorded and accurate comparisons between developing and industrialized countries can be subject to errors.

period effect An effect which has a simultaneous effect on all age groups of the population in a particular period of time, for example antismoking legalization introduced into the workplace (in contrast to a cohort effect).

phenotype The outer biological characteristic or trait exhibited by an individual presumed to be the result of the genotype and that individual's environment.

population Population in general use this refers to the whole collection of individuals within a given geographical area or country. In statistical usage the population refers to the *universe* from which a sample is drawn and which enables a population parameter to be estimated.

population attributable risk The proportion of the disease which can, in a given population, be attributable to a particular risk factor. In contrast the **attributable risk** usually refers to a particular sub population under study conditions.
A population attributable risk depends on the incidence and prevalence of a disease in the general population.

population prevalence studies Studies which examine all established cases of disease in a given population.

population prevention Prevention of disease by reducing risk factors for disease in the general population rather than in particular *high risk* sub groups.

positive predictive value In relation to screening, the proportion of individuals who test positive on the screening test that truly have the disease or condition. Unlike sensitivity and specificity this test depends on the incidence of a disease in a given population.

post-neonatal mortality Mortality after the first 28 days of life and up to the end of the first year expressed as a rate per 1000 live births.

power (of a test) Is the probability of rejecting the null hypothesis when it is false. Factors which influence the power are the study design, effect size and sample size. Power calculations indicate whether a study can show an effect if one exists.

prescriptive This refers to a screening test which is offered to an individual as being of potential benefit to them.

prevalence – cumulative The total number of cases counted in a given population during a specified time period typically ranging from one year to a lifetime. The time period is usually specified.

prevalence – period Total number of cases of a particular disease within a given time period (most commonly during one year).

prevalence – point The number of cases existing in a given population at any particular point in time. Commonly this usage is termed simply prevalence.

prevalence 'rate', 'ratio', proportion or percentage Number of cases of a particular disease as a proportion of the population at risk of the disease in a given time period. Strictly this is not a rate but is more accurately termed a ratio, proportion or percentage.

prevalence round This usually refers to population examinations carried out at intervals to examine trends in particular diseases or risk factors in the general population.

prevention Actions aimed at eradicating or eliminating diseases **(primary prevention)** or minimizing the impact of diseases and disability **(secondary prevention)** or if these are not possible then retarding the progress of disease or disability **(tertiary)**.

prospective or longitudinal study Study in which individuals are recruited and followed for outcome events during a specified period.

P-**value** The probability of the observed value of the test statistic, together with any other equally extreme or more extreme values that might have occurred, calculated assuming that the null hypotheses is true. If it is less than the significance level of the test then the null hypothesis is rejected.

qualitative study An exploratory study in which psychological or sociological variables are defined in broad terms with the underlying purpose of understanding health related behaviours or of developing variables which may be used in a future quantitative study.

quality of life An elusive and essentially subjective phenomenon, but typically measured in epidemiological and clinical studies using scales of physical and mental functioning and well-being, derived from preliminary qualitative studies and incorporating the patient's perspective.

quality-adjusted life-years (QALYs) Used to adjust for the presence of chronic disease to comparing the effects (and costs) of different medical interventions. Weighting factors are used (to represent the quality of life), as in the case of DALYs.

quantitative Describes any variable or study in which measurements are made or ranked.

quarantine A public-health action in which individuals with a particular disease and their possible contacts are isolated from the general population for a period, which depends on the probable incubation period of the particular disease.

quasi-experimental A study in which true experimental design has not been used (often for practical reasons) but which attempts to reproduce the features of an experimental study.

Quetelet's index The most commonly used index of body mass or body fat, weight (kilograms) divided by height squared (metres), described by the Belgian scientist Quetelet in the nineteenth century.

randomized controlled trial (RCT) An experiment in which a new treatment or intervention and a placebo or existing treatment are allocated randomly. This process minimizes the risk of bias in the allocation of treatment. Double-blind RCTs are the study design of choice in which both patient and outcome assessors are unaware of the treatment allocation.

random In probability theory, governed completely by chance. A statistically designed survey should involve elements of random selection. Similarly in randomized trials, treatments are allocated at random to patients.

rank Arrange in a meaningful order by number or severity etc.

rate of an event (incidence rate) The measure of the frequency of occurrence of a disease or trait usually expressed as the number of a disease events in a specified period divided by the population at risk during that period. The population denominator is usually expressed in multiples of 10.

rate ratio The ratio produced by dividing the rate in an exposed group by the rate in the unexposed population.

recall bias The systematic error due to differences in the accuracy of the recall of past exposures by subjects with and without a disease.

receiver operator characteristic A graphical method of describing the ability of a screening test to discriminate between healthy and diseased persons. A plot of the sensitivity versus 1 – specificity for various cut-points of a diagnostic or screening test.

reference population A large well studied population used as a 'gold' standard for particular variables. The values may be compared in other populations typically at different levels of industrial or economic development.

reference standards Values which have been derived from reference populations that are believed to represent optimal health status.

regression analysis A general term used to describe methods of analysis which model the relationship between an explanatory variable (exposure) and an outcome variable. Simple linear regression models a quantitative outcome with a single quantitative explanatory variable; in multiple regressions there are several explanatory variables. In binary logistic regression the outcome variable is binary.

regression coefficients The slope of a linear relationship between the outcome variable and an explanatory variable in a linear regression.

regression modelling See regression analysis.

relative hazard (synonym hazard ratio) A measure of the probability of a disease event or death at a particular point in time in an exposed group compared to a non-exposed group. Hazard ratios are typically used to summarize results from a Cox's proportional hazard regression method.

relative risk The ratio of the risk of disease or death among an exposed group compared with that among an unexposed group (see Chapter 3).

response rate The percentage of a sample which participates in a survey or study in relation to the total eligible sample.

retrospective Describes a study which looks backwards towards a history of exposures obtained typically using recall interview techniques.

retrospective case–control study A study in which subjects with the disease (cases) and subjects without the disease (controls) are defined and exposures are obtained, typically by recall using interview or questionnaire.

retrospective cohort study A study in which the **outcomes** in terms of disease events are known for an entire cohort in which exposures can be obtained from historical records.

risk The probability of the occurrence of a future adverse event such as death, a disease, condition or trait, or a complication of disease. For a categorical outcome variable logistic regression tends to be used; for survival (time-to-event) Cox regression and, for rates and counts, Poisson regression is used.

risk difference (synonym excess risk) The absolute difference between the risks in two subgroups.

risk factor Used in the specific sense of an exposure that has been linked causally with a particular disease, but often used more loosely in the sense of a factor which may be associated with risk of disease.

risk marker A factor which has been shown to be closely associated with risk of a disease but is believed not to be associated causally with the disease.

risk ratio The ratio of risk in the exposed group compared to that in the unexposed group.

sample Any group of individuals or observations derived from a larger group or population and which may be used to characterize the population.

sampling The process of selecting individuals or observations from a larger group.

sampling distribution The distribution of a statistic calculated for all possible samples of some given size from a population.

sampling error The level of error predicted for a particular sample drawn from a wider population often described by 95% confidence intervals.

sampling frame A list of all items in the population from which a sample can be drawn, sometimes divided into units and sub units, for example geographical regions, counties and wards.

scatter diagram A graphical representation of the association between two (usually continuous) variables.

screening – mandatory A compulsory test usually taken as a requirement in certain occupational groups which is designed to protect other individuals rather than the person under test.

screening – mass A screening programme aimed at preventing disease in the general population although it may be confined to a particular age and sex groups (cf. screening of high risk populations).

screening – multiphasic Screening using several screening tests on the same occasion.

secondary prevention Prevention of the recurrence of a disease.

selection bias A type of bias in which the method by which the subjects or patients were selected leads to unrepresentativeness. This usually arises when the method of selection does not include *all* groups from the population.

sensitivity In relation to a screening or diagnostic test, it is the percentage of individuals with the disease who are classified as having the disease by the test.

sensitivity analysis An analysis in which a repeat analysis of a data set is carried out using a different range of values or set of assumptions to determine how much the conclusions of the analysis are affected.

sentinel general practice A general practice from which data are obtained from routine consultations and blood samples etc and used to monitor trends in particular diseases and to predict epidemics of infectious disease, such as influenza.

sickness The disease state as perceived by an individual.

sickness absence Absence from work duties either self reported or reported for statutory purposes by an individual's general practitioner.

significance level The P-value from a hypothesis test is compared to the significance level, usually 0.05 (or 5 per cent). If $P < 0.05$, the null hypothesis is rejected, otherwise, the null hypothesis is retained.

significance testing The process of applying tests of statistical significance

to samples to make inferences about the populations from which the samples were drawn.

skewness If a distribution is not symmetric, it is said to be skewed. When the long tail is towards the right side the distribution is described as positively skewed. When the long tail is towards the left side the distribution is described as negatively skewed.

specificity In relationship to a screening or diagnostic test, it is the percentage of individuals without the disease who are classified as being free of the disease by the test.

stakeholder Any individual or organization that has a possible role in the organization, delivery or outcome of a component of health care.

standard deviation A measure of the variation or dispersion of a particular set of results about a central value.

standard error The standard deviation of the sampling distribution of some statistic. It is used as a measure of sampling error in the calculation of test statistics and confidence limits. It reduces with increasing sample size, for example the standard error of the mean is the standard deviation divided by the square root of the sample size.

standardized mortality ratio (SMR) The ratio of the number of deaths observed in a group relative to the number of deaths expected were the group to experience the death rates of some standard population.

statistic May refer to the summary value for a sample (e.g. mean, proportion), or the result of a statistical test.

statistical inference The process of inferring the characteristics of a population from sample data. It takes two forms: estimation and hypothesis testing.

stepwise selection In regression analyses the process of both adding and removing variables one at a time on the basis of their individual contributions to the regression. Backward elimination and forward selection are simpler alternative approaches.

stratified sampling When the population is divided into strata and a sample is taken from each stratum. It can be used to ensure appropriate or adequate representation of each stratum in the sample.

study population The group of individuals or results from which the sample is selected.

surveillance – passive The routine collection of data to establish trends in the incidence of infectious or chronic disease.

surveillance – active Implementation of non-routine measures such as special surveys, data collection and analysis to establish a trend in an infectious or chronic disease or to study an outbreak.

syndrome A group of symptoms and/or clinical signs which may define a separate clinical disorder.

systems approach Any formal analysis which investigates a particular pathway from the beginning to the end of a particular set of events in a given system.

target population The population at which a particular study is directed. The study intervention may be observational or interventional in nature.

teratogen A substance which causes developmental abnormalities in the embryo or fetus.

tertiary prevention Maintenance of optimal possible quality of life once a disease state has become established, for example rehabilitation after stroke or myocardial infarction.

test statistic The result of a particular statistical test for a specific group of observations.

total period fertility rate (TPFR) An estimate of the average number of children per fertile women (aged 15–45 years) in a given population calculated from the age-specific fertility rates in that particular population.

track This is usually used to describe the persistence of a characteristic or condition, for example high blood pressure, over a period of time if an individual is followed during a prospective study.

trait Any characteristic quality or property of an individual usually existing as a permanent feature.

twin/adoption studies Studies based on monozygotic and dizygotic twins which aim to distinguish genetic and environmental causes of disease. Studies of adopted twins raised in different environments represent an extension of this approach.

uniphasic Operating at a single point in time.

validity Accuracy of epidemiological measurements either made in relation to diagnostic or screening tests, or those made by questionnaire designed to evaluate clinical symptoms or quality of life, for example. **Measurement validity** can be further defined as construct, content and criterion validity. **Study validity** evaluates the extent to which the conclusions drawn from a study can be supported; internal (consisting of the results within the study) and external (consistency of the results in comparison with external studies) validity represent the major approaches to examining this systematically.

variable It represents a property or characteristic of an individual and can be one of several different types: categorical, continuous, discrete.

vector In the epidemiology of infectious disease any living carrier of an infectious agent which transmits the disease organism to the ultimate human host.

vital statistics The recording of life events such as births, deaths, marriages.

World and European standard populations Standard weighting factors which represent the proportions of individuals in sequential age groups in the total available world population (which contain a high proportion of younger individuals) and in Europe (which contains a more uniform distribution of individuals throughout the age range of the population). These weights are used to adjust, or standardize, disease rates across populations with different age structures.

yellow card A system used in the UK to notify potential complications of drugs, vaccines, or other therapies that have already been licensed for use.

z-score A measurement based on standard deviation units which enables comparisons characteristics of variables measured in different units. **= (variable value – sample mean) / sample standard deviation.**

Index

Note: page numbers in *italics* refer to Figures and Tables, whilst those in **bold** refer to entries in Boxes and Glossaries.